Early Pregnancy Loss

Mechanisms and Treatment

Edited by
R. W. Beard and F. Sharp

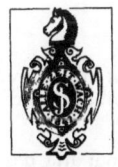

Springer-Verlag
London Berlin Heidelberg New York
Paris Tokyo

Professor Frank Sharp, MD, FRCOG
Department of Obstetrics and Gynaecology, Northern General Hospital,
Herries Road, Sheffield S5 7AU

Professor Richard W. Beard, MB, BChir(Cantab), MD, FRCOG
Department of Obstetrics and Gynaecology, St Mary's Hospital,
Praed Street, London W2 1PG

ISBN-13:978-1-4471-1660-8   e-ISBN-13:978-1-4471-1658-5
DOI: 10.1007/978-1-4471-1658-5

British Library Cataloguing in Publication Data
Royal College of Obstetricians and Gynaecologists, *Study Group. (18th: 1987).*
Early pregnancy loss. 1. Women. Miscarriages I. Title II. Beard, Richard W. (Richard
William) III. Sharp, F. (Frank), *1938-* . 618.3'92
ISBN-13:978-1-4471-1660-8

Library of Congress Cataloging-in-Publication Data
Royal College of Obstetricians and Gynaecologists (Great Britain). Study Group (18: 1987)
Early pregnancy loss.
Includes bibliographies.
1. Miscarriage—Congresses. I. Beard, Richard W. II. Sharp, F. (Frank) III. Title. [DLNM:
1. Abortion—congresses. 2. Fetal Death—congresses. WQ 225 R8884 1987e] RG648.R67
1987 618.3'92 88-16070
ISBN-13:978-1-4471-1660-8

2128/3916-543210

Preface

The first few months of any pregnancy are of supreme importance to the success of that pregnancy. This statement is so obvious as to be almost a platitude, yet it must be said that no aspect of pregnancy has been more neglected in the human than the first three months. Little is known of the morphological changes that occur at that time and our knowledge of the mechanisms that control this vital stage of pregnancy is almost non-existent. The explanation for this neglect of what is an obvious area for study is the difficulty of obtaining normal material. It is rare to have material to study from a healthy first trimester pregnancy and the study by Hertig and Rock[1] of early conception found by chance in hysterectomy specimens must be unique.

The information that we do have about early pregnancy is mostly gained from animal studies or single miscarriages in humans. Chromosomal defects are common but are not an explanation for the majority of recurrent miscarriages. Obstetricians have hypothesised many causes for this condition and have developed numerous methods for treating it, but the studies have been poorly controlled so that our understanding of the cause(s) has not advanced.

Treatment of women with a history of recurrent miscarriage by paternal leucocyte infusion (immunotherapy) may be yet another form of treatment that is hailed as a new advance only to be rejected when subject to rigorous testing. However, the encouraging results from many centres have had the effect of stimulating new and intense interest in early pregnancy. The Study Group, the deliberations of which are reported in this book, is the product of that interest. Scientists and clinicians have come together to examine the evidence to decide whether knowledge has been advanced. Whether this is so or not must be left to the reader to decide, but the editors, and all those who participated, present the data in the hope that a small flame will be lit to illuminate the gloom that has surrounded the subject of early pregnancy for so long.

We are grateful to the co-editors for their valuable assistance in editing the papers and discussions for their particular section, together with Diane Morgan, the Publications Officer and Beryl Stevens and staff of the Postgraduate Education Department of the RCOG for their assistance in organising the Study Group and its publication.

REFERENCE
1. Hertig AT, Rock J. A series of potentially abortive ova recovered from fertile women prior to the first missed menstrual period. *Amer J Obstet Gynec* 1949; **58**: 968-993.

London
May, 1988

Professor Richard W. Beard
Professor Frank Sharp

Participants

Professor E. Alberman
Department of Clinical Epidemiology
The London Hospital Medical College
London E1 1BB

Dr. S. Alexander
Université Libre de Bruxelles
Laboratoire d'Epidémiologie et de
  Médicine Sociale
Campus Erasme CP 590/5
808, route de Lennik
1070 Brussels, Belgium

Dr. W.R. Allen
The Thoroughbred Breeders'
  Association
Equine Fertility Unit
Animal Research Station
307 Huntingdon Road
Cambridge CB3 0JO

Dr. D.F. Antczak
James A. Baker Institute for
  Animal Health
New York State College of
  Veterinary Medicine
Cornell University
Ithaca, NY 14853, U.S.A.

Professor R.W. Beard
Department of Obstetric and
  Gynaecology
St. Mary's Hospital Medical School
Praed Street
London W2 1PG

Professor A.E. Beer
Department of Obstetrics/Gynecology
  and Microbiology and Immunology
University of Health Sciences
The Chicago Medical School
3333 Green Bay Road
North Chicago, IL 60064, U.S.A.

Dr. S.C. Bell
Department of Obstetrics and
  Gynaecology
University of Leicester
Clinical Sciences Building
Leicester Royal Infirmary
P.O. Box 65
Leicester LE2 7LX

Dr. W.D. Billington
Department of Pathology
University of Bristol
The Medical School
University Walk
Bristol BS8 1TD

Dr. J.M. Bulmer
Department of Pathology
University of Leeds
Leeds LS2 9JT

Dr. H.J.A. Carp
Department of Obstetrics and
  Gynaecology
Sheba Medical Centre
Tel Hashomer, Israel

Dr. G. Chaouat
Clinique Universitaire Baudelocque
INSERM U262
123 Bd. de Port Royal
75674 Paris Cedex 14, France

Mr. M.G. Chapman
Department of Obstetrics and
  Gynaecology
Guy's Hospital
St. Thomas Street
London SE1 9RT

Professor D.A. Clark
Department of Medicine
McMaster University
1200 Main Street West
Hamilton, Ontario L8N 3Z5
Canada

Dr. M.R. Creasy
Regional Cytogenetics Laboratory
East Birmingham Hospital
Bordesley Green East
Birmingham B9 5ST

Dr. A. Croy
Department of Biomedical Sciences
University of Guelph
Ontario Veterinary College
Guelph, Ontario N1G 2W1
Canada

Dr. S. Daya
Department of Obstetrics and
  Gynaecology
McMaster University
1200 Main Street West
Hamilton, Ontario L8N 3Z5
Canada

Mr. D.K. Edmonds
Department of Obstetrics and
  Gynaecology
Queen Charlotte's Maternity Hospital
Goldhawk Road
London W6 0XG

Professor T.J. Gill
Department of Pathology
School of Medicine
University of Pittsburgh
716a Scaife Hall
Pittsburgh, PA 15261
U.S.A.

Professor J.G. Grudzinskas
Department of Obstetrics and
  Gynaecology
Holland Wing
The London Hospital Medical College
London E1 1BB

Dr. E.N. Harris
Division of Rheumatology
Department of Medicine
University of Louisville
Louisville, Kentucky
U.S.A.

Professor R. Harris
Department of Medical Genetics
St. Mary's Hospital
Hathersage Road
Manchester M13 0JH

Professor R.F. Harrison
Department of Obstetrics and
  Gynaecology
Maternity Unit
St James' Hospital
Dublin 8, Ireland

Dr. R.B. Heap
AFRC Institute of Animal Physiology
  and Genetics Research
Cambridge Research Station
Babraham Hall
Cambridge CB2 4AT

Mr. G. Hill
Department of Obstetrics and
  Gynaecology
Pembury Hospital
Pembury
Tunbridge Wells TN2 4QJ

Professor P. Howie
Department of Obstetrics and
  Gynaecology
University of Dundee
Ninewells Hospital
Dundee DD1 9SY

Professor D.M. Jenkins
Department of Obstetrics and
  Gynaecology
Erinville Hospital
Western Road
Cork, Ireland

Professor P.M. Johnson
University Department of Immunology
Royal Liverpool Hospital
P.O. Box 147
Liverpool L69 3BX

Professor T.G. Kennedy
Department of Obstetrics and
  Gynaecology
University of Western Ontario
339 Windermere Road
London, Ontario N6A 5A5
Canada

Professor J. Klein
Max Planck-Institut für Biologie
Abteilung Immungenetik
Corrensstrasse 42
D-7400 Tübingen 1
F.R.G.

Dr. Y.W. Loke
Cambridge University Department of
  Pathology
Cellular Pathology Division
Tennis Court Road
Cambridge CB2 1QP

Mr. M. Michel
Department of Obstetrics and
  Gynaecology
St. Mary's Hospital Medical School
Praed Street
London W2 1PG

Dr. W.J. Modle
Senior Medical Officer
Department of Health and
  Social Security
Room D1017, Alexander Fleming
  House
Elephant and Castle
London SE1 6BY

Professor J.F. Mowbray
Department of Experimental Pathology
St. Mary's Hospital Medical School
Praed Street
London W2 1PG

Dr. W. Page Faulk
Department of Experimental Pathology
Methodist Center for Reproduction
  and Transplantation Immunology
1701 North Senate Blvd.
Indianapolis, IN 46202
U.S.A.

Mr. G.D. Pinker
(President RCOG)
Department of Obstetrics and
  Gynaecology
St. Mary's Hospital Medical School
Praed Street
London W2 1PG

Dr. C.W.G. Redman
Nuffield Department of Obstetrics
  and Gynaecology
John Radcliffe Hospital
Headington
Oxford OX3 9DU

Miss L. Regan
Department of Obstetrics and
  Gynaecology
The Rosie Maternity Hospital
Robinson Way
Cambridge CB2 2SW

Dr. C. Renard
Institut Nationale de Recherche
  Agronomique
Laboratoire de Radiobiologie,
  Appliquée
78350 Jouy-en-Josas
Versailles, France

Dr. M.F. Reznikoff-Etievant
CNTS Foundation
Etablissement Cabanel
6, rue Alexandre Cabanel
75739 Paris, Cedex 15, France

Dr. L. Rhodes
Department of Clinical Sciences
Cornell University
New York State College of
  Veterinary Medicine
Ithaca, NY 14853
U.S.A.

Professor W.B. Robertson
The Royal College of Pathologists
2 Carlton House Terrace
London SW1Y 5AF

Dr. D.I. Rushton
The Birmingham Maternity Hospital
Queen Elizabeth Medical Centre
Edgbaston
Birmingham B15 2TG

Professor J.S. Scott
Department of Obstetrics and
  Gynaecology
University of Leeds
Clarendon Wing
Belmont Grove
Leeds LS2 9NS

Dr. A.E. Semprini
Obstetric and Gynaecology Clinic
Ospedale San Paolo
Via A. di Rudini 8
20142 Milan, Italy

Dr. B. Stray-Pederson
Department of Obstetrics and
  Gynaecology
Aker Hospital
University of Oslo
Oslo 0514, Norway

Dr. S. Stray-Pederson
Department of Obstetrics and
  Gynaecology
National Hospital
University of Oslo
Oslo, 0514, Norway

Professor G. Stirrat
Department of Obstetrics and
  Gynaecology
Bristol Maternity Hospital
Southwell Street
Bristol BS2 8EG

Professor A.E. Szulman
Department of Pathology
Magee Womens' Hospital
Forbes Avenue and Halket Street
Pittsburgh, PA 15213
U.S.A.

Dr. C. Taylor
Department of Haematology
Pembury Hospital
Pembury
Tunbridge Wells TN2 4QJ

Dr. M. Unander
Department of Obstetrics and
  Gynaecology
Sahlgren's Hospital
S-413 45 Gothenburg, Sweden

Ms. J. Underwood
Department of Experimental Pathology
St. Mary's Hospital Medical School
Praed Street
London W2 1PG

Additional Contributors

Dr. P.R. Apps
Pembury Hospital
Pembury
Tunbridge Wells TN2 4QJ

Professor S. Campbell
Department of Obstetrics and
  Gynaecology
King's College Hospital Medical School
Denmark Hill
London SE5 9RS

Mr. M.A. Crepeau
Department of Biomedical Sciences
University of Guelph
Ontario Veterinary College
Guelph, Ontario N1G 2W1
Canada

Dr. M. Debruyere
Université Catholique de Louvain
Cliniques Saint Luc
Avenue Hippocrate, 10
1200 Brussels, Belgium

Professeur E. Dupont
Département d'Immunologie
Hôpital Erasme
808, route de Lennik
1070 Brussels, Belgium

Mrs. I. Durieux
Unité CHP/INTS
23 rue Crozatier
75012 Paris, France

Dr. F. Figueroa
Max-Planck-Institut für Biologie
Abteilung Immungenetik
Correnstrasse 42
D-7400 Tübingen
F.R.G.

Dr. Walter Gottlieb
Obstetrics and Gynaecology
Hôpital Erasme
808, route de Lennik
1070 Brussels, Belgium

Dr. Hong-Nerng Ho
Department of Obstetrics and
  Gynaecology
National Taiwan University Hospital
1 Chang-Te Street
Taipei, Taiwan 10016
Republic of China

Dr. J. Huchet
Centre d'Hémobiologie Périnatale
  (CHP)
Hôpital St. Antoine
Paris, France

Dr. A. Kanbour
University of Pittsburgh
School of Medicine
Department of Pathology
716a Scaife Hall
Pittsburgh, PA 15261
U.S.A.

Dr. M. Kasahara
Department of Microbiology and
  Immunology
University of Miami School of Medicine
Miami, FL 33101
U.S.A.

Dr. H.W. Kunz
University of Pittsburgh
School of Medicine
Department of Pathology
716a Scaife Hall
Pittsburgh, PA 15261
U.S.A.

Dr. D. Latinne
Université Catholique de Louvain
Cliniques Saint Luc
Avenue Hippocrate, 10
1200 Brussels, Belgium

Dr. N.A. Maclachlan
Pembury Hospital
Pembury
Tunbridge Wells TN2 4QJ

Dr. T.A. Macpherson
University of Pittsburgh
School of Medicine
Department of Pathology
716a Scaife Hall
Pittsburgh, PA 15261
U.S.A.

Dr. J.A. McIntyre
Methodist Center for Reproduction
    and Transplantation Immunology
Methodist Hospital of Indiana
Indianapolis, IN 46202
U.S.A.

Dr. D.N. Misra
University of Pittsburgh
School of Medicine
Department of Pathology
716a Scaife Hall
Pittsburgh, PA 15261
U.S.A.

Professor A. Netter
Hôpital Saint Louis
Paris, France

Miss A. Ritson
Department of Pathology
University of Leeds
Leeds LS2 9JT

Dr. M.F. Robards
Pembury Hospital
Pembury
Tunbridge Wells TN2 4QJ

Professor C. Salmon
Institut National de Transfusion
    Sanguine (INTS)
Paris, France

Dr. I. Stabile
Academic Unit of Obstetrics and
    Gynaecology
The London Hospital Medical College
London E1 1BB

Dr. K. Thomas
Université Catholique de Louvain
Département d'Obstétrique
Avenue Hippocrate, 10
1200 Brussels, Belgium

Dr. V. Vincek
Max-Planck-Institut für Biologie
Abteilung Immungenetik
Corrensstrasse 42
D-7400 Tübingen
F.R.G.

Dr. T.G. Wegmann
Medical Research Council of Canada
Immunology Group
University of Alberta
Edmonton, Alberta
Canada

Dr. J.K. Wilson
Pembury Hospital
Pembury
Tunbridge Wells TN2 4QJ

Dr. S. Yamashiro
Department of Biomedical Sciences
University of Guelph
Ontario Veterinary College
Guelph, Ontario N1G 2W1
Canada

Contents

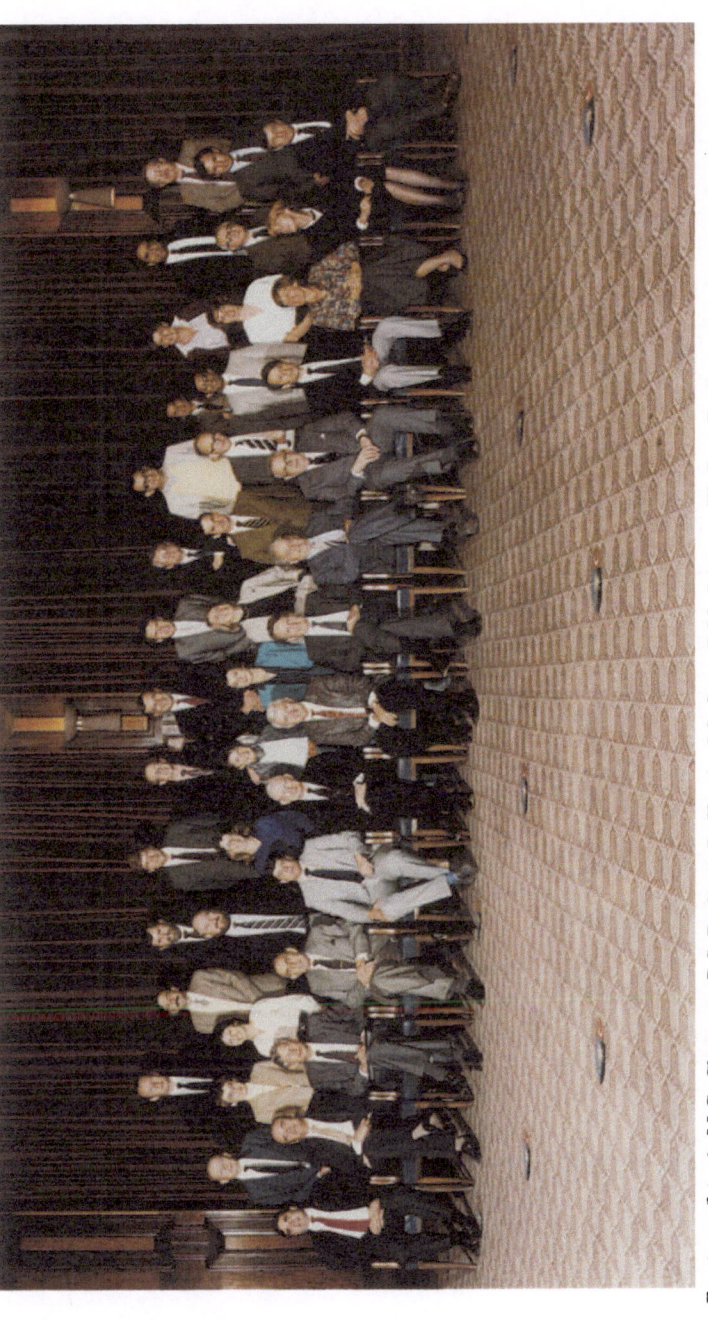

Front row (l to r): M.G. Chapman, D.I. Rushton, R. Harris, J.S. Scott, P.M. Johnson, W. Page Faulk, A. Beer, R.W. Beard, J.F. Mowbray, T.J. Gill, C.W.G. Redman, M.F. Reznikoff-Etievant, S. Alexander, W.R. Allen.

Middle row (l to r): R.F. Harrison, A. Croy, J.M. Bulmer, H.J.A. Carp, L. Rhodes, C. Renard, L. Regan, M. Unander, D.F. Antczak, G. Hill, S. Daya, J. Kydd, A.E. Szulman, A.E. Semprini.

Back row (l to r): D.K. Edmonds, S.C. Bell, T.G. Kennedy, S. Stray-Pedersen, W.D. Billington, G. Stirrat, P. Howie, D.M. Jenkins, G. Chaouat, Y.W. Loke, J. Underwood, M. Michel, D.A. Clark.

ERRATUM

See Page 197

Should read as follows:

REFERENCES

1. Fox H. Perivillous fibrin deposition in the human placenta. *Am J Obstet Gynecol* 1967; **98:** 245-251.
2. Moe N, Jorgensen L. Fibrin deposits on the syncytium of the normal human placenta: evidence for their thrombogenic origin. *Acta Path Microbiol Scand* 1968; **72:** 519-541.
3. Moe N. Deposits of fibrin and plasma proteins in the normal human placenta: an immunofluorescence study. *Acta Path Microbiol Scand* 1969; **76:** 74-88.
4. Stirling Y, Woolf L, North WRS, Seghatchian MJ, Meade TW. Haemotasis in normal pregnancy. *Thromb Haemost* 1984; **52:** 176-180.
5. Kruithof EKD, Tran-Thang C, Gudinchet A, Hauert J, Nicolosco G, Genton C, Welti H, Bachmann F. Fibrinolysis in pregnancy: a study of plasminogen activator inhibitors. *Blood* 1987; **69:** 460-466.
6. Boyd JD, Hamilton WJ. *The Human Placenta.* London: Heffer, 1970.
7. Faulk WP, Johnson PM. Immunological studies of human placentae: identification and distribution of proteins in mature chorionic villi. *Clin Exp Immunol* 1977; **27:** 365-375.
8. Faulk WP, Hsi BL. Immunopathology of human pregnancy. In: *Haines & Taylor's Obstetrical and Gynaecological Pathology.* Ed. H Fox. Edinburgh: Churchill Livingstone, 1987.
9. Faulk WP, Hijmans W. Recent developments in immunofluorescence. *Prog Allergy* 1972; **16:** 9-39.
10. Faulk WP, Jarret R, Keane M, Johnson PM, Boackle RS. Immunological studies of human placentae: complement components in immature and mature chorionic villi. *Clin Exp Immunol* 1980; **40:** 229-305.
11. Dawes J, James K, Micklem LR, Pepper DS, Prowse CV. Monoclonal antibodies directed against human alpha-thrombin and the thrombin-antithrombin III complex. *Thromb Res* 1984; **36:** 397-409.
12. Wun T-C, Capuano A. Initiation and regulation of fibrinolysis in human plasma at the plasminogen activator level. *Blood* 1987; **69:** 1354-1362.
13. Matter L, Faulk WP. Fibrinogen degradation products and Factor VIII consumption in normal pregnancy and pre-eclampsia: role of the placenta. In: *Hypertension in Pregnancy.* Eds. J Bonnar, I McGillivray, EM Symonds, 1980; Lancaster: MTP Press. pp.357-369.
14. Johnson PM, Faulk WP. Immunological studies of human placentae: identification and distribution of proteins in mature chorionic villi. *Immunol* 1978; **34:** 1027-1035.
15. Galbraith RM, Sinha DP, Galbraith GMP, Faulk WP. Immunohistological studies of placentae from insulin dependent diabetic women. In: *Carbohydrate Metabolism in Pregnancy and the Newborn.* Eds. HW Sutherland, JM Stowers. Edinburgh: Churchill Livingstone, 1984; pp.23-33.
16. Sinha DP, Wells M, Faulk WP. Immunological studies of human placentae: complement components in pre-eclamptic chorionic villi. *Clin Exp Immunol* 1984; **56:** 175-184.
17. Faulk WP, Fox H. Reproductive immunology. In: *Clinical Aspects of Immunology* 4th edition. Eds. P Lachmann, K Peters. Oxford: Blackwell Scientific Publications, 1981; pp.1104-1150.
18. Hsi BL, Faulk WP, Yeh CJG, McIntyre JA. Immunohistology of clotting factor V in human extra-embryonic membranes. *Placenta;* In press.
19. Esmon CT. The regulation of natural anticoagulant pathways. *Science* 1987; **235:** 1348-1351.
20. Comp PC, Thurnau GR, Welsh J, Esmon CT. Functional and immunologic Protein S levels are decreased during pregnancy. *Blood* 1986; **68:** 881-885.
21. Astedt B, Lecander I, Brodin T, Lundblad A, Low K. Purification of a specific placental plasminogen activator inhibitor by monoclonal antibody and its complex formation with plasminogen activator. *Thromb Haemost* 1985; **53:** 122-126.
22. Faulk WP, McIntyre JA. Trophoblast survival. *Transpl* 1981; **32:** 1-5.

23. Faulk WP, McIntyre JA. Immunological studies of human trophoblast: markers, subsets and functions. *Immunol Rev* 1983; **75:** 372-408.
24. Rothberger H, Zimmerman TS, Vaughan JH. Increased production and expression of tissue thromboplastin-like procoagulant activity in vitro by allogeneically stimulated human leucocytes. *J Clin Invest* 1972; **68:** 649-655.
25. Cochrane CG. Initiating events in immune complex injury. In: *Progress in Immunology.* Ed. B Amos. New York: Academic Press, 1971. pp.143-153.
26. Schorer AE, Kaplan ME, Rao GHR, Moldow CF. Interleukin-1 stimulates endothelial cell tissue factor production and expression by a prostaglandin-independent mechanism. *Thromb Haemost* 1986; **56:** 256-259.
27. Colucci M, Balconi G, Lorenzet R, Pietra A, Locati D, Donati MB, Semararo N. Cultured human endothelial cells generate tissue factor in response to endotoxin. *J Clin Invest* 1983; **71:** 1893-1896.
28. Camussi G, Aglietta M, Malavasi F, Tetta C, Piacibello W, Sanavio F, Bussolino F. The release of platelet-activating factor from human endothelial cells in culture. *J Immunol* 1983; **131:** 2397-2403.
29. Prescott SM, Zimmerman GA, McIntyre TM. Human endothelial cells in culture produce platlet-activating factor (1-alkyl-2-acetyl-sn-glycerol-3-phosphoryl-choline) when stimulated with thrombin. *Proc Nat Acad Sci USA* 1984; **81:** 3534-3538.
30. Van Hinsbergh VWM, Sprengers ED, Kooistra T. Effects·of thrombin on the production of plasminogen activators and PA inhibitor-1 by human foreskin microvascular endothelial cells. *Thromb Haemost* 1987; **57:** 148-153.

ERRATUM

See Page 340

Studies quoted in Table 1 are referenced as follows:

STUDY	REFERENCE
Faulk	Taylor C, Faulk WP. Prevention of recurrent abortions with leukocyte transfusions. *Lancet* 1983; **2:** 8237
Mowbray	Mowbray JF, Gibbings C, Liddell H, Reginald PW, Underwood JL, Beard RW. Controlled trial of treatment of recurrent spontaneous abortion by immunization with paternal cells. *Lancet* 1985; **1:** 941.
Beer	Beer AE, Semprini AE, Zhu X, Quebbeman JF. Pregnancy outcome in human couples with recurrent spontaneous abortions: 1) HLA antigen profiles; 2) HLA antigen sharing; 3) Female serum MLR blocking factors and 4) Paternal leukocyte immunization. *Exp Clin Immunogenet* 1985; **2:** 137.
Beer	Beer AE, Quebbeman JF, Zhu X. Nonpaternal leukocyte immunization in women previously immunized with paternal leukocytes: Immune responses and subsequent pregnancy outcome. In: *Reproductive Immunology 1986.* Eds. DA Clark, BA Croy. Amsterdam: Elsevier Science Publications, 1987; p. 261.
Johnson	Johnson PM, Chia KV, Risk JM. Immunologic question marks in recurrent spontaneous abortion. In: *Reproductive Immunology 1986.* Eds. DA Clark, BA Croy. Amsterdam: Elsevier Science Publishers, 1987; p. 239.
Reginald	Reginald PW, Beard RW, Chapple J, Forbes BP, Liddell HS. Anticoagulant in pregnancy. *Br J Obstet Gynaecol* 1984; **91:** 357.
Carp	(Unpublished; personal communication)
Unander	Unander AM, Linholm A. Transfusions of leukocyte-rich erythrocyte concentrater: A successful treatment in selected cases of habitual abortion. Am J Obstet Gynecol 1986; 154;516.
Stray-Pederson	Stray-Pederson B, Stray-Pederson S. Etiologic factors and subsequent reproductive performance in 195 couples with a prior history of habitual abortion. *Am·J Obstet Gynecol* 1984; **148:** 140.

SECTION 1

THE CLINICAL PROBLEM

Clinical associations of recurrent miscarriage

R. W. Beard

INTRODUCTION

Recurrent miscarriage is defined as three or more pregnancies ending before 28 weeks from the date of the last menstrual period. It is important to distinguish between a miscarriage which is a single isolated event in a woman's reproductive history, and miscarriage which recurs repeatedly in women who have either had no pregnancies beyond 28 weeks (primary or 1° miscarriers) or, less commonly, have had at the most one or two pregnancies after 28 weeks (secondary or 2° miscarriers). A single miscarriage is common ($\approx$ 15%), frequently being associated with a non-recurrent chromosomal abnormality of the conceptus.[1] Recurrent miscarriage is much less common (probably less than 1% in the population), and as such is likely to be due to a single cause which may have a variable influence on the wellbeing of the conceptus at all stages of pregnancy. This latter concept is borne out by the study of 2° miscarriers by Reginald et al[2] which revealed a high prevalence of small for gestational age babies, preterm delivery and perinatal mortality amongst these women when they became pregnant. These findings support those of earlier studies on women who have had two or three miscarriages.[3,4,5] There was no evidence for an increase in the prevalence of fetal abnormalities.

Thus it seems that pregnancies of 2° miscarriers are less stable and less supportive of fetal growth than normal—what is sometimes referred to by clinicians by the collective description of 'placental insufficiency'. This leads one to hypothesise that the common causative link between these cases may be defective implantation of the conceptus in early pregnancy.

The purpose of this paper is to investigate possible causes of recurrent miscarriage by reviewing the obstetric histories of women before and after treatment for recurrent miscarriage.

METHODS

The results of two studies undertaken in our department are presented:-
1. A retrospective survey of the outcome of 175 pregnancies progressing beyond 28 weeks of gestation in 162 2° miscarriers considered suitable for immunotherapy who had three or more miscarriages and who had attended the

3

Recurrent Miscarriage Clinic at the Samaritan Hospital for Women, London between 1981-86. These studies only include women who have not been treated by immunotherapy.[6]
2. A progressive survey of 156 recurrent miscarriers who became pregnant after immunisation with paternal lymphocytes.[7,8] One hundred and twelve (72%) had a successful pregnancy after treatment and we have obtained a full clinical history from 82 of them.

RESULTS

Relationship between the number of miscarriages and obstetric outcome

Table 1 shows that there is a highly significant increase in the incidence of babies that are small for gestational age, preterm delivery, and perinatal mortality among untreated recurrent miscarriers. However, there is no significant difference in the prevalence of these complications of pregnancy between women who have only had 3 miscarriages compared with those who have had 4 or more.

Table 1

Comparison of rates for small for gestational age (SGA), preterm delivery (PTD) and perinatal mortality (PNM—expressed as a rate per 1000 births)

	SGA	PTD	PNM
General Obstetric Population	7%	10%	19.3—10.1*
3 miscarriages only (n = 53)	26%	24%	188
4 or more miscarriages (n = 65, range 4—11 miscarriages)	33%	31%	138

*national perinatal mortality rates between 1975-84.

Partner Specificity

Twenty-one women had been pregnant by two partners. Only two of the 21 (10%) babies born to this group from their first partners had been small for gestational age, one was preterm, and all the babies had survived, whereas with the second partner all the pregnancies had ended in miscarriages. These findings suggest that recurrent miscarriage is a partner-specific condition. The obstetric outcome was essentially normal, but with the second partner some as yet undetermined factor caused all pregnancies to end in miscarriage.

Characteristics of Stillbirths and Neonatal Deaths

Figure I shows the weights of 21 perinatal deaths of 171 2° miscarriers plotted onto a weight gestation chart. It reveals that i) 13 (62%) of the babies were below the tenth centile for their gestational age, ii) 15 (71%) were preterm ($\leq$ 37 weeks gestation), and ii) only 2 (10%) had a malformation. These results confirm that placental insufficiency is the commonest cause of perinatal death amongst women with a history of 2° miscarriage.

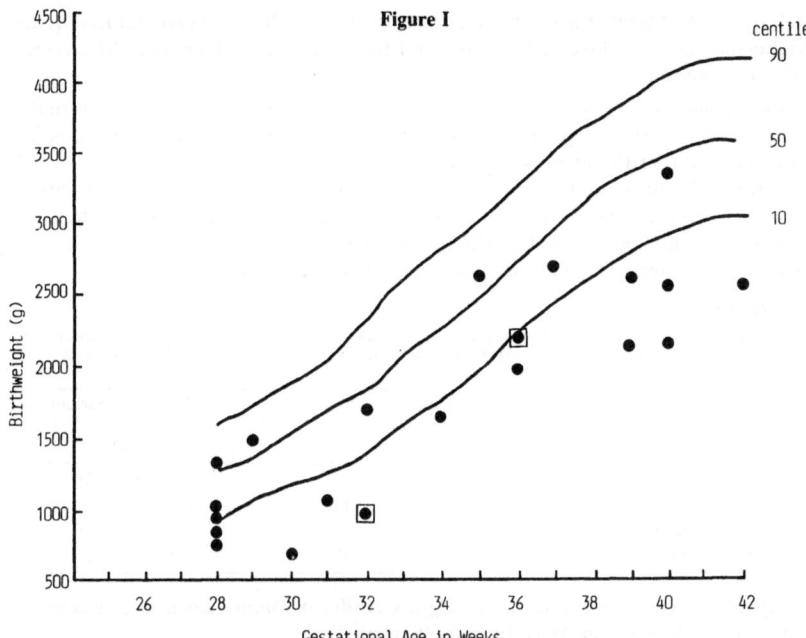

Gestational Age in Weeks

Distribution of weights of stillbirths and neonatal deaths of the 175 babies born to 162 2°
recurrent miscarriers. ▣ major malformation.

Complications of Pregnancy in Untreated and Treated Miscarriers

Table 2 is a comparison of the relative risk of hypertension and bleeding in pregnancy among untreated and treated 1° and 2° miscarriers. The results show that hypertension in pregnancy is no more common amongst untreated recurrent miscarriers than amongst the general obstetric population. However, bleeding at any stage of the pregnancies of these women is significantly increased with a relative risk of 2.94. The conclusions also apply to pregnancies of recurrent miscarriers following immunotherapy with no increase in hypertension although there is still a significant increase in the incidence of bleeding during pregnancy (relative risk 2.16).

Table 2

Relative risk of pregnancy hypertension and of bleeding at any time in pregnancy in untreated and treated recurrent miscarriers compared with the general obstetric population[9] *p < 0.05 ***p < 0.001. Figures in brackets refer to numbers of affected women in the group.

| | Relative Risk | | | |
	Untreated Recurrent Miscarriers (162)		Treated Recurrent Miscarriers (88)	
Pregnancy hypertension	1.0	26	0.75	(11)
Bleeding in pregnancy	2.94***	(50)	2.16*	(20)

Relative Risk of Small for Gestational Age, Preterm Delivery, Perinatal Death, and Malformations in Untreated Recurrent Miscarriers and Recurrent Miscarriers after Immunotherapy

Table 3 compares the relative risk of an adverse outcome in treated and untreated recurrent miscarriers. Again, it is not a longitudinal study so that it is not possible to be certain that the groups are comparable. However, the results show clearly that while the untreated recurrent miscarriers have the expected rate of various adverse outcomes, those treated by immunotherapy have similar rates of small for gestational age babies and perinatal death to that of the general obstetric population, leaving a small but significant increase in preterm delivery.

Table 3

Relative risk of adverse outcome of pregnancy in treated and untreated recurrent miscarriers. *p < 0.05 **p < 0.01 ***p < 0.0001. Figures in brackets refer to number of pregnancies.

	Untreated Recurrent Miscarriers (175)		Treated Recurrent Miscarriers (92)	
Small for Gestational Age	2.97**	(50)	0.33	(3)
Preterm Delivery	2.78**	(45)	1.48*	(13)
Perinatal Death	12.0***	(21)	1.0	(1)
Fetal Malformation	1.14	(5)	1.0	(2)

Longitudinal Comparison of Birthweight Centiles of Babies Born to 2° Recurrent Miscarriers Before and After Immunotherapy

Figure II shows the birthweight centiles of babies of 16 secondary recurrent miscarriers before and after immunotherapy. In 7, the weight centile of the baby increased, in 5 there was no change, and in 4 there was a fall. These preliminary results cannot be interpreted as showing any significant change, but there is a trend towards improved centile birthweight after immunotherapy.

DISCUSSION

These results confirm the high rate of pregnancy complications amongst untreated 2° miscarriers. Bleeding in pregnancy, preterm labour, fetal growth retardation, and a high perinatal mortality are all significantly increased compared with the general obstetric population. The likelihood that these conditions are linked by 'placental insufficiency' is further strengthened by the finding that 62% of the babies that were stillborn or neonatal deaths of these women were growth retarded with only one having a major malformation. The cause of 'placental insufficiency' is unknown, but the finding that during pregnancy there was a high prevalence of bleeding throughout and a low prevalence of hypertension amongst these women suggests that implantation was defective in some way.

Sant-Cassia[10] suggested that "it would be reasonable to suspect a genetic base for recurrent abortion". This statement needs to be questioned. While it is important to exclude the possibility of a lethal gene causing repeated miscarriage, experience of the treatment of recurrent miscarriage, which has achieved a successful outcome of pregnancy in around 78% of cases,[7,11] suggests that neither

Figure II

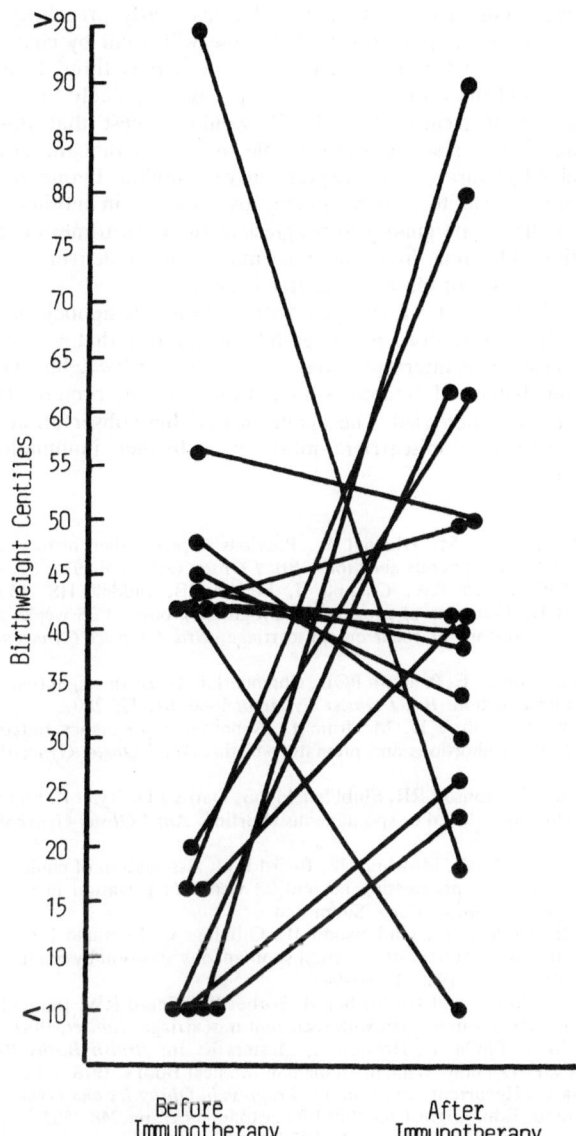

Birthweight centiles of babies born to 16 recurrent miscarriers before and after immunotherapy.

a lethal gene nor a chromosomal abnormality is a common cause of recurrent miscarriage. A non-recurring cause is likely to be responsible for the great majority of single miscarriages. However, because early pregnancy loss is so common in the general population, such a cause will occur by chance in some women who have two miscarriages and even a few who have three. Nonetheless, a woman who has had three or more miscarriages is most likely to have a single recurring cause. Our treatment studies[7,8] would suggest that this cause is immunological. If that is so, it is reasonable to suggest that the effect of this immunological defect varies from one pregnancy to another. In one, implantation may be so poor as to lead to early pregnancy loss, whereas in another, it may just be sufficient to allow a pregnancy to progress to the third trimester, albeit with fetal retardation, bleeding from the placenta, preterm delivery or perinatal death—all the products of placental insufficiency.

Treatment of recurrent miscarriage with paternal lymphocytes before or immediately after conception, is successful for reasons that are, at present, entirely speculative. It is interesting that whereas the birthweights and perinatal mortality of the babies of treated women were normal, preterm labour and vaginal bleeding were increased. The significance of these observations and those on untreated recurrent miscarriers must await further immunological and placental studies.

REFERENCES

1. Alberman E, Elliot M, Dhadial R. Previous reproductive history in mothers presenting with spontaneous abortions. *Brit J Obstet Gynaecol* 1975; **82:** 366-373.
2. Reginald PW, Beard RW, Chapple J, Forbes PB, Liddell HS, Mowbray JF, Underwood JL. Outcome of pregnancies progressing beyond 28 weeks gestation in women with a history of recurrent miscarriage. *Brit J Obstet Gynaecol* 1987; **94:** 643-648.
3. Alberman E, Roman E, Pharoah POD, Chamberlain G. Birthweight before and after a spontaneous abortion. *Brit J Obstet Gynaecol* 1980; **87:** 275-280.
4. Funderburk SJ, Guthrie D, Meldrum D. Suboptimal pregnancy outcome among women with prior abortions and premature births. *Am J Obstet Gynecol* 1976; **126:** 55-60.
5. Schoenbaum SC, Monson RR, Stubblefield PG, Darny PD, Ryan K. Outcome of the delivery following induced or spontaneous abortion. *Am J Obstet Gynecol* 1980; **136:** 19-24.
6. Forbes PB, Michel MZ, Mowbray JF, Beard RW. Association of clinical features of previous pregnancies progressing beyond 28 weeks of gestation in women with a history of recurrent miscarriage. Submitted.
7. Mowbray JF, Liddell HS, Underwood JL, Gibbings C, Reginald PW, Beard RW. Controlled trial of treatment of recurrent spontaneous abortion by immunisation with paternal cells. *Lancet,* 1985; **1:** 941-943.
8. Mowbray JF, Underwood JL, Michel M, Forbes PB, Beard RW. Immunisation with paternal lymphocytes in women with recurrent miscarriage. *Lancet,* 1987; **2:** 679-680.
9. Chamberlain G, Phillip E, Howlett B, Masters K. In: *British Births 1970,* vol. 2. Obstetric Care. London: William Heineman Medical Books. 1978; p.84.
10. Sant-Cassia LJ. Recurrent Abortion. In: *Progress in Obstetrics and Gynaecology,* vol. 5. Ed: J Studd. Edinburgh: Churchill Livingstone. 1985; pp.248-258.
11. Stray-Pederson B, Stray-Pederson S. Etiologic factors and subsequent reproductive performance in 195 couples with a prior history of habitual abortion. *Am J Obstet Gynecol* 1984; **148:** 140-146.

The epidemiology of repeated abortion

E. Alberman

INTRODUCTION

It is generally accepted that about 15% of all recognised pregnancies are miscarried, or aborted before the 28th week, most before the 12th week, and if we were able to measure embryonic death rates immediately after fertilisation this proportion would be considerably higher. There is a large number of causes for such losses, including anomalies of the embryonic or fetal karyotype; major fetal malformations; fetal infections; the presence of chronic maternal illness; maternal uterine anomalies and hormonal or immunological problems.

Many of these causes are to be explored later, but I will concentrate on that group of mothers who have repeated abortions, specifically those who have had at least three abortions, who are thought by some to comprise a fairly homogenous subgroup of as yet doubtful pathogenesis.

DEFINITIONS

There remain problems of definition which need to be considered before describing the epidemiology of this group. First of all, it must be acknowledged that since the stage at which a pregnancy is recognised will vary from woman to woman, there will be many affected women who may not be aware that they have had three or more early fetal losses. Moreover, there will be others, theoretically eligible, who will stop trying, or fail to become pregnant after one or two recognised losses. Researchers sometimes include and sometimes exclude those women who have had, in addition to at least three losses, some normal or abnormal pregnancies lasting at least 28 weeks. It will be shown later that this makes a difference to the incidence of the condition and probably to the prognosis also. Moreover, many retrospective studies of this condition will only enrol[1] mothers who have at least one registrable pregnancy, and others depend for their ascertainment on the women who seek medical care to help them achieve a successful pregnancy.

It follows, firstly, that there are many recognisable recurrent aborters who will not come to the notice of researchers, for there have been few if any, surveys of unselected female populations with a history of three recognised reproductive losses, and even these would not include women with unrecognised losses. On the

9

other hand, the women that come for help may not be a representative group, probably including an unduly high proportion of Social Class I, or women with serious medical problems.

INCIDENCE

The incidence of three or more consecutive fetal losses is quoted as occurring in about 1%[1] of the child-bearing population, twice or three times as commonly as one would expect if the risk to three consecutive recognised pregnancies was constant at about 15%. In a sample of Gravidae 3 women doctors who were asked to report retrospectively on any pregnancies they had experienced only 4 mothers out of 742 (0.5%) reported only fetal losses. Five out of 355 (1.4%) Gravidae 4 mothers in the same study reported 3 or more consecutive losses (Figures I and II).

Figure I

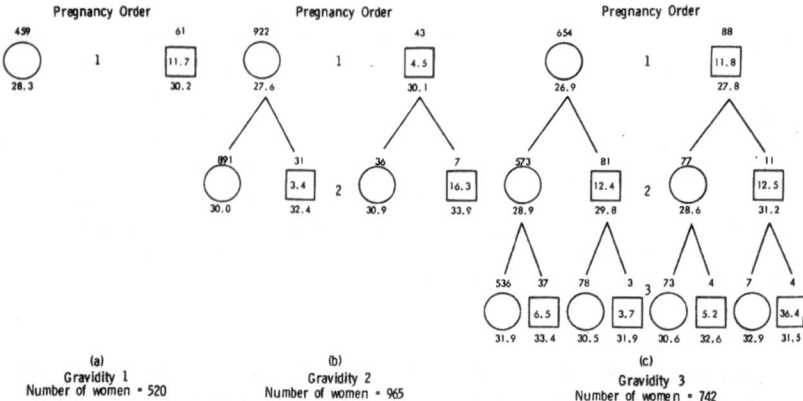

(a)
Gravidity 1
Number of women = 520

(b)
Gravidity 2
Number of women = 965

(c)
Gravidity 3
Number of women = 742

Classification of pregnancy histories by gravidity, pregnancy order and previous outcome.[2] **[Circles represent live births; squares spontaneous abortions. Numbers above represent number of women; below represent mean maternal age; inside symbols represent % spontaneous abortions].**

Taking all gravidities together, over 1% of the 2786 women whose pregnancy sequences were studied reported up to 3 spontaneous abortions as well as at least one live birth. In this particular analysis, mothers who had stillbirths or terminations of pregnancy were excluded.

The increasing risk of abortions to pregnancies following one, two or three spontaneous abortions was evident (Figure II), and it is these findings which suggest that some women may throughout their reproductive life, be at greater risk than others from recurrent fetal losses.

It is the purpose of the present account to describe, largely from the literature, what epidemiological findings there are in regard to women having recurrent abortions.

Figure II

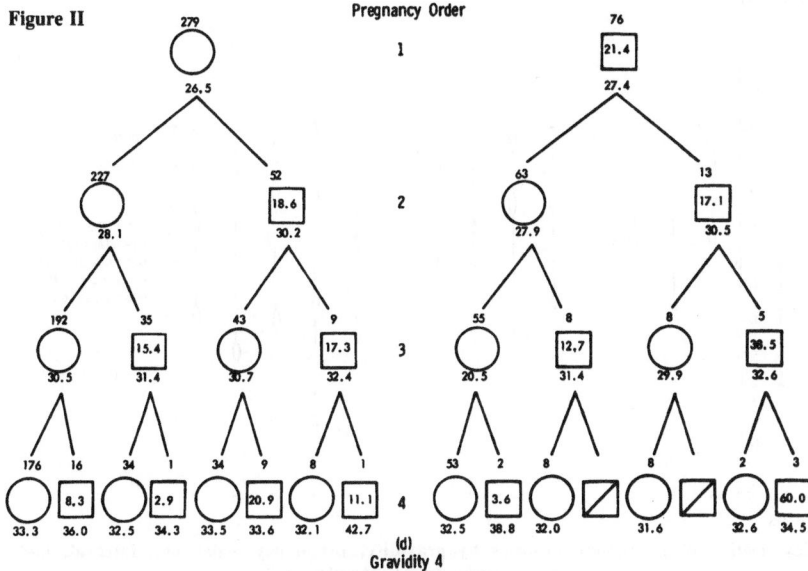

(d)
Gravidity 4
Number of women = 355

Classification of pregnancy histories by pregnancy order and previous outcome of only gravidity 4 mothers.[2]
[Circles represent live births; squares spontaneous abortions. Numbers above represent number of women; below represent mean maternal age; inside symbols represent % spontaneous abortions].

MATERNAL AGE AND PREGNANCY INTERVAL

The study of women doctors already mentioned investigated mean maternal age in pregnancy sequences with and without abortions. After controlling for pregnancy order, women who had a sequence of abortions were consistently older than others of the same gravidity. These findings vary a little with gravidity, but Figure II shows that in mothers of gravidity 4, those destined to become recurrent aborters started reproduction later, and data from individual sequences suggested that the intervals before conceiving a pregnancy destined to abort were longer than before the conception of a live birth. This is illustrated in Figure III showing other gravidities also. Others[3] have also found delays before the conception of pregnancies which were to abort.

MATERNAL RISK FACTORS

Warburton and Strobino[3] reviewed the literature on likely risk factors to be associated with recurrent abortion. They found no convincing or systematic association with maternal diabetes, epilepsy, or progesterone deficiency.

Figure III

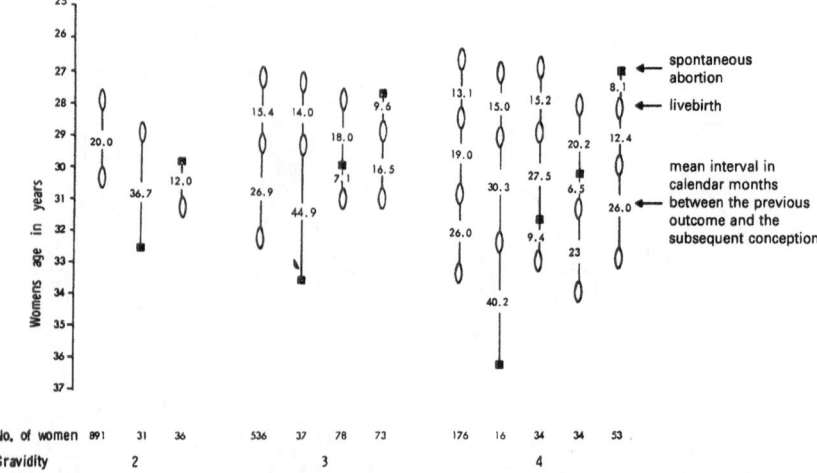

Classification of pregnancy histories by gravidity, pregnancy order and interval, and previous and subsequent outcome.[2]

However, some increase in the incidence of abortions has been reported in women before and after a diagnosis of systematic lupus erythematosus.[4] The question of the role of cervical incompetence remained equivocal. Table 1 taken from their review suggests that this and other uterine abnormalities have been reported more commonly in women who have had repeated abortions,[5-11] but causality in the sense that it is preventable by surgical measures, has yet to be established in the case of cervical incompetence. There has been no controlled study of an association with endometriosis, although this has been reported in the

Table 1

Abnormalities of uterus and cervix per 1000 women

Ref. No.	Dates	Incompetent cervix	Abnormality of uterus
Ascertained through sporadic abortion			
7	1959	—	4.1
8	1973	6.7	2.2
9	1976	15.7	3.2
Ascertained through multiple abortions			
10	1963	117.6	58.8
11	1979	40.0	100.0
5	1986	105.2	—
6	1984	128.0	97.4

adapted from Warburton and Strobino[3]

literature.[12] Similarly, slightly equivocal findings were reported in relation to maternal infections including chlamydia, cytomegalovirus, candida, brucella, toxoplasmosis gondii, herpes virus and mycoplasma.

ENVIRONMENTAL EXPOSURE
Both smoking and the consumption of alcohol in pregnancy have been found to be associated with an increased risk of abortion, and both could contribute towards the occurrence of repeated abortion. Although occupational exposure to certain agents including anaesthetic gases has been suspected to increase abortion rates,[13] this can only rarely be the cause of three or more repeated abortions.

CHROMOSOMAL CONSTITUTION OF PARENTS
The presence of chromosomal rearrangements in couples who have had recurrent abortions has been repeatedly investigated[14] and Table 2 shows the results as summarised by Warburton and Strobino.[3] They point out that the results are similar whether the number of recurrent abortions comprise two or three, or whether couples who have had other types of reproductive failure are included or not. The increased rate of balanced translocations in the female member of the couple involved has been found in other studies, and may reflect a difference in the segregation behaviour of translocations in males and females, or selection against them in male and female gametes. However, only rarely is there a clear causal relationship between the chromosomal constitution of the parents and that of any karyotyped abortions. In a New York study quoted by Warburton and Strobino[3] this was shown to be the case in only 6 out of 2500 karyotyped abortions, sporadic or recurrent.

Table 2
Percentage of parents found to have chromosomal rearrangement

Parents of recurrent aborters		Newborn surveys
Mothers	Fathers	
2.8	1.2	0.2

taken from Warburton and Strobino[3]

CHROMOSOMAL CONSTITUTION OF THE ABORTION
It is well known that a high proportion of all spontaneous abortions can be demonstrated to have a chromosomal anomaly. However, this is more common in sporadic than recurrent abortions. In the New York study, of 69 repeaters in whom the products of conception were karyotyped, only 17.4% were chromosomally abnormal, compared with 33.2% of sporadic abortions. In keeping with this the mean gestational age of recurrent abortions tends to be longer than that of the sporadic abortions, whose early gestational age is probably accounted for by the high proportion of abnormal constitution. It is known that these are more likely to be lost earlier than conceptions of normal consitution (Table 3).

Table 3

Gestational age of abortions in NY Series

	Recurrent (184)	Sporadic (741)
Mean gestation (days)	101.9	88.0

Warburton and Strobino[3]

A special case of the role of chromosomal constitution in repeated abortions is in the small group of sibships where there seems to be a familial tendency towards certain types of anomaly. Such repeated chromosomally anomalous abortions are often of different specific constitution, showing that this is unlikely to be directly inherited, but the phenomenon may be related to a familial tendency to non-dysjunction. Table 4 shows the frequency of reports of karyotypes of more than one abortion with the same couple, and their general outcome, and Table 5 the examples of such repeated abortion series. There are very few reports of three or more of such a series, and to my knowledge none where three or more were abnormal without a corresponding anomaly in one parent.

Table 4

Chromosome analysis of 125 pairs of consecutive spontaneous abortions

First abortion	Second abortion			Total
	Normal	*Trisomy*	*Other abnormal*	
Normal	55	6	7	68
Trisomy	8	24	2	34
Other abnormal	9	8	6	23
Total	72	38	15	125

Adapted from Hassold et al[15]

Table 5

Examples of chromosome analysis of recurrent spontaneous abortions

No. in series	Abortion I	Abortion II	Abortion III
2	46,XY	46,XY	46,XX
23	45,X	47,XY+7	
25	45,XY−21	45,X	
27	47,XY+9	48,XY+18+21	
30	47,XX+18	47,XX+D	

Adapted from Hassold et al[15]

CHARACTERISTICS OF LIVEBORN SIBLINGS OF RECURRENT ABORTIONS

In the study of women doctors it was found that birthweight of live born siblings born after a series of two or more abortions was lower than that found in other live born siblings of women who had had a single spontaneous abortion (Figure IV). Interestingly, the birthweight of live births preceding a spontaneous abortion also tended to be lower than those preceding a live birth (Figure V). These findings, which have been confirmed by other similar analyses[17] suggest that parents of such sibships may have joint adverse characteristics, possibly of an immunological nature, which affect more than one of their pregnancies.

Figure IV

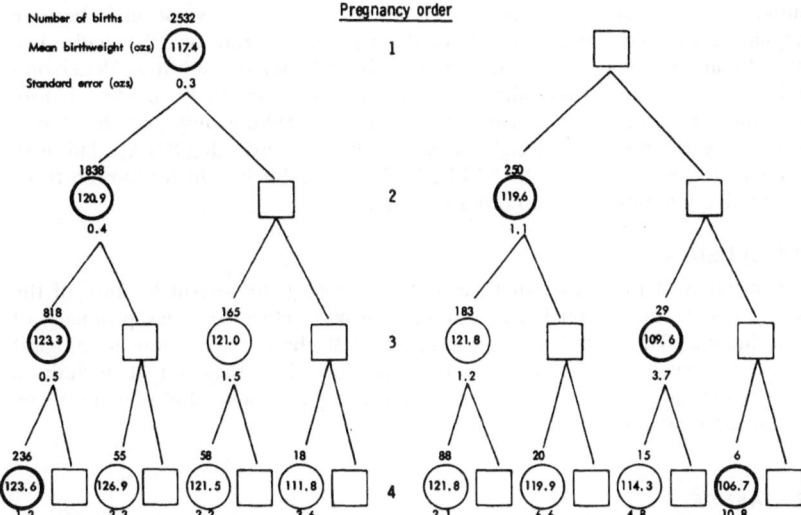

Mean birthweight by pregnancy order, and previous outcome.[16]

Figure V

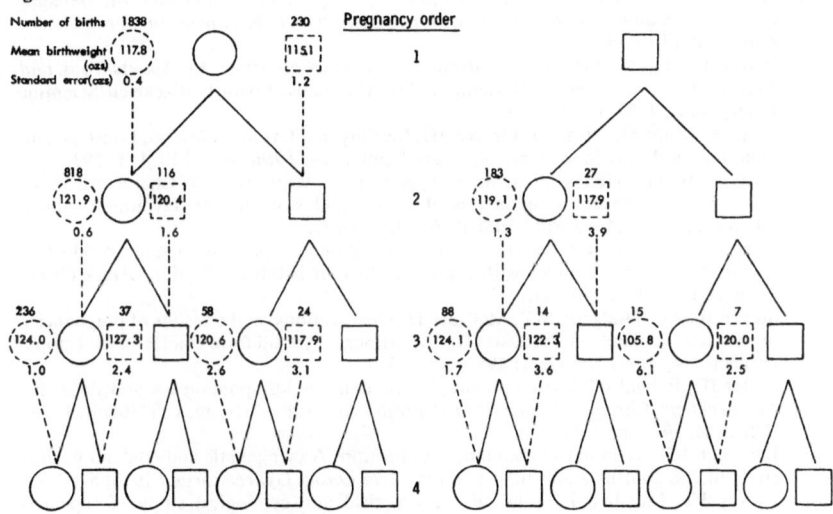

Mean birthweight by pregnancy and subsequent outcome.[16]

PROGNOSIS AFTER THREE OR MORE SPONTANEOUS ABORTIONS

In view of the current attempts to improve the chance of a live born conception after a sequence of abortions, it is important to look at the available outcomes before the current immunological treatment is given. In the women doctors study, 10 women out of 14 who had had three fetal losses, went on to become pregnant for a fourth time, and six of them (a success rate of 60%) had a live birth. Similar success rates are reported by Stray-Pederson and Stray-Pederson[6] and Graves.[18] These and other comparable data need to be studied before assessing the success rate of current treatment.[19] Taking only gravidae 4 it is notable that the mean birthweight of these babies was overall 2.821 kg. This is to be compared with a mean of 3.518 kg in those live births which followed three consecutive live births and no other outcome.

CONCLUSION

The question of the causes of recurrent abortions is important because of the misery it can cause, and because it may provide clues to other problems of reproduction. Their epidemiology suggests that there are several aetiological subgroups, even in this fairly rare condition, but they might include a homogenous group in whom therapy may be efficacious. This remains to be convincingly proven.

REFERENCES
1. Coulam CB. Recurrent pregnancy loss (foreword). In: *Clinical Obstetrics and Gynecology*, Volume 29, No. 4. Ed. C Greenshaw. Philadelphia: Harper and Row, 1986; pp.863-864.
2. Roman E. Maternal age, pregnancy interval and spontaneous abortion. In: *Spontaneous abortion and its relationship to various maternal and obstetric factors*, PhD Thesis. University of London.
3. Warburton D, Strobino B. Recurrent spontaneous abortion. In: *Spontaneous and Recurrent Abortion*. Eds. MJ Bennett, DK Edmonds. Oxford: Blackwell Scientific Publications, 1987, pp.193-213.
4. Fraga A, Mintz G, Orozco J, Orozco JH. Sterility and fertility rates, fetal wastage and maternal morbidity in systemic lupus erythematosus. *J Rheumatol* 1974; **1:** 293.
5. Strobino B, Fox HE, Kline J, Stein Z, Susser M, Warburton D. Characteristics of women with recurrent spontaneous abortions and women with favourable reproductive histories. *Am J Publ Hlth* 1986; **76:** 986-991.
6. Stray-Pederson B, Stray-Pederson S. Etiological factors and subsequent reproductive performance in 195 couples with a prior history of habitual abortion. *Am J Obstet Gynecol* 1984; **148:** 140-146.
7. Stevenson AC, Dudgeon MY, McClure H. Observations on the results of pregnancies in women resident in Belfast. II. Abortions, hydatidiform moles and ectopic pregnancies. *Ann Hum Genet* 1959; **23:** 395.
8. Miller JR, Poland BJ. Some epidemiological data on 902 spontaneous abortions. In: *Les Accidents Chromosomique de la Réproduction*. Eds. A Boué, C Thibault. Paris: INSERM, 1973, pp.289.
9. Lauristen JG. Aetiology of spontaneous abortion. A cytogenetic and epidemiological study of 288 abortuses and their parents. *Acta Obstet Gynecol Scand* 1976; **52:** 1-29.
10. Rowey PT, Marshall R, Ellis JR. A genetical and cytological study of repeated spontaneous abortion. *Ann Hum Genet* 1963; **27:** 87.

11. Phung TT, Byrd JR, McDonough PG. Etiologies and subsequent reproductive performance of 100 couples with recurrent abortions. *Fertil Steril* 1979; **32**: 389-395.
12. Wheeler JM, Johnston BM, Malinak LR. The relationship of endometriosis to spontaneous abortion. *Fertil Steril* 1983; **39**: 656-660.
13. Pharoah POD, Alberman E, Doyle P, Chamberlain G. Outcome of pregnancy among women in anaesthetic practice. *Lancet* 1977; **1**: 34-36.
14. Tharapel AT, Tharapel SA, Bannerman RM. Recurrent pregnancy losses and parental chromosome abnormalities: a review. *Brit J Obstet Gynaecol* 1985; **92**: 899-914.
15. Hassold TJ. A cytogenetic study of repeated spontaneous abortions. *Am J Hum Genet* 1980; **32**: 723-730.
16. Alberman E, Roman E, Pharoah POD, Chamberlain G. Birth weight before and after a spontaneous abortion. *Brit J Obstet Gynaecol* 1980; **87**: 275-280.
17. Reginald PW, Beard RW, Chapple J, Forbes PB, Liddel HS, Mowbray JF, Underwood JL. Outcome of pregnancies progressing beyond 28 weeks gestation in women with a history of recurrent miscarriage. *Brit J Obstet Gynaecol* 1987; **94**: 643-648.
18. Graves WL. Psychological Aspects of Spontaneous Abortions. In: *Spontaneous and Recurrent Abortion*. Eds. MJ Bennett, DK Edmonds. Oxford: Blackwell Scientific Publications, 1987; pp.214-235.
19. Mowbray JF, Underwood JL, Michel M, Forbes PB, Beard RW. Immunisation with paternal lymphocytes in women with recurrent miscarriage. *Lancet* 1987; **2**: 679-680 (letter).

Discussion

Chairman: Professor R. W. Beard

Dr REDMAN: I have a question about the presentation of the results of recurrent miscarriers. Were these patients a clinic population self-selected from afar by their need for specialist treatment?

Professor BEARD: Yes.

Dr REDMAN: So could it be that their poor obstetric history in the past is a bias of the way they came in?

Professor BEARD: It could well be. But of course they are not being referred primarily because of their poor obstetric history. They are being referred to us because they have had three or more miscarriages.

Dr REDMAN: But the pressure would be there from the woman herself because of her poor previous history, the perinatal death or whatever.

Professor BEARD: No. Our experience has been that they come to us primarily because they are having repeated miscarriages, so that whether or not they have had a poor obstetric history does not seem to influence whether they come to us.

Dr REDMAN: Then the comparison of the outcomes of the pregnancy is a before and after. Is that right? Where the data show poor results without treatment and the much better results after treatment, is that in the same cohort of women?

Professor BEARD: No. The poor results before are those of the women who have come to the clinic and is culled from their histories. The results after treatment are obtained from another group of women (although they contain quite a few from the first study), that we have looked at prospectively after treatment with immunotherapy. In addition, however, there is the small group of 17 women before and after the treatment.

Dr REDMAN: What is the method of ascertainment? As I understand the workings of the clinic, people come in from very far distances and then go back to their home base to conceive and have their pregnancies subsequently? How would one determine exactly what happens subsequently from this vast and spread out group of women?

Professor BEARD: Miss Underwood has a system whereby all those living in the UK keep in contact with her. In general, those who live abroad are not included in our results unless by chance they happen to contact us, but the great majority of those living in the UK keep us informed of their outcome.

Miss UNDERWOOD: After immunisation, on the whole, most of them make contact, and especially from abroad the gynaecologists or the obstetricians do write to us and give us information on the pregnancies and on the babies born. We get a bit of both from people abroad and in England.

Dr REDMAN: Would they be followed up if you did not hear from them?

Miss UNDERWOOD: Yes. We write to them. Every year or couple of years we write to those we have not heard from; which is a small minority actually.

Dr REDMAN: And what proportion of the total are never heard from again?

Miss UNDERWOOD: A small proportion. We had two women who fell out because they divorced and one who had adopted children decided not to go on.

Dr DAYA: My question is to try to put Professor Beard's data into perspective in Canada because of differences in definition. We use the definition of recurrent abortion for any abortion that occurs after 20 weeks, whereas in the UK you use 28 weeks. If those between 20 and 28 weeks were to be excluded from the data, how would that affect the obstetrical outcome that we were shown?

Professor BEARD: I did not show the data, but looked at the effect of gestational age of the pre-treatment group on outcome and could find no relationship between the two. A woman was just as likely to have a growth retarded baby if she had miscarried at 12 weeks as if she had miscarried at 28 weeks; but the numbers after 20 weeks are relatively small.

Dr CHAOUAT: A lower birthweight was reported by Professor Alberman in spontaneous abortion. Is anything known about placental weight in the recurrent aborters before and after treatment, and placental proteins pre-treatment, or any of the other markers of placental function in recurrent abortion?

Professor BEARD: The only data that we have on placental weight concerns the perinatal deaths. The great majority of the perinatal deaths that were growth-retarded had small placentas.

Dr B STRAY-PEDERSON: Professor Alberman used female doctors in her material. Being a female doctor myself I do not think that that is very representative. We looked at it too and found that their age when becoming pregnant is higher than the general population; their workload is different from the general population because they do a lot of night duty. On the other hand, they may diagnose their pregnancy earlier than the general population and they may do something with their abortions, their miscarriages, before the general population. So the frequency of 0.4% is unlikely to be representative.

This material was ten years old. Today we have better methods of diagnosing pregnancy; we have more sensitive methods. In our opinion, the frequency of recurrent abortions is in the range of 0.5 to 1.0, and in our own material 0.7% among those who conceived.

Professor ALBERMAN: Of course Dr Stray-Pederson is right. One of the reasons we picked women doctors was that we hoped they would tell us more about their history. I do not think that alters the general pattern of our findings.

Dr B. STRAY-PEDERSON: I agree with your pattern.

Professor ALBERMAN: The 0.4 proportion quoted was only of gravidae three, and it was only of women who had no other outcomes.

Dr B. STRAY-PEDERSON: That is what I meant too; our material, 0.7.

Professor ALBERMAN: That is possible. But I wanted to make the point that if I had included later gravidae, or if I had included women that had other outcomes the proportion goes up, and the highest proportion we had was >1%, as other people reported.

I agree that it does not really matter because I think that every population would be different. The Norwegian population will have one figure and ours will have another. So I agree.

Professor GILL: Was there some implication that there might be a vascular aetiology for recurrent spontaneous abortion and that the immunisation may make the decidua more receptive and more vascularised?

Professor BEARD: I did not actually imply anything on purpose on that data. But one could hypothesise that with poor implantation there is a tendency for the placenta to separate earlier in pregnancy thereby resulting in bleeding. But the data is not sufficiently strong; it needs a prospective study to look at it before one gets into the realm of hypothesis.

Professor BEER: Is there any data on second pregnancies in the control group and the immunised group, whether they were re-immunised or untreated?

Professor BEARD: We do have some.

Professor BEER: I am talking about a second live birth.

Professor BEARD: Second live births in women after treatment?

Professor BEER: And also second live births in the control group that were untreated. Three spontaneous abortions, a live birth, and now a subsequent live birth.

Professor MOWBRAY: I do not think we have any examples of the latter.

Professor BEER: How good is the cure?

Professor MOWBRAY: If we are talking about the treated group, first let me express the slight difference between Professor Beard and myself concerning these two groups. The immunised group is a highly selected group out of those attending the clinic. It is not all of the patients. The results that he showed are of patients attending the clinic who had a live child or more, and a small number were not cytotoxic antibody negative.

Professor BEER: The reason I bring it up is that that has not been our finding. If one now looks at the index pregnancy following immunisation and a group that has not been immunised versus a group that has been immunised, it appears that the couple reverts to the previous pattern of recurrent spontaneous abortion.

Professor BEARD: The implication being that the effect of immunisation does not last into a second pregnancy?

Professor BEER: Groups of immunised patients who have experienced a live birth entering now their second pregnancy. In the group studied, one group of the couples were immunised again and the other went on with no further treatment. The incidence of a subsequent loss was far greater in those not re-immunised.

Professor BEARD: We have not yet analysed our data fully but it is not our impression that that was the case.

Dr RUSHTON: I am a little worried about using the term rejection straight off, although I am not sure whether it has been used as a general term or based on definite immunological rejection.

Professor BEARD: The general term.

Dr RUSHTON: In relation to hypertension and bleeding, as we found—and I know Professor Robertson has found—there is good evidence that a significant number of the later abortions have lesions in their placental beds which are identical to the lesion we see in pre-eclampsia, and therefore I personally have the theory that many of these are lost because they abort before they develop eclampsia or pre-eclampsia. In other words, the abortion terminates a process that we know probably begins very much earlier.

Dr S. STRAY-PEDERSON: I missed Professor Beard's comment on the definition of a spontaneous abortion. We all know that we now have new diagnostic methods for the early detection of pregnancy and we know that it is very difficult during the first days after missed menstruation to make that pregnancy diagnosis. It is an important question and we have to be clear what we are talking about if we are talking about spontaneous abortion.

Professor BEARD: I said that we were dating it from the first day of the last menstrual period. I accept that ultrasound dating is more precise, but we were looking at a population many of whom had had pregnancies before ultrasound was available for dating pregnancies.

Dr S. STRAY-PEDERSON: But what about those who show up as positive for some days? Do we define them as pregnant or not?

Professor BEARD: I agree with the implied criticism but maybe that should be applied to prospective studies from now on.

A prospective study of spontaneous abortion

L. Regan

> ". . . I recall nothing which in times past has caused me
> more anxiety and doubt, or in regard to which I have found
> it more difficult to get any satisfactory rules from
> books, than the treatment of abortion"
>
> T. G. Thomas M.D.
> 1894

INTRODUCTION

Spontaneous abortion is the commonest complication of pregnancy, for it is estimated that 1 in 4 women who become pregnant experience an abortion during their reproductive career.[1] Hence, establishing the cause and assessing the risk of a subsequent pregnancy loss for women presenting with a history of an early abortion is a persistent problem in clinical practice. But despite the recent advances in reproductive medicine, most people working in this field still find themselves unable to answer satisfactorily the two fundamental questions that an affected woman will pose to her doctor. Firstly, "Why did it happen?", and secondly, "What is the chance of it happening again?" Answers to these apparently simple questions have proved difficult to establish, confusion and controversy surrounding every aspect of the problem. There are inconsistencies in the terminology used and an absence of generally accepted figures for the number of individuals affected. Furthermore, since frequently the aetiology of the abortion is not understood, the implementation of treatment becomes empirical, is often uncontrolled and the results from such regimes thereby rendered equivocal and inconclusive.

The term "abortion" was coined originally to describe a pregnancy that terminated at a gestational age before which the fetus was viable. Fetal viability varies, not only amongst individual pregnancies but also with the neonatal services available to that patient. In 1977, the World Health Organisation defined abortion as 'the expulsion or extraction from its mother of a fetus or an embryo weighing 500g or less', which approximates to 20-22 completed weeks of gestation.[2] As the incidence of abortion reaches its lowest level between 20-27 weeks, most epidemiological data will correspond reasonably well to the WHO definition. Hence, in this account, spontaneous abortion will be defined as the

23

spontaneous loss of a pregnancy before 20 weeks gestation and recurrent abortion as the loss of 3 or more consecutive conceptuses before 20 weeks gestation.

Although in the few instances a well defined cause for the abortion may exist, in the vast majority of spontaneous abortions, the clinician's investigative checklist fails to elucidate the cause, and the aetiology remains unknown. Frequently fetal chromosome anomalies are cited as accounting for 50-60% of first trimester losses,[3,4,5] but it is important to remember that only 10-20% of products of conception yield successful culture. Hence the percentages quoted are a percentage of those karyotyped successfully. Moreover, the risk of a second abortion, following the abortion of a fetus with an abnormal karyotype, is less than the risk incurred by women who have had karyotypically normal abortuses.[3,4,5] The finding of a balanced reciprocal translocation in one of the patients affects the prognosis for, and the management of, a subsequent pregnancy, but the incidence rarely exceeds 5%,[6] even in those couples who have experienced repeated abortions. Structural abnormalities of the genital tract are an important group to identify, since they are potentially remediable,[7] but their contribution to the overall spontaneous abortion rate is small[8]. Similarly, maternal domestic disorders during the reproductive years are uncommon, and in particular little evidence exists to support the frequent implication of both diabetes[9] and thyroid disease[10] that is reported in the literature. An infectious agent is frequently sought, but rarely found in cases of recurrent abortion. The possibility that a disturbed endocrine environment is the causative factor is an attractive one,[11] but the studies to date have concluded that the administration of exogenous hormones (such as hCG and progesterone) in an attempt to increase *corpus luteum* efficiency, have no proven beneficial effect.[12]

More recently, it has been suggested that all the aforesaid possibilities account for only a small percentage of recurrent abortions, and that the commonest aetiology in this group of women is an immunological alteration which prevents them from mounting an appropriate protective response towards their fetal allograft.[13,14] The exact nature of this putative maternal immune response has yet to be established, but the hypothesis that it is a cause of recurrent abortion, has suggested to some that it may be remediable. As a result, immunological therapy is already being explored,[15,16] further emphasising the need to document accurately the incidence of recurrent abortion and identify those women for whom therapy might be beneficial.

INCIDENCE OF SPONTANEOUS ABORTION

It is frequently quoted that 15% of clinically recognised pregnancies abort spontaneously,[1,17-20] although the use of highly sensitive hCG assays, detecting implantation before the first missed period,[21] has led some authors to suggest that the rate of conceptual loss is in the region of 60%.[22,23] This figure may be an overestimate, and is being investigated currently with the aid of newly introduced monoclonal antibodies that do not crossreact with luteinising hormone.

There is some evidence to suggest that abortion is a more common outcome of first pregnancies than later pregnancies.[24] That there is an increased risk of abortion after a previous abortion is reported consistently,[1,4,18,19] but no generally accepted figures for the risks of recurrence are available. Huisjes[25] has applied a statistical hypothesis arguing that all abortions can be considered attributable to random factors and that a large percentage of recurrent abortions will therefore be a purely fortuitous event. Using the previous estimates that 15% of the clinically recognised pregnancies will abort, he calculates that 2.3% of women will abort two successive pregnancies and similarly that 0.34% of this group would be expected to abort three consecutive pregnancies. Malpas' theoretical formulation of 1938 estimated the same figure at 73%,[26] and although this has now been disproven, it is recognised that not all women have the same propensity to abort, the risks for any individual being higher or lower depending on her specific circumstances, for example, her age, parity and biological variables such as chromosome abnormality of the conceptus.[4,27-29] Moreover, abortion does tend to recur in the same women and the reproductive characteristics of "repeaters" are well documented.[6,30] In summary, there do seem to be factors distinguishing women with repeated abortion from others, suggesting that in addition to random causes, specific components are involved in this type of reproductive failure and that 'recurrent abortion' is a distinct entity.

Table 1

Probability of Spontaneous Abortion

Percentage of women aborting in relation to number of previous abortions.

	Number of previous abortions			
Type of study	0	1	2	3+
Retrospective studies				
Stevenson *et al* (1959)[46]		16.8	19.2	26.2
Warburton and Fraser (1964)[1]	12.3	26.2	32.2	30.2
Leridon (1976)[47]	15.2	22.0	35.3	
Poland *et al* (1977)[19]		19.0	35.0	47.0
Naylor and Warburton (1978)[36]	11.0	20.3	29.2	37.0
Cohort studies				
Shapiro *et al* (1970)[48]	10.9	18.0		
Awan (1974)[49]	10.4	22.1	27.4	
Prospective studies				
Boué *et al* (1975)[3]		13.8		24.9
Harger *et al* (1983)[50]			17.4	29.2
Fitzsimmons *et al* (1983)[38]			31.3	45.7

STUDIES OF RECURRENCE RISKS

Estimates for the occurrence of an abortion where there is no previous history of an unsuccessful pregnancy average about 12% (Table 1), whereas values ranging from 25-50% are quoted for those women who have aborted on 3 previous occasions. Although there are numerous studies which attempt to put figures on the recurrence risk of an abortion after the first, second, third or subsequent pregnancy loss experienced by a woman, the results are at considerable variance because they are directly dependent on the population sample and the method of data analysis employed. For example, the study of Warburton and Fraser[1] was undertaken by interviewing personally over 2000 women consulting a medical genetics unit, and analysing retrospectively 10,000 of their accumulated pregnancies. Their figures include all women with previous abortions, irrespective of whether a successful pregnancy intervened. On the other hand, Poland *et al*[19] collated their data from hospital records alone, noting the subsequent pregnancy outcome of 472 patients who had only experienced successive abortions, which probably accounts for their higher figures. By definition a retrospective study can provide no meaningful information about first pregnancies. Very early abortions will be under-represented because they are centred most frequently around hospital populations and the woman with less pronounced symptoms is less likely to seek specialist help. The prospective studies performed to date have not included primigravidae, nor have they enrolled the women pre-conceptually.

Nevertheless, despite the shortcomings of existing studies, it is notable that most authors have found the likelihood of a successful pregnancy following three previous abortions, to be in the region of 60%, which leads many gynaecologists to question whether the implementation of any treatment is justifiable. However, the woman who has aborted repeatedly is desperately seeking help, and is not prepared to accept that she has been the victim of chance. Frequently the doctor is pushed into investigating and implementing treatment in a patient for whom no cause for the repeated losses can be demonstrated, and it may be argued, has been statistically unlucky.[31] This point has been well illustrated by the public demand that has been developed for 'immunotherapy' over the last couple of years, and further emphasises the need to establish accurate recurrent abortion rates, in order for the clinician to be able to justify or refute the implementation of any form of treatment, be it immunologically based or not.

IMMUNOTHERAPY

The belief that some women who abort recurrently may have an immune deficiency which prevents them from mounting the appropriate protective response towards their fetus, has already been mentioned and will be discussed at length by other authors in these proceedings. Reports of successful pregnancy outcome after immunisation treatment using whole blood donor or partner's lymphocytes are accumulating steadily in the literature.[15,16,32,33,34] Success rates for the subsequent pregnancy outcome in all these centres have been consistently high, averaging 75-80%, although it must be pointed out that in the only two groups including control subjects, the subsequent successful pregnancy outcomes in the centres were 64% (Beer *et al* 1985)[32] and 34% (Mowbray *et al*)[16], compared with 72% and 78% respectively for treated patients.

The mechanism whereby immunisation confers its apparently beneficial effect is not clearly understood, but is presumed to be secondary to the maternal immunological response stimulated by the infusion of allogeneic (paternal) lymphocytes. Some workers believe that the production of an anti-paternal cytotoxic antibody after treatment is a good prognostic factor for the subsequent pregnancy[16,35] and the majority of centres offering immunisation insist that their patients are negative for anti-paternal cytotoxic antibody prior to treatment. The

use of this inclusion criterion presumes that the absence of the antibody (the presence of which by definition demonstrates that the mother has immunologically recognised the paternal component of her fetus) is of significance in the aetiology of her recurrent abortions. The most recent report from Mowbray *et al*[35] states that "only women with no antibodies to paternal T and B lymphocytes were offered treatment, on the basis that they had not shown the normal antibody response to repeated pregnancies". These authors go on to suggest that women who seroconvert after their white cell infusion have an improved outcome in a subsequent pregnancy, and that this immunological protection remains for up to one year after treatment. In contrast, patients who remain negative for cytotoxic antibodies and conceive more than 80 days after treatment, are likely to miscarry again and should be offered booster injections. If the development of cytotoxic antibody is an essential prerequisite for successful pregnancy outcome, why then do a significant percentage of immunised women who go on to have successful pregnancies never produce detectable antibody? The literature lacks detailed documentation of the incidence and significance of such antibodies in normal pregnancy rendering unjustifiable the clinical assumptions described above. The Cambridge study was initiated to resolve some of these unanswered questions about the role of cytotoxic antibody and its diagnostic value. We have recruited a prospective, representative group of pregnant women, including primigravidae, in order to:-
1) establish the spontaneous abortion rate in the community,
2) assess the risks of recurrent abortion, and
3) examine some immunological parameters in normal human pregnancies
so as to be able to compare and contrast them with those implicated in recurrent aborters, with particular reference to the incidence and time of development of anti-paternal cytotoxic antibody.

CAMBRIDGE EARLY PREGNANCY LOSS STUDY

The Cambridge catchment area offers a unique opportunity to study pregnancy prospectively, since patients receive all their maternity care at one single hospital. In order to recruit a representative cross-section of the community, a radio and poster appeal was started in February 1986, asking women who were contemplating a pregnancy in the near future to come forward. In addition, recruits were drawn from the infertility, general gynaecology and postnatal clinics, together with women who had suffered recent miscarriages within the confines of the maternity hospital.

All the volunteers were seen individually to explain the purpose of the study and agreed to provide a pre-pregnancy blood sample and to return as soon as pregnancy occurred. As soon as the pregnancy was declared the women were seen again to obtain an early serum sample and make arrangements for the serial pregnancy blood samples to be collected. Ninety-five percent of the pregnancies were confirmed by ultrasound before the completion of the eighth gestational week and having confirmed and dated the pregnancy, subsequent blood samples were taken at the time of antenatal clinic booking (between 10 and 12 weeks gestation in this hospital) followed by samples at 18, 28, 32 weeks of gestation and at the time of delivery. After delivery, arrangements were made to see the woman and her partner four weeks post-partum in order to collect the final maternal serum sample and obtain fresh paternal blood for the cytotoxic testing, the details of which will be described subsequently. The recruitment programme was started in February 1986 and remains ongoing. For the purposes of this account the results obtained during the interval between February 1986 and August 1987 will be discussed. During this period a total of 456 non-pregnant women contemplating pregnancy in the near future were enrolled into the study. 234 pregnancies have already been declared, of which 17 came as a result of the radio and poster appeal, 44 were drawn from the infertility clinic (of which about half were participating in the *in vitro* fertilisation programme) and 73 had suffered a recent spontaneous abortion.

PREGNANCY OUTCOME

Of these 234 women, 8 cannot be included because they are still in the first trimester, and thus are not yet classifiable. The outcome of the 226 pregnancies is shown in Figure I. There have been 130 live births, 23 spontaneous abortions, 1 therapeutic termination for fetal abnormality diagnosed at 20 weeks gestation, 2 ectopic gestations have occurred and 70 pregnancies remain ongoing beyond 20 weeks gestation.

The gestational ages at which the 23 abortions occurred are displayed in Figure II. Since all the abortions in this population occurred before 14 weeks gestation, all patients that had completed 20 weeks gestation have been included in the ensuing calculations since the chances of someone aborting in our population after this date are minimal. Moreover, this cut-off point complies with the WHO definition of spontaneous abortion described earlier. Hence from this point onwards, the data presented will include all 70 of the pregnancies that had reached 20 weeks gestation as potentially live births, and compares them to the 23 abortions. As the correct classification for the ectopic pregnancies and the termination is debatable and there were only 3 women involved, they have been excluded from the subsequent calculations.

Table 2

Outcome of 223 pregnancies by gravidity

Outcome of Indexed Pregnancy	1st Pregnancy	2nd Pregnancy	3rd Pregnancy	≥ 4th Pregnancy	Total
Live	51	65	45	41	200
Abortion	3	4	8		23
Total	54	69	53	49	223
Spontaneous Abortion Rate	5.6%	5.8%	15.1%	16.3%	10.3%

The outcome of 223 pregnancies of which 200 were potentially live births, is shown in Table 2. Although the crude spontaneous abortion rate for this population was 10.3%, it can be seen that there is a direct relationship between gravidity and abortion rate, (taking no account of the outcome of any previous

Figure I

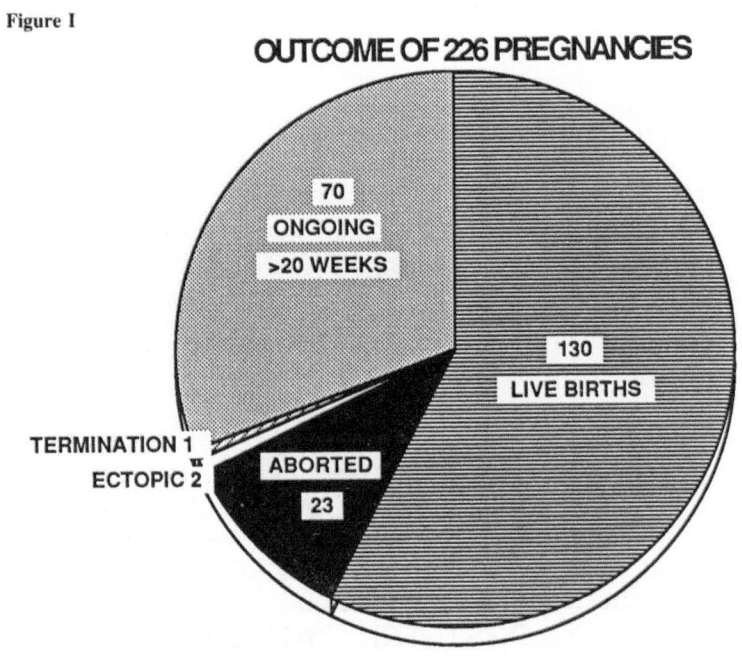

OUTCOME OF 226 PREGNANCIES

70
ONGOING
>20 WEEKS

130
LIVE BIRTHS

TERMINATION 1
ECTOPIC 2

ABORTED
23

Figure II

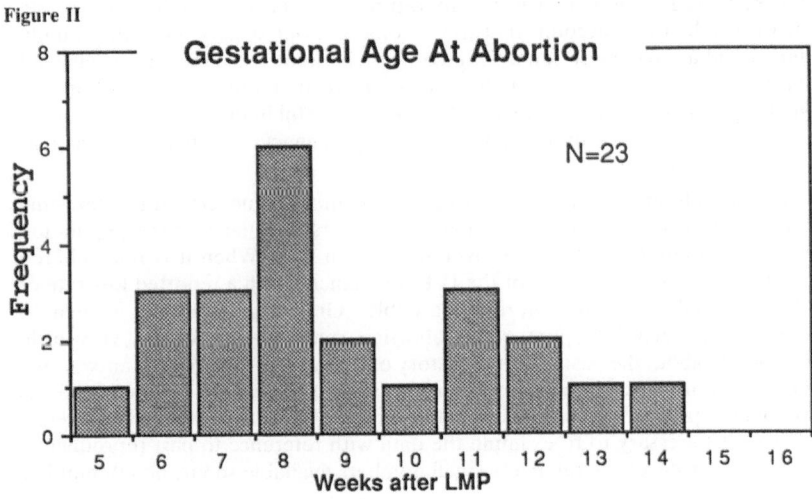

Gestational Age At Abortion

N=23

Figure IIIa

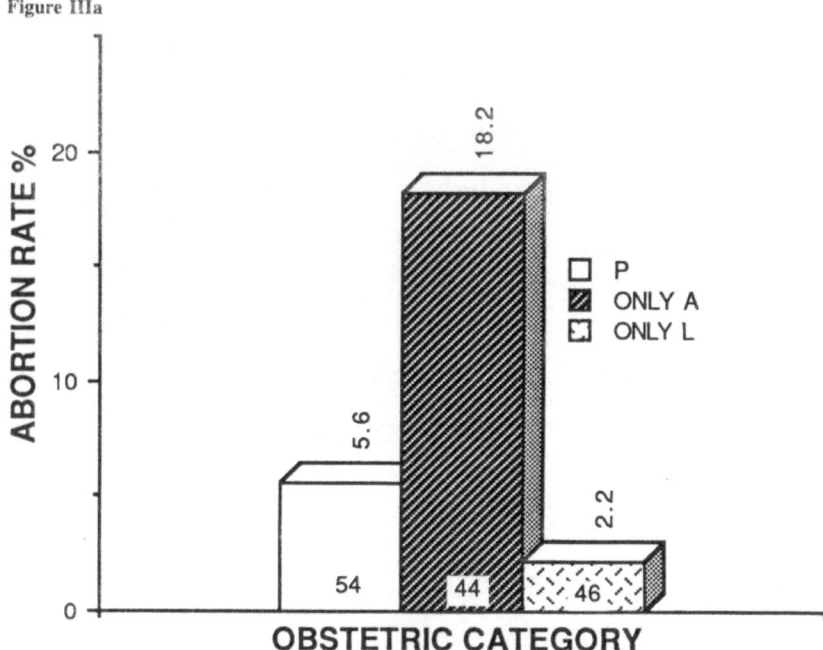

a. Histogram showing the abortion rate in primigravidae (P) and that for women who had
    only aborted (ONLY A) and only had live births (ONLY L).

pregnancy), an effect which is most marked after the second pregnancy. This
increase is well documented in the literature,[1,28,36] and is a predictable finding
when it is taken into account that most women in our society limit their family
number and are aiming for an average of two children. Once they have achieved
their reproductive goal, they usually discontinue further attempts at pregnancy.[37]
On the other hand, women who have been unsuccessful in the past will embark on
more pregnancies to achieve their aim, and pregnancy will therefore occur at
progressively older ages.[37,38]

Since the literature lacks prospective data on first pregnancies, it is interesting
to note that the loss rate among women having a first pregnancy in this population
was considerably lower than the overall abortion rate. When it is remembered
that this group included some of the IVF pregnancies with a reported loss rate of
25%, the finding is even more remarkable. Gravidity therefore, is seen to
influence the recorded spontaneous abortion rate, but it provides very little
information about the past obstetric history of the woman. In order to answer one
of the questions posed initially—what advice should be given to a woman who has
experienced pregnancy losses and is planning to embark on further pregnancies?—
it becomes necessary to re-examine the data with reference to past reproductive
outcome. In view of the relatively small numbers available so far, no attempt has

Figure IIIb

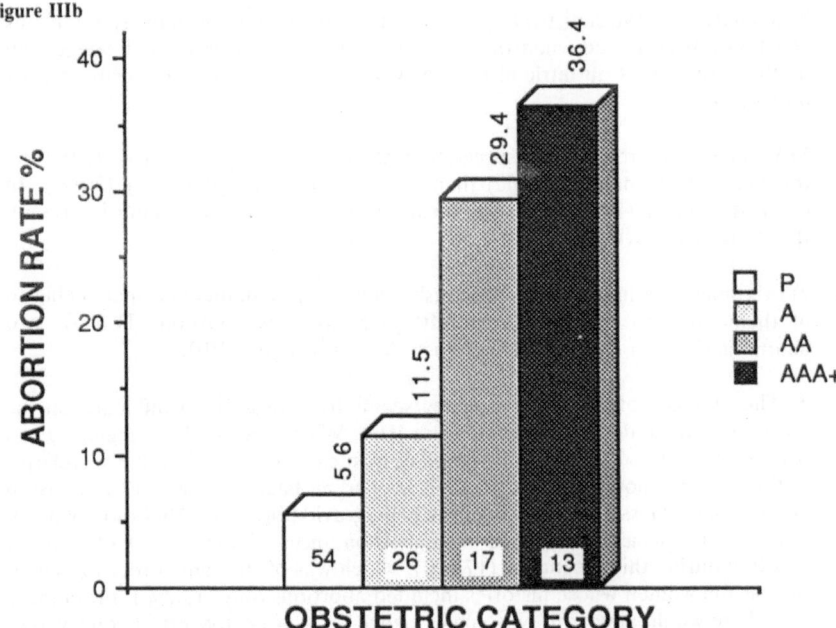

b. Histogram showing the primigravid abortion rate (P) together with the abortion rate in women with a history of only 1 abortion (A), 2 abortions (AA), and 3 or more abortions (AAA+).

Figure IIIc

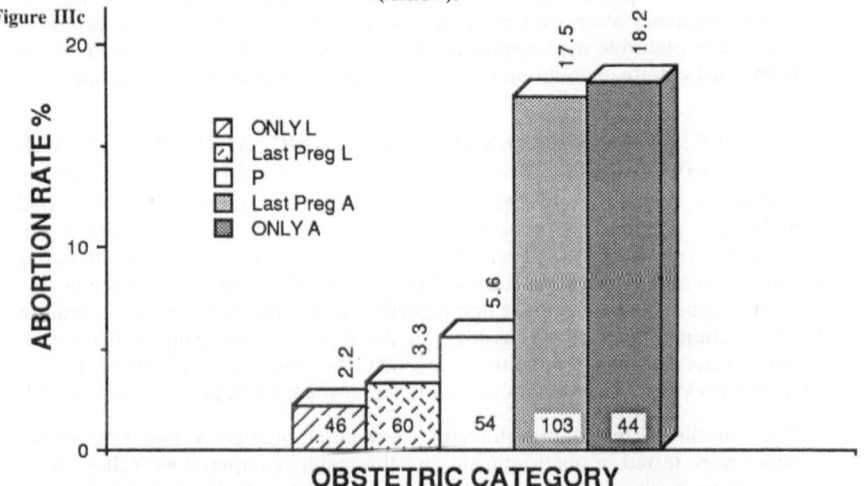

c. Histogram showing the abortion rate in women with a history of only live births (ONLY L), when the last pregnancy had a live outcome (Last Preg L), when the last pregnancy was aborted (Last Preg A), and when all previous pregnancies ended in abortion (ONLY A), compared and contrasted to the primigravid abortion rate.
The numbers of patients in each group are shown at the bottom of each column and the abortion rate (%) above each column.

been made to derive statistical significance from the variations in the spontaneous abortion rate observed when the pregnancies were subgrouped and categorised on the basis of past obstetric history. Nevertheless, some very interesting trends do emerge.

1) Women with previously unsuccessful histories were at greater risk of aborting this indexed pregnancy (18.2%) than those in their first pregnancy (5.6%). In contrast, women with previous live births enjoyed an even lower abortion rate in the study (2.2%) (Figure IIIa).

2) In women who had aborted previously, there was a cumulatively higher chance of them aborting this pregnancy with one previous abortion (11.5%), two abortions (29.4%) and three abortions (36.4%), (Figure IIIb).

3) The outcome of the last pregnancy seems to have a direct influence on the outcome of the index pregnancy (Figure IIIc). Women whose last pregnancy had been successful had a comparably good outcome on this occasion (3.3%) relative to the women whose previous pregnancies had all been successful (2.2%). Both groups aborted less frequently than the primigravid population, but those women whose last pregnancy had resulted in an abortion, incurred a higher risk of a further abortion during this pregnancy (17.5%), which was of the same order of magnitude as the women whose histories included abortions only (18.2%). From these data there would appear to be some evidence for a protective effect conveyed to the indexed pregnancy, when the last pregnancy resulted in a live child. Conversely, a detrimental effect was observed if the previous pregnancy had been unsuccessful. The possibility that an immunological event occurring during the previous pregnancy offers protection against abortion in a subsequent pregnancy, provides one plausible explanation of this observation and leads us to measure anti-paternal cytotoxic antibodies as one way of investigating this possibility.

INCIDENCE OF ANTI-PATERNAL CYTOTOXIC ANTIBODY IN THE COMPLETED PREGNANCIES

The cytotoxic antibody results presented here include all those patients who had completed a pregnancy (successful or aborted) and reached the postpartum interval by the end of August 1987—120 live births and 21 spontaneous abortions—a total of 141 pregnancies. The method of testing used was the microdroplet lymphocytotoxicity assay first described by Mittal *et al*[39] and standardised by the National Institute of Health. All the stored serum samples from each patient were tested retrospectively against the respective partner's freshly prepared peripheral blood lymphocytes taken at the 4 week postpartum interval.

Each of the maternal pre-pregnant, sequential pregnancy and postpartum samples were tested in quadruplicate and the results compared with those from one of known positive and negative control sera. The results for each patient were read by two independent observers and positive results recorded when lymphocytotoxicity levels in excess of 20% above the background negative control were present. Only 38% of the women who had live births ever produced detectable antibody (Table 3), which is considerably lower than the figure of 64% found by Beard *et al*[40] and argues against an absolute necessity for anti-paternal cytotoxic antibody to allow successful pregnancy outcome. Although Gelabert *et al*[41] found that women with spontaneous abortions had a higher prevalence of positive sera than do primigravidae, the percentage of positive antibody results in our women who subsequently aborted was only 9.5%, which might at first be interpreted as supportive evidence implicating causally the lack of antibody in abortion. However, it must be remembered that the 21 abortions discussed here all occurred before 14 weeks gestation (Figure II). Hence an equally plausible explanation for the low incidence of antibody in this aborting group would be that the appearance of detectable cytotoxic antibody does not occur until later in pregnancy.

Table 3

Incidence of Antipaternal Cytotoxic Antibody in 441 Completed Pregnancies

Indexed Pregnancy Outcome	Number of Patients	Number Antibody Positive	Percentage Antibody Positive
Live	120	46	38.3
Abortion	21	2	9.5
Total	141	48	34.0

TIME COURSE OF DEVELOPMENT OF ANTI-PATERNAL CYTOTOXIC ANTIBODY

The possibility that cytotoxic antibody production is a time-dependent event was confirmed by examining the gestational intervals at which the 120 women with live births developed antibody for the first time (Figure IV). Only 4 women had antibody present in their pre-pregnant serum. Two of these women had received blood transfusions in the past and 1 woman had undergone an ectopic gestation, suggesting that all 3 had been 'sensitised' previously. In the index pregnancy, 1 woman developed antibody at 5 weeks, 1 at 8 weeks, and 2 became positive at 14 and 18 weeks respectively. The suggestion that early antibody production correlates with a past history of abortion[41] could not be confirmed, since the majority of positive results were found only after the pregnancy had reached the third trimester, the frequency rising steadily from 28 weeks gestation and peaking around the time of delivery. This contrasts with previous studies which have shown that antibody is boosted in the first trimester and falls towards term.[42] In 8 of the live births antibody was only detectable in the 4 week postpartum serum.

Three important points are emphasised from an examination of the cumulative frequency of positive antibody results for the 120 live births. Firstly, only 4 women developed antibody before 14 weeks, the time by which all the abortions in this study group had occurred. Secondly, the overall incidence of antibody production in the total population of live births involved only one-third of the

Figure IV

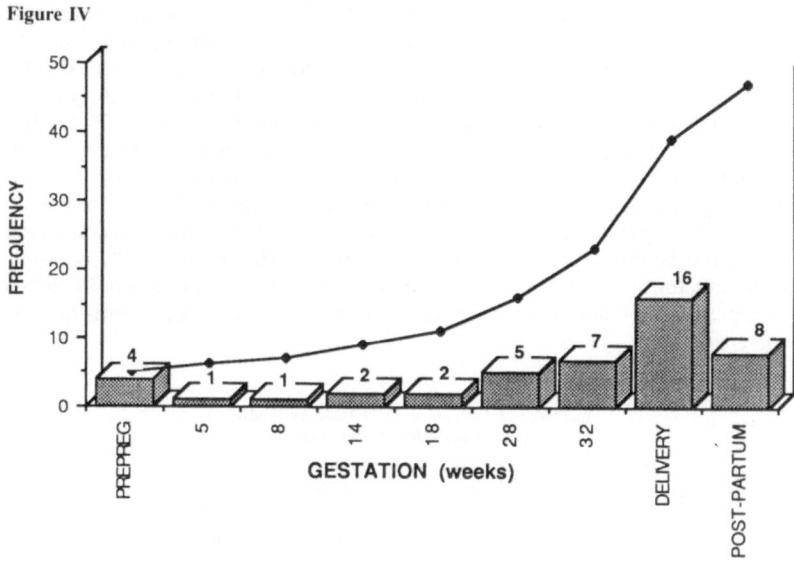

Histogram showing the time of first detection of anti-paternal cytotoxic antibody in 120 women having a live birth. The number of women with positive tests at each gestational time interval is denoted above each histogram bar. The cumulative frequency of anti-paternal cytotoxic antibody is shown by the solid line (————).

women. Thirdly, of those women who did produce antibody, the majority only became positive after completing 28 weeks of gestation. In addition, it can be inferred from the finding of only 4 positive pre-pregnant serum samples that this antibody is a transient and pregnancy-related phenomenon.

INCIDENCE OF ANTIBODY BY GRAVIDITY

In contrast to a previously held belief that the incidence of antibody positive women increases with cumulative successful pregnancies,[43,44] the percentage of antibody-positive women in groups analysed by maternal gravidity, appeared to share no such relationship (Table 4). Even when it is taken into account that the 3rd and 4th gravidity groups included women who had aborted in the past, and would therefore be less likely to have produced antibody, the percentages show little increase above the 38% incidence of positive results for live births in this pregnancy. Interestingly, the primigravidae in this population shared a similar incidence of antibody production to that found in the multiparous women. Moreover, if women with a history of infertility are considered separately, since not all fall into the primigravid grouping, 55% of the 31 women so far tested became antibody positive during the pregnancy study.

Table 4
Incidence of anti-paternal cytotoxic antibody
in 141 completed pregnancies by gravidity

Outcome Indexed Pregnancy	1st Pregnancy	2nd Pregnancy	3rd Pregnancy	4th Pregnancy	Total
Live	36.7%	42.4%	40.0%	31.8%	38.3%
	(11/30)	(14/33)	(14/35)	(7/22)	(46/120)
Abortion	33.3%	0	0	14.3%	9.5%
	(1/3)	(0/4)	(0/7)	(1/7)	(2/21)
Total	36.4%	37.8%	33.3%	27.6%	34.3%

CONCLUSIONS

It is possible to draw some conclusions from the study data so far analysed. The overall incidence of spontaneous abortion in this prospective study is considerably lower than those reported in previous studies (10.3% overall; 5.6% for primigravidae), possibly reflecting the fact that this population has been recruited prospectively and pre-conceptually. Alternatively, it may reflect the fact that because they were a well motivated group of women, they have an inherently lower risk of spontaneous abortion. The pregnancy loss rate increased with gravidity, in agreement with previously cited studies, and the outcome of the previous pregnancy was associated with an effect on the outcome of a future pregnancy, suggesting that a previously successful pregnancy may offer some protective effect.

Sixty-two percent of the women who had live births never produced detectable cytotoxic antibody during their pregnancy, but the corresponding figure for the women in the aborting group was 90.5%. However, this result should not be interpreted as supportive evidence for lack of antibody being causally related to a woman's tendency to abort recurrently, because all of these women suffered pregnancy losses prior to 14 weeks, and the majority of positive antibody results in the live birth group occurred after 28 weeks gestation. Thus the relatively low incidence of antibody present in the spontaneously aborting group arose simply because they had insufficiently long gestation to produce a response.

Finally, the results from this study suggest that detectable circulating anti-paternal cytotoxic antibody is not necessary for the maintenance of pregnancy, neither does this antibody provide a reliable marker for a pregnancy that is destined to be successful.[45] It may now be concluded that the absence of anti-paternal cytotoxic antibody is not related causally to a woman's tendency to abort repeatedly, and the temptation to use this antibody to monitor immunisation treatment and predict future pregnancy outcome should be resisted until the significance of its presence is fully understood.

ACKNOWLEDGEMENTS

I would like to thank Peter Braude and Martin Johnson for their practical help and advice and Dan Hill, Janet Currie, Anne Cant and Soo Pickering for their technical assistance. This work is being supported by an MRC programme grant awarded to Doctors M. H. Johnson and P. R. Braude.

REFERENCES

1. Warburton D, Fraser FC. Spontaneous abortion risks in man: data from reproductive histories collected in a medical genetics unit. *Hum Genet* 1964; **16:** 1-25.
2. WHO Recommended definitions, terminology and format for statistical tables related to the perinatal period. *Acta Obstet Gynecol Scand* 1977; **56:** 247-253.
3. Boué J, Boué A, Lazar P. Retrospective and prospective epidemiological studies of 1500 karyotyped spontaneous human abortions. *Teratology* 1975; **12:** 11-26.
4. Lauritsen JG. Aetiology of spontaneous abortion. A cytogenetic and epidemiological study of 288 abortuses and their parents. *Acta Obstet Gynecol Scand* 1976; **52:** 1-29.
5. Geisler M, Kleinebrecht J, Cytogenetic and histological analyses of spontaneous abortions, *Hum Genet* 1978; **45:** 239-251.
6. Warburton D, Strobino B. Recurrent spontaneous abortion. In: *Spontaneous and recurrent abortion.* Eds. MJ Bennett and DK Edmonds. Oxford: Blackwell Scientific Publications, 1987; pp.193-213,
7. McDonald IA. Cervical cerclage. *Clin Obstet Gynecol* 1980; **7:** 461-479.
8. Phung TT, Byrd JR, McDonough PG. Etiologies and subsequent reproductive performance of 100 couples with recurrent abortion. *Fertil Steril* 1979; **32:** 389-395.
9. Crane JP, Wahl N. The role of maternal diabetes in repetitive spontaneous abortion. *Fertil Steril* 1981; **36:** 477-479.
10. Prout TE. Thyroid disease in pregnancy. *Am J Obstet Gynecol* 1975; **122:** 669-676.
11. Horta JL, Fernandez JG, Soto de Leon B, Cortes-Gallegos V. Direct evidence of luteal insufficiency in women with habitual abortion. *Obstet Gynecol* 1977; **49:** 705-708.
12. Goldzieher JW. Double blind trial of a progestin in habitual abortion. *J Am Med Assoc* 1964; **188:** 651-654.
13. Mowbray JF, Underwood JL. Immunology of abortion. *Clin Exp Immunol* 1985; **60:** 1-7.
14. Beer AE, Quebbeman JF, Semprini AE. Immunopathological factors contributing to recurrent spontaneous abortion in humans. In: *Spontaneous and recurrent abortion.* Eds. MJ Bennett, DK Edmonds. Oxford: Blackwell Scientific Publications, 1987; pp.90-108.
15. Taylor C and Faulk WP. Prevention of recurrent abortion with leucocyte transfusions. *Lancet* 1981; **2:** 68-70.
16. Mowbray JF, Gibbings C, Liddell H, Reginald PW, Underwood JL, Beard RW. Controlled trial of treatment of recurrent spontaneous abortion with paternal cells. *Lancet* 1985; 1: 941-943.
17. Roth DB. The frequency of spontaneous abortion. *Int J Fertil* 1963; **8:** 434.
18. Petersson F. *Epidemiology of early pregnancy wastage.* Svenska Bokforlaget, Norstedts 1968.
19. Poland BJ, Miller JR, Jones DC, Trimble BK. Reproductive counseling in patients who have had a spontaneous abortion. *Am J Obstet Gynecol* 1977; **127:** 685-691.
20. Stray-Pederson B, Stray-Pederson S. Etiologic factors and subsequent reproductive performance in 195 couples with a prior history of habitual abortion. *Am J Obstet Gynecol* 1984; **148:** 140-146.
21. Tamada T, Fukwai Z. Early detection of pregnancy around the first missed menstrual period by 2 hour haemagglutination test. *Acta Obstet Gynaecol Jpn* 1976; **23:** 23-26.
22. Edmonds DK, Lindsay KS, Miller JF, Williamson E, Wood PJ. Early embryonic mortality in women. *Fertil Steril* 1982; **38:** 447-453.
23. Miller JF, Williamson E, Gordon YB, Grudzinskas JG, Sykes A. Fetal loss after implantation. *Lancet* 1980; **2:** 554-556.
24. Glass RH, Golbus MS. Habitual abortion. *Fertil Steril* 1978; **29:** 257-265.
25. Huisjes HJ. *Spontaneous abortion.* Edinburgh: Churchill Livingstone, 1984.
26. Malpas P. A study of abortion sequences. *J Obstet Gynaecol Br Empire* 1938; **45:** 932-949.

27. James WH. Notes towards an epidemiology of spontaneous abortion. *Am J Hum Genet* 1963; **15:** 223-240.
28. Roman EA, Alberman E, Pharoah POD. Pregnancy order and reproductive loss. *Br Med J* 1980; **280:** 715.
29. Alberman E, Elliott M, Creasy M, Dhadial R. Previous reproductive history in mothers presenting with spontaneous abortions. *Br J Obstet Gynaecol* **82:** 366-373.
30. Fitzsimmons J, Jackson D, Wapner R, Jackson L. Subsequent reproductive outcome in couples with repeated pregnancy loss. *Am J Med Genet* 1983; **16:** 583-587.
31. Vlaanderen W. Het begrip 'habituele abortus', een fictie? *Ned Tijdschr Geneeskd* 1977; **121:** 439-442.
32. Beer AE, Semprini AE, Zhu Z, Quebberman JF. Pregnancy outcome in human couples with recurrent spontaneous abortions: 1) HLA antigen profiles; 2) HLA antigen sharing; Female serum MLR blocking factors; and 3) paternal leukocyte immunisation. *Exp Clin Immunogenet* 1985; **2:** 137-153.
33. Unander AM, Lindholm A, Olding LB. Blood transfusions generate/increase previously absent/weak blocking antibody in women with habitual abortion. *Fertil Steril* 1985; **44:** 766-771.
34. Taylor CG, Faulk WP, McIntyre JA. Prevention of recurrent spontaneous abortions by leukocyte transfusions. *J R Soc Med* 1985; **78:** 623-627.
35. Mowbray JF, Underwood JL, Michel M, Forbes PB, Beard RW. Immunisation with paternal lymphocytes in women with recurrent miscarriage. *Lancet* 1987; **2:** 679-680.
36. Naylor AF. Warburton D. Sequential analysis of spontaneous abortion. II. Collaborative study data show that gravidity determines a very substantial increase in risk. *Fertil Steril* 1979; **31:** 282-286.
37. James WH. Spontaneous abortion and birth order. *J Biosoc Sci* 1974; **6:** 23-41.
38. Resseguie LJ. Pregnancy wastage and age of mother among the Amish. *Hum Biol* 1974; **46:** 633-639.
39. Mittal KM, Mickey MR, Singal PP, Terasaki PI. Serotyping for homotransplantation XVIII. Refinement of microdroplet lymphocyte cytotoxicity test. *Transplantation* 1969; **6:** 904-912.
40. Beard RW, Braude P, Mowbray JF, Underwood JL. Protective antibodies and spontaneous abortion. *Lancet* 1983; **2:** 1090.
41. Gelabert A, Balasch J, Ercilla G, Vanrell JA, Vives J, González-Merlo J, Castillo R. Abortion may sensitize the mother to HLA antigens. *Tissue Antigens* 1981; **17:** 353-356.
42. Vives J, Gelabert A, Castillo R. HLA antibodies and period of gestation: decline in frequency of positive sera during last trimester. *Tissue Antigens* 1976; **7:** 209-212.
43. Van Rood JJ, Eernisse JG, Van Leeuwen A. Leucocyte antibodies in sera from pregnant women. *Nature* 1958; **181:** 1735-1736.
44. Ahrons S. Leukocyte antibodies: occurrence in primigravidae. *Tissue Antigens* 1973; **1:** 178-183.
45. Regan L, Braude PR. Is antipaternal cytotoxic antibody a valid marker in the management of recurrent abortion? *Lancet* 1987; **2:** 1280.
46. Stevenson AC, Dudgeon MY, McClure H. Observations on the results of pregnancies in women resident in Belfast. II. Abortions, hydatidiform moles and ectopic pregnancies. *Ann Hum Genet* 1959; **23:** 395.
47. Leridon H. Facts and artefacts in the study of intrauterine mortality: a reconsideration from pregnancy histories. *Population Studies* 1976; **30:** 319-335.
48. Shapiro S, Levine HS, Abramivicz M. Factors associated with early and late fetal loss. In: *Advances in Planned Parenthood VI*. Proceedings of the VIII Annual Meeting of the AAPP, no. 45. Excerpta Medica International Congress Series, Number 224.
49. Awan AK. Some biologic correlates of pregnancy wastage. *Am J Obstet Gynecol* 1974; **119:** 525-531.
50. Harger JH, Archer DF, Marchese SG, Muracca-Clemens M, Gawer KL. Etiology of recurrent pregnancy losses and outcome of subsequent pregnancies. *Obstet Gynecol* 1983; **62:** 574-581.

Discussion

Chairman: Professor R. W. Beard

Professor BEER: Early in the presentation the pie-shaped wedge of people who had previous abortions was removed, yet the group of patients that were undergoing *in vitro* fertilisation was left in as a normal part of the study population. That troubled me and I should like to know how that was permissible.

Miss REGAN: I removed 35 patients who self-referred themselves saying that they were recurrent miscarriers and they wished for treatment. We had another group of women who were, by definition recurrent miscarriers; they had had three or more consecutive miscarriages, but those patients for some reason considered themselves to be relatively normal, and I have left them in.

I take the point about the *in vitro* fertilisation patients. When we looked at the primigravid population, of which there were 57 who had pregnancies with us, as I said earlier, over half of them came from the poster or radio appeal. Obviously by definition of their being primigravidae there was no past history; they just came as normals from the general population. Less than half of them were infertility patients and about one-quarter of them were from the *in vitro* fertilisation programme.

Of note is the fact that in our infertility group there was only one abortion and one ectopic in the general infertility group, and there was one termination—sadly for fetal abnormality and not diagnosed until 20 weeks—and one ectopic in our IVF group. And I believe that in the absence of them having a very markedly high abortion rate, they are a reasonable group to include in the primigravid population.

Professor BEARD: That can only be determined by looking at their outcome and results in relation to the normals.

Miss REGAN: Yes. And the percentage did not change.

Professor JENKINS: Are people, when they are talking about previous abortion, talking about histologically confirmed abortion or not? I have a clinical impression, which is probably shared by other clinicians, that if patients complain of recurrent abortion they exaggerate the number of abortions that they have had and they do not have histological confirmation for many of the abortions that they complain of having had. So what are we talking about precisely when we talk about a past recurrent abortion history?

39

Miss REGAN: I am talking about a woman who has had a clinically recognised pregnancy, by which I mean that the doctor and the patient know that she has been pregnant.

Professor BEARD: Can I reply to that for our group? It has not been our impression on the large number that we have that women over-estimate. If anything they under-estimate the number of miscarriages they have had. Our group consisted of either histologically or biochemically determined or ultrasound diagnosed.

Dr CARP: For our group, a pregnancy is defined either histologically, ultrasonically or biochemically. We do not include patients who have very low beta-hCG levels, but there has to be objectivity.

Professor HARRIS: When looking at cytotoxic antibodies, in a way one is setting ground rules for discussions of immunology later in our proceedings. The presence of an antibody using the cytotoxicity test is a very crude measure and it may well be that many of those who have found antibodies have used a more sensitive test. Secondly, the specificity of the antibodies, we know that they are against terminal antigens but are they against Class I or Class II? Thirdly, what about all the cellular immunological events that must be going on? I am not asking for answers to those questions but some of them quite clearly need to be addressed.

Miss REGAN: I take the point. Obviously that is something that we have to move on to and examine as well.

Professor GILL: The data in the literature show that the percentage of cytotoxic antibodies found in pregnant women appears to increase from the postpartum period after the first pregnancy to the fifth pregnancy, when it is about 35 or 38%, and it stays constant. Does Miss Regan have any idea why her group got roughly 35% from the first pregnancy on?

Miss REGAN: We included some women who did not have successful pregnancies, which would account for some of it. I do not know why in our population we seem to have a much lower incidence of cytotoxic antibodies than all of the people who have reported data before. But then no one has done it prospectively and sequentially before.

Dr DAYA: How would one account for the very high prevalence of recurrent abortion in this group of patients? I know that they were excluded from the analysis, but if we were to include them just to look at their effect, it comes to almost 8% of the population that was sampled as having recurrent abortions, which is enormously higher than the general population results would indicate.

Does that mean that in Cambridge there is a much higher incidence of recurrent abortion, or is that again a pre-selected population of patients?

Miss REGAN: They are most definitely pre-selected. They are referring themselves. Some of them will come from just outside, from the borders of our catchment area, which if you work in the East Anglian Health Authority you know is a pretty substantial catchment area. It covers the North of Norwich territory as well. So yes, they are a very pre-selected group.

Dr CARP: Could I comment again about some of the results. I also want to comment on some of our results.

Our results agree very much with yours. We see a much lower incidence of cytotoxic antibodies, 11% in primary aborters, 24% in secondary aborters and 32% in our parous population. But we do seem to see some differences. In the patients who are parous, their antipaternal antibodies seem to be polymorphic, they seem to be directed against Class II and Class I antigens. What we have seen in our primary aborter population is that they only seem to be directed against Class I antigens.

In patients whom we have immunised—I do not want to speak about immunisation, but those patients who have produced antibodies, again they seem to be directed against Class I and Class II antigens overall.

We do not yet have large enough figures to do statistical analysis, but if we look at the results of the following pregnancies, the primary aborters with antibody who have not been immunised, or who have been immunised, all seem to do very badly in their following pregnancies. It is as if the recurrent aborter who produces antibody is producing one which acts *in vivo* possibly very differently to a patient with successful pregnancies who produces antibodies.

Let me say something else. Miss Regan mentioned that immunologically her group takes 20% of cell kill as being the criterion. We have taken a 50% cell kill as being our criterion; we have also noted down those who have had less than 50%. What seems to be very strange is that three patients who have had <50% in their antibodies, but do have some concentration of antibody present, seem to have successful pregnancies. It seems to be a very strange story that the patient with abortions and a full dose of antibody aborts. The patient with a very small dose of antibody seems to have successful pregnancies.

It may be that in this very gross test we are simply not defining which antibodies we are looking at.

Miss REGAN: I accept that point. My experience of immunisation patients, and one of the reasons that this study was started, was that in the first 30 or 40 that we immunised in our recurrent abortion clinic we found that less than half of the women who had successful pregnancy outcomes after their immunisation treatment ever produced detectable antibody. Conversely, over half of the women who aborted again did produce antibody, which was one of the starting points for wanting to assess what the incidence was in the normal population.

Dr CARP: That is not our experience, as we have discussed in the past.

Dr ANTCZAK: We must be much more precise about the antibodies we are discussing.

Professor ALBERMAN: I should like to query whether bearing a pregnancy which is chromosomally abnormal and may be lost very early is likely to give the same sort of picture as bearing a pregnancy that is chromosomally normal.

Dr ALLEN: In the 23 first-time aborters in the primigravidae, was any delay in conception noticed in those compared with the others in the prospective group? Did they conceive as readily—and I assume equal mating opportunities? Did they have any pathology about the uterus? Were they suspected of having other than immunological pathological reasons?

Miss REGAN: We still have to do the endometrial biopsy study—but I have no specific data to give now. I have not analysed the time sequence, how many months it took for those women who had aborted in the past and came to us because of their previous miscarriages and those women who were primips.

My impression is that the women who were primigravidae stopped using their contraception and fell pregnant immediately.

Dr ALLEN: Including the 23 aborters?

Miss REGAN: Yes.

Dr B. STRAY-PEDERSON: The risk of a further abortion following three successive abortions was discussed and a number of references were cited. But they all include people who have been treated. My problem is assessing the risk of abortion in a woman who has had three or more successive abortions and has had no treatment.

Miss REGAN: That is my question too, which is why I am trying, little by little, to establish the data.

Professor HARRIS: Is anyone collecting information on a family history of abortion; for example, did the woman's mother have spontaneous abortions? Is anyone collecting that sort of data?

Miss REGAN: I am doing it retrospectively. I am ashamed to say that when I started the study I did not think of including that, so now every time I contact a patient again I try and obtain that data.

Professor JOHNSON: In the series that we have investigated in Liverpool we have been collecting information on both family size and family history. Clearly with an absolute family history the patient would not be there in the first place, and therefore the definition of a family history is an arbitrary point. But we have taken any patient who has a blood relative with three or more spontaneous abortions, not necessarily consecutive, and there is a mildly but statistically significant increase of a family history in the primary recurrent spontaneous abortion group.

Interestingly, though the figures are still quite small, that was not the case in the secondary recurrent spontaneous abortion group.

Clinical and immunological significance of anti-phospholipid antibodies

E. N. Harris

Anti-phospholipid antibodies are a family of autoantibodies detected by standard tests for syphilis (STS), the lupus anticoagulant (LA) test or by solid phase anti-cardiolipin (aCL) antibody tests. These antibodies have attracted much attention in recent years because their occurrence has been associated with both venous and arterial thrombosis, recurrent fetal loss and thrombo-cytopenia.[1-5] In addition, some clinicians have reported an increased frequency of livedo reticularis,[6,7] migraine headaches,[7] endocardial lesions,[8] chorea,[9,10,11] positive Coombs test,[12] decreased complement,[13] and type 5 antimitochondrial antibodies[13,14] in affected patients. However, it is yet to be determined whether these additional features reflect an underlying autoimmune disorder or are directly related to the presence of anti-phospholipid antibodies.[15]

HISTORICAL

Anti-phospholipid antibodies were probably first detected by Wasserman in 1906, and for several years were important as a means of diagnosing syphilis.[16] In the 1940s it was noted that some patients had positive standard tests for syphilis (STS), but did not have the clinical features of syphilis and their sera gave negative results in the newly introduced treponemal immobilisation (TPI) test.[16,17] These unusual patients were subsequently defined as having a biological false positive test for syphilis (BFP-STS).[17] Investigators of the time also found that many patients with the BFP-STS had an underlying autoimmune disorder, systemic lupus erythematosus (SLE) usually, and that a positive test could precede the onset of these autoimmune disorders by several years.[16-20] Beginning with the work of Mary Pangborn,[21] it was ascertained in the 1950s and 60s that a positive standard test for syphilis was caused by antibodies that bound a phospho-lipid molecule named cardiolipin.[22,23]

At the time that the first series of patients with the BFP-STS were being reported,[17] Conley and Hartmann described two patients with SLE who presented with bleeding, prolonged prothrombin and whole blood clotting time as well as a positive BFP-STS.[24] The prolonged prothrombin time could not be corrected by mixing with normal plasma, suggesting that this abnormality was not due to a clotting factor deficiency. Other reports of similar patients started appearing in the literature, and these patients invariably had a BFP-STS.[25] In 1957, Laurell and Nilsson found that pre-incubation of these patients' plasma with the Kahn antigen, which contained cardiolipin, corrected the prolonged prothrombin time.[26] By the 1970s, several haematologists firmly believed that this abnormal "anticoagulant", detected primarily in patients with SLE and now termed the "lupus anticoagulant",[27] was due to an anti-phospholipid antibody.[27,28] That the lupus coagulant phenomenon may be caused by anti-phospholipid antibodies was confirmed during the last few years, and work leading to this conclusion will be discussed later.

Although the lupus anticoagulant prolongs clotting time *in vitro*, investigators reported that affected patients seldom had bleeding disorders, even when undergoing surgery.[25,26-29] Not only was bleeding rare, but Bowie and colleagues reported in 1963, that of eight patients with the lupus anticoagulant, four had had episodes of venous thrombosis in the past.[30] In 1977, Johansson and colleagues reported 8 patients with the BFP-STS, lupus anticoagulant and thrombosis.[31] The report that eventually attracted the attention of the general medical community was that of Mueh and colleagues who described eight patients with the lupus anticoagulant who had venous or arterial thrombosis.[32] The interest of obstetricians in these unusual patients was stimulated by three separate reports appearing during the period of 1975 to 1980. In 1975, Inga Marie Nilsson reported the case of one woman with an "anti-thromboplastin" (the old name for the lupus anticoagulant) who had suffered several abortions.[33] Then in 1982, Firkin in Australia[34] and Soulier and Boffa in France[35] each reported four women with the lupus anticoagulant who had had frequent abortions. Since then, there have been several series of patients reported with the lupus anticoagulant and recurrent fetal loss.[12,36-47] More importantly, as will be discussed later, it has been reported that treatment of affected women during pregnancy with steroids and aspirin may result in successful pregnancy outcome.[37]

Because the lupus anticoagulant tests lacked specificity and varied between laboratories, it became necessary to find some alternative means of detecting and characterising these antibodies. Reasoning that patients with the lupus anti-coagulant frequently had a BFP-STS and because cardiolipin is the antigen detected in the STS, Harris, Gharavi and co-workers devised a sensitive solid phase radioimmunoassay test to detect antibodies to cardiolipin.[48] In an initial series of 65 SLE patients, they found that patients with the lupus anticoagulant invariably had a positive anticardiolipin antibody test, and in this particular patient group, the presence of anticardiolipin antibodies was strongly associated with a history of thrombosis.[48] Since that time there have been several improvements in the performance of the anticardiolipin test, and standard sera have been introduced to calibrate the assay.[49,50] Besides providing an additional means of identifying patients with antiphospholipid antibodies who may be prone to thrombosis and fetal loss, the anticardiolipin assay has enabled better characterisation of anti-phospholipid antibodies.

OCCURRENCE

As interest has increased in anti-phospholipid antibodies, the disease conditions in which they appear to be present have grown considerably. This is particularly true of the anticardiolipin test, which because of its sensitivity, has been found to be positive in a variety of autoimmune,[2] infectious,[51,52] drug induced[53] and other miscellaneous disorders. The Acquired Immunodeficiency Syndrome (AIDS) has been added recently to the list of disease conditions in which anti-cardiolipin antibodies occur.[54] The lupus anticoagulant phenomenon, too, has been reported in patients with a variety of diseases,[29,32,55] and the same has been true of the BFP-STS.[16,17,20] Because anti-phospholipid antibodies can occur in so many disorders, in most instances without any readily apparent sequelae, investigators are currently turning their attention to determining the subset of patients with anti-phospholipid antibodies who are most prone to thrombosis and fetal loss.[12,15]

THROMBOSIS

About 25-33% of unselected patients with the lupus anticoagulant appear to be prone to venous or arterial thrombosis.[56,57,58] In a population composed mainly of patients with rheumatological disorders, we have found thrombosis in about 50% of patients with anticardiolipin antibodies.[12] We have found a history of thrombosis in greater than 75% of patients who have high levels of IgG anti-cardiolipin antibodies.[12] Affected patients usually have these antibodies over prolonged periods of time, hence a diagnosis of "anti-phospholipid related thrombosis or fetal loss" should be based on more than one positive test performed several weeks apart.

Thrombosis may occur elsewhere in the vascular system, and patients may present in a variety of ways depending on where the site of the occlusion occurs. Thrombosis in the arterial circulation is about half as frequent as that in the venous system,[12,57,59,60] but the consequences of arterial occlusion are probably more serious.[60,61] Patients may present with deep vein thrombosis, thrombo-phlebitis, or recurrent pulmonary emboli.[32,34-36,40-42,48,51,56-64] Other presentations include stroke or transient ischaemic attacks, multi-infarct dementia,[17] myocardial infarction,[72,73] gangrene of the extremities[74] and decreased vision.[75] These complications are particularly tragic when one considers that the majority of affected patients are young.[1-3] Documented sites of venous thrombosis include the superficial[76] and deep veins of the legs,[32,34-36,40-42,48,51,56-64] renal,[77] hepatic,[78,79] axillary[60] and intracranial veins,[80] as well as the inferior vena cava.[60] Arterial sites include the cranial,[65-70] coronary,[72,73] retinal,[75] mesenteric,[81] and peripheral arteries.[74] Small vessels such as the glomerulus of the kidney[60] and placental vessels[37,44,82] may also be affected. Placental vessel thrombosis resulting in placental infarction or placental insufficiency may be the mechanism by which fetal loss occurs.[36,83] A few patients with these antibodies have presented with pulmonary hypertension, either because of recurrent pulmonary emboli or because of thrombosis within the pulmonary vasculature.[84] In the few instances where histology has been available, thrombosis of vessel walls appears to occur without any underlying atherosclerosis or cellular infiltration of the vessel wall characteristic of a vasculitis.[74]

Since thrombosis appears to be associated with anti-phospholipid antibodies independent of the underlying disease condition,[1-4] it would be reasonable to propose that these antibodies may play some role in causing thrombosis. However, there is no proof that this is true. The thrombotic process involves an interplay of clotting factors and their physiological inhibitors, fibrinolytic proteins, platelets and endothelial cells. Almost every one of these systems has been reported to be abnormal in patients with the lupus anticoagulant. Proposed mechanisms include increased platelet aggregation secondary to decreased prostacyclin production by vascular endothelium; the endothelium presumably being damaged by anti-phospholipid antibodies.[36,83] Schorer and Watson recently reported that lupus anticoagulant plasma markedly reduced thrombin-stimulated release of prostacyclin from endothelial cells.[85] On the other hand, several groups have been unable to demonstrate specific binding of anti-phospholipid antibodies to cultured endothelial cells.[86,87] Other mechanisms by which these antibodies have been proposed to cause thrombosis include inhibition of fibrinolytic activity,[88] inhibition of prekallikrein activity,[89] inhibition of antithrombin III activity,[90] inhibition of protein C activation,[91] and inhibition of thrombomodulin.[92] It is also conceivable that these antibodies can bind phospholipids in platelet membranes so causing their activation, aggregation and thrombosis.[93]

On the basis of retrospective studies, thrombosis appears to to recur in patients with anti-phospholipid antibodies.[47,57,62] This observation is used as the main reason for prolonged prophylactic treatment with oral anticoagulants of patients with anti-phospholipid antibodies who have had a previous episode of thrombosis.[94] Treatment of patients with arterial thrombosis is less certain, but either warfarin or aspirin and dipyridamole have been used in small numbers of affected patients with varying success.[57,71] Because warfarin therapy appears to be effective in preventing recurrent thrombosis,[41,57,62] and since patients may be at risk for several years, the use of steroids and immunosuppressive agents to suppress antibody production is usually not recommended. However, when thrombosis occurs despite adequate anticoagulant therapy or in life-threatening situations, steroids and/or immunosuppressive agents should be considered. Only some patients with the lupus anticoagulant or anticardiolipin antibodies appear to be subject to thrombosis, hence there is no justification for administering prophylactic treatment to patients who have had no previous history of thrombosis.

FETAL LOSS

Perhaps the greatest benefit to be derived from work on anti-phospholipid antibodies will be the identification of women with a treatable cause of recurrent fetal loss.

Based on retrospective studies, most authorities agree that the majority of women with the lupus anticoagulant are subject to recurrent fetal loss. In a survey of the published literature, Branch and colleagues reported that 89% of 43 women had one or more fetal losses. In their own series of 28 women, they found a perinatal survival rate of only 14%.[43] Elias and Eldor reported that of 26 pregnancies in seven women with the lupus anticoagulant, only one was successful.[41] Lubbe and colleagues reported that one of 36 pregnancies in 12 women with the lupus anticoagulant was successful.[37] Not all reports paint as gloomy a picture with respect to pregnancy outcome in lupus anticoagulant positive mothers. Ros and colleagues found that only 3 of 10 women with the lupus anticoagulant had a history of fetal loss.[39] In a recent retrospective study of pregnant women with the lupus anticoagulant, Lockshin and colleagues reported that six of 12 affected women had good pregnancy outcome.[95]

Fetal loss in women with anti-cardiolipin antibodies probably depends on antibody level[12,95] and isotype.[95] Derue and colleagues[44] first reported an association between anti-cardiolipin antibodies and fetal loss in a study of 40 women, most of whom had SLE and 23 of whom had a history of fetal loss. Sixteen of the 23 had anti-cardiolipin antibodies while only 3 of 17 women with normal pregnancy outcome had these antibodies. In two studies of women with SLE who became pregnant, Lockshin and colleagues found a high correlation between positive anticardiolipin tests and fetal death.[45,95] In another study of 121 patients with varying IgG anti-cardiolipin levels, Harris and colleagues found that the percentage of women with fetal loss tended to increase as the level of IgG anti-cardiolipin increased.[12] Elucidation of antibody level and isotype as well as the importance of lupus anticoagulant activity in determining pregnancy outcome, must await appropriate prospective studies.

In an unselected population of women with recurrent fetal loss, the number with anti-phospholipid antibodies may be quite small. In an unpublished survey of over 600 women with first trimester fetal loss, we found few who were anti-cardiolipin positive. Lockwood and colleagues reported that of 55 women with poor obstetric outcome, 15 (27%) had a positive anti-cardiolipin test and four had a positive lupus anticoagulant test.[96] Tincani and colleagues surveyed 103 women with a history of three or more fetal losses and found eight (7%) who had positive lupus anticoagulant or anti-cardiolipin tests.[97] Petri and colleagues surveyed 40 idiopathic habitual aborters and found the lupus anticoagulant in 9% and anti-cardiolipin in 11%.[98] In surveying sera of large populations of women with fetal loss, it is important that antibody level and isotype as well as lupus anticoagulant activity be considered in terms of defining a patient as having "anti-phospholipid related fetal loss".[12,15] This author reviewed the data published in the Petri study,[98] and suggests that only 2/40 patients with the highest anti-cardiolipin levels (both also had lupus anticoagulant activity and histories of venous thrombosis) had "anti-phospholipid related fetal loss" rather than the 5/40 stated by Petri and colleagues.[98] Similarly, in the Lockwood study,[96] this author's view in contrast to that of Lockwood and colleagues is that only the 5 patients with the highest IgG anti-cardiolipin levels, all of whom had the lupus anticoagulant, plus the single patient with the very high IgM levels (total of six patients) should have been considered as having "anti-phospholipid related fetal loss", rather than all 15 anti-cardiolipin positive patients. Guidelines for selection of patients as having "anti-phospholipid related fetal loss" (the "Anti-Phospholipid Syndrome") are shown in Table 1. Until proper prospective studies are performed, it seems wise not to consider treating all patients with fetal loss who have positive anti-cardiolipin or lupus anticoagulant tests, particularly if these tests are borderline positive. It might be better to repeat these tests, if possible, over several weeks, since it appears that patients who best fit the diagnosis of "Anti-Phospholipid Syndrome" frequently have positive tests over long periods of time.

Table 1

Anti-Phospholipid Syndrome

Clinical	Serology
Venous thrombosis	IgG anti-cardiolipin antibody (>10 GLP Units)
Arterial thrombosis	*Positive Lupus anticoagulant Test
Recurrent fetal loss	IgM anti-cardiolipin antibody (>10 MLP Units) + positive LA test

Patients with Anti-Phospholipid Syndrome would be defined as having at least one clinical and one serological feature at some time in their disease course. An anti-phospholipid test should be positive on at least two occasions, more than eight weeks apart.

*Lupus anticoagulant should be confirmed by demonstrating inhibition by phospholipids or by free thawed platelets.

Fetal loss can occur at any stage of pregnancy in women with anti-phospholipid antibodies. Derue and colleagues reported that of 60 fetal losses in 23 women, 22 occurred in the first trimester, 31 in the second and 7 in third.[44] Of 36 fetal losses in 12 women, Lubbe and colleagues reported 24 occurring in the first, and 12 in the second and third trimesters of pregnancy.[99] Branch and colleagues in their series of 28 women reported 51% losses in the first, 29% in the second and 19% in the third trimester.[43] On the basis of this data, it would appear reasonable to recommend that treatment be instituted early in pregnancy.

In 1983, Lubbe and colleagues reported that treatment of 6 women with lupus anticoagulant activity and histories of fetal loss resulted in live births in 5.[37] These women were treated with prednisone, in doses sufficient to decrease lupus anticoagulant activity to normal (doses of about 40mg/day were required), and aspirin 75mg/day.[37] Lubbe and colleagues have extended their series to 16 treated pregnancies in 12 women, with live births in 10.[99] A number of other centres have used the same treatment regimens for similarly affected women with varying results. Farquharson and colleagues[100] and Vermylen and colleagues[3] reported successful pregnancy outcome in 2 and in 4 similarly affected women respectively, after treatment with prednisone and aspirin. Branch and colleagues treated 8 affected women with steroids and aspirin, five of whom had successful pregnancy outcome.[43] Of these 5, however, 2 had persistent lupus anticoagulant activity throughout pregnancy despite treatment with steroids. Given the somewhat uncertain results of the Branch study, and questions raised by other investigators,[38,39,101] it is becoming increasingly evident to several investigators that prospective randomised trials of therapy need to be initiated. To find sufficient numbers of patients, such trials will need to involve several centres. Alternatives to steroids would be welcome since these drugs have a long list of side-effects including Cushingoid facies,[99,43] acne,[43] impaired wound healing,[43] infection and adrenal insufficiency.[43] There are a few aspects of successful pregnancy outcome after treatment of lupus anticoagulant positive women with steroids and azathioprine,[97,102,103] and we know of one case of successful pregnancy outcome after treatment with aspirin and dipyridamole alone (NA MacLachlan, unpublished). There is an instance, too, of a woman with lupus anticoagulant activity, high anti-cardiolipin levels and five fetal losses, who was given no treatment during her sixth pregnancy and had successful pregnancy outcome despite persistence of anti-phospholipid antibodies (Waveny Charles, personal communication).

The mechanism by which anti-phospholipid antibodies influence fetal loss is unknown. The most popular explanation is that these antibodies may cause thrombosis of placental vessels resulting in placental infarction and fetal death.[44,82,83] Thrombosis of fetal vessels and placental infarction do not appear to be uniform findings in placentae of aborted fetuses of women with anti-phospholipid antibodies,[45,95] nor are such findings specific to patients with these antibodies. Several investigators have argued that autoantibodies other than anti-phospholipid antibodies may play a role in fetal loss,[97,98,104-108] and this possibility needs further investigation.

THROMBOCYTOPENIA

Some studies have found that thrombocytopenia occurs frequently in patients with the lupus anticoagulant[32,35,40,41,59,62] and/or with anti-cardiolipin antibodies.[12,93,109] The mechanism by which thrombocytopenia occurs is unknown. However, the frequency of thrombocytopenia in these patients makes it tempting to speculate that anti-phospholipid antibodies may cause thrombosis through a platelet-mediated mechanism.[93] Platelet membranes contain phospholipids, some of which may be bound by anti-phospholipid antibodies. It is conceivable that by binding platelets, these antibodies can cause platelet activation, aggregation and resulting thrombosis. A recently completed study in our laboratory (Khamashta *et al*, unpublished) showed that anti-phospholipid antibodies bind only partially disrupted but not intact platelets. This led us to conclude that if these antibodies do indeed bind platelets *in vivo*, some conformational change of the platelet membrane must first take place to "expose" target phospholipids on the platelet surface before antibody binding.

THE "ANTI-PHOSPHOLIPID SYNDROME"

Some authorities have suggested that patients with anti-phospholipid antibodies (the lupus anticoagulant and/or anti-cardiolipin antibodies) constitute a separate diagnostic entity, the clinical features of which include thrombosis, fetal loss, thrombocytopenia and neurological disorders.[1] More recently, livedo reticularis,[6,7] migraine headaches,[7] endocardial lesions,[8] chorea,[9-11] and multi-infarct dementia[65] have been suggested as possible additional features. That such a disease entity exists is arguable,[15] but it may be useful to group these patients under the title "Anti-Phospholipid Syndrome" using defined criteria, so that prospective studies may be performed (Table 1). Using the criteria listed in Table 1, we have identified 28 patients in our series who might be classified under the heading of the "Anti-Phospholipid Syndrome". Only half had the classical features of systemic lupus, but the patients in the non-lupus group often had one or more clinical or laboratory feature that suggested an underlying autoimmune disorder (Harris et al, in preparation). It will be important to determine what clinical and laboratory features are directly related to the presence of anti-phospholipid antibodies and what features are coincidental, reflecting factors (other than anti-phospholipid antibodies) associated with an underlying autoimmune disorder.

IMMUNOLOGICAL CHARACTERISTICS

The Lupus Anticoagulant

The lupus anticoagulant is recognised by its ability to prolong phospholipid dependent clotting tests.[29] It is believed to inhibit or delay formation of the so-called "prothrombin activator complex" by competing with factors Xa and prothrombin for the phospholipid template on which this complex is formed (Figure I). Tests commonly used for the lupus anticoagulant include the Russell Viper Venom time (RVVT),[29] Kaolin clotting time (KCT)[110,111] (these two tests believed by some haematologists to be the most sensitive means of detecting the lupus anticoagulant,[29,111] as well as the activated partial thromboplastin time (aPTT),[29,112]) the thromboplastin inhibition test (a prothrombin time test with dilute thromboplastin),[15,112] and the prothrombin time (usually prolonged only when there is accompanying prothrombon deficiency).[29] A number of variations of these tests have been devised by various authors.[113,122] In general, the use of platelet-poor plasma, and reagents low in phospholipids[111]—particularly phosphatidylserine[114]—are believed to enhance the sensitivity of the test. Addition of freeze-thawed platelets neutralises the test,[112,115,116] possibly because platelet phospholipids absorb out anti-phospholipid antibodies. Since various clotting factor deficiencies can prolong these tests, confirmation of the presence of the lupus anticoagulant is established by mixing patient plasma with an equal volume of normal plasma. If the anticoagulant is present, the clotting time remains prolonged after mixing with normal plasma. The lupus anticoagulant acts immediately and its effect is not increased if the mixture is incubated at 37C. On the other hand, the effect of other inhibitors, such as the Factor VIII inhibitor, increases with incubation time.[29]

Although most lupus anticoagulant positive plasma conform to the general rules listed above, more careful study has shown wide variability in behaviour.[117-119] In addition, the degree of prolongation of clotting tests for various patients' plasma may vary deeply depending on the type of test performed and the reagents used.[120-124] A decrease in the abnormally prolonged clotting time after addition of freeze-thawed platelets[112] or after addition of phosphatidyl serine liposomes may help confirm the presence of the lupus anti-coagulant.[114]

Figure I

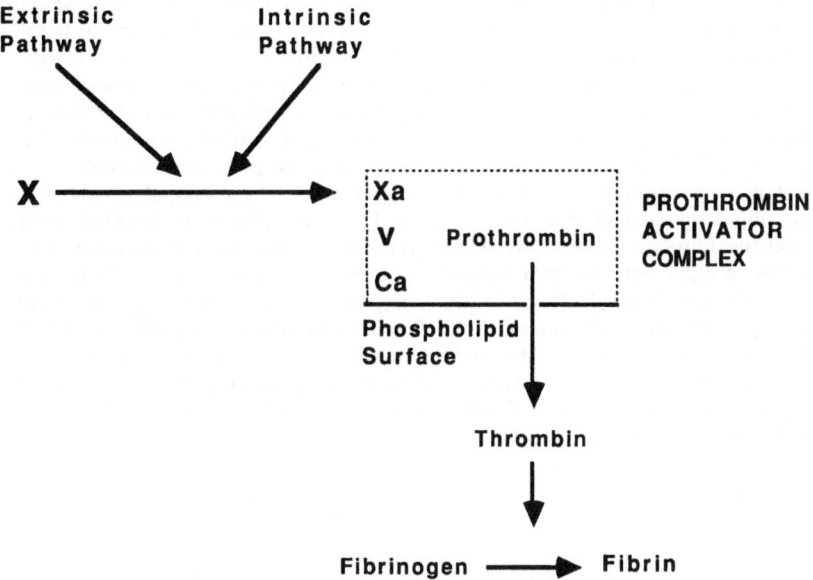

Lupus anticoagulant activity is believed to occur because of competition between anti-phospholipid antibodies and factor Xa for the phospholipid template on which the *prothrombin activator complex* is formed. Delay in formation of this complex results in prolongation of clotting *in vitro*. All clotting tests which require the activation of Factor X to Xa to go to completion (fibrin formation) should theoretically be prolonged by presence of the lupus anticoagulant. Tests that will be prolonged include the partial thromboplastin time (intrinsic pathway), prothrombin time (extrinsic pathway) and Russell Viper Venom Time (direct conversion of X to Xa). The thrombin time (direct activation of prothrombin) is usually not prolonged.

Yin and Gaston[123] and Lechner[124,125] established that the lupus anticoagulant is an antibody either of the IgG or IgM class. Although various authorities suspected that the lupus anticoagulant was an anti-phospholipid antibody, firm evidence to this effect came only when Thiagarajan and colleagues demonstrated that an IgM monoclonal antibody with lupus anticoagulant activity cross-reacted with negatively charged phospholipids.[126] With the development of the anti-cardiolipin antibody assay, Harris and colleagues demonstrated that the great majority of lupus anticoagulant-positive plasma gave a positive anti-cardiolipin test.[48] Anti-cardiolipin antibodies like the lupus anticoagulant cross-reacted with negatively charged phospholipid antibodies.[127,128] Affinity purified anti-cardiolipin antibodies have been shown to have lupus anticoagulant activity.[128-130] Affinity purified anti-cardiolipin antibodies and F(ab)₂ fragments of these preparations inhibited the calcium-dependent binding of prothrombin and factor

X to phosphatidylserine and to cardiolipin coated surfaces.[130] Taken together, this evidence suggests that the antibodies responsible for lupus coagulant activity share similar specificities to that of the antibodies detected by anti-cardiolipin antibodies.[128-130] However, several investigators have reported patients whose plasma samples had lupus anticoagulant activity but were anticardiolipin negative.[95,131] There are also reports of patients treated with steroids where the lupus anticoagulant activity decreased, but where anti-cardiolipin antibodies have persisted.[131] If one assumes that the population of anti-phospholipid antibodies in any given patient plasma is heterogenous and that only a subpopulation accounts for lupus anticoagulant activity, while a larger population is detected by the sensitive anti-cardiolipin assay (Figure II), one can understand why changes can occur in lupus anticoagulant without significant observable changes in the anti-cardiolipin assay result. It will be important to determine which subgroup of anti-phospholipid antibodies are most closely related to thrombosis and recurrent fetal loss. It should be recalled that only about 30% of lupus anticoagulant positive patients are subject to thrombosis, whereas the percentage of anticardiolipin-positive patients subject to thrombosis may be much higher than 70% in the subgroup with high IgG levels.[12,49]

Figure II

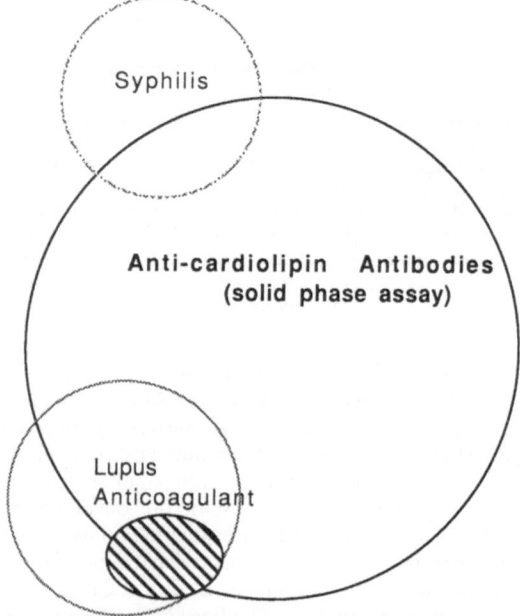

Venn diagram to show relationship of three groups of anti-phospholipid antibodies. It will be important to determine which is the thrombotic/fetal loss subset (shaded area) of anti-phospholipid antibodies and how large this group is.

Anti-cardiolipin antibodies

All antibodies detected in the anti-cardiolipin assay are not identical. Some evidence for this is the lack of complete concordance between lupus anticoagulant and anti-cardiolipin test results, as discussed previously. Even more interesting are the anti-phospholipid antibodies of syphilis which can also give a positive anti-cardiolipin test.[51,52,132] Syphilis plasma usually does not give a positive lupus anticoagulant test, and anti-phospholipid antibodies of syphilis do not appear to predispose patients to thrombosis or fetal loss. In a series of recently performed experiments, we have demonstrated, using a VDRL-ELISA assay, that syphilis serum binds cardiolipin best when it is mixed with phosphatidylcholine (PC) and cholesterol (Chol).[132] In contrast, autoimmune anti-cardiolipin antibodies exhibit greatest avidity for cardiolipin alone; mixing cardiolipin with PC and cholesterol reduces binding. In other experiments, we found as we had previously, that autoimmune anti-cardiolipin antibodies cross-react with negatively charged phospholipids. In contrast, the anti-cardiolipin antibodies of syphilis are limited primarily to binding cardiolipin, and exhibit much less cross-reactivity with negatively charged phospholipids.[52] These findings may explain why autoimmune anti-cardiolipin (and not syphilis anti-cardiolipin) antibodies may potentially bind negatively charged phospholipids on cell surfaces and possibly alter cell function, with resulting thrombosis and fetal loss. These findings also suggest that the origins of the anti-phospholipid antibodies of syphilis and of autoimmune disorders are probably quite different.[52]

Several monoclonal anti-DNA antibodies raised in mouse-mouse[133,134] and human-human[135] hybridomas have been shown to cross-react with cardiolipin, and monoclonal anti-cardiolipin antibodies have been shown to bind DNA.[136] Our own studies, confirmed by several other groups, find that autoimmune anti-cardiolipin antibodies are specific for negatively charged phospholipids and exhibit little binding to DNA.[127,128,137-138]

FURTHER STUDIES

Relatively little is known about anti-phospholipid antibodies or about the nature of their association with thrombosis and fetal loss. The most immediate problem to be addressed is how best to treat women who have recurrent fetal loss with these antibodies, and how best to manage patients with recurrent thrombosis, particularly arterial thrombosis. Since most centres have only a few patients, prospective, randomised, therapeutic trials will have to be multi-centre to find sufficient numbers of patients. Adoption of criteria for defining the "Anti-Phospholipid Syndrome" (Table 1) and standardised tests[49] will provide some of the groundwork for such studies. The study of anti-phospholipid antibodies may provide vital clues to the nature of the autoimmune disease process. These antibodies may also prove to be useful tools to study the phospholipid composition of cell membranes and to understand more about clotting processes.

54   *Study Group: Early Pregnancy Loss*

REFERENCES
1. Hughes GRV. Thrombosis, abortion, cerebral disease and lupus anticoagulant. *Br Med J* 1983; **287:** 1088-1089.
2. Harris EN, Gharavi AE, Hughes GRV. Anti-phospholipid antibodies. *Clin Rheum Dis* 1985; **11:** 591-609.
3. Vermylen J, Blockmans D, Spitz B, Deckmyn H. Thrombosis and immune disorders. *Clin Haematol* 1986; **15:** 1-9.
4. Feinstein DI. Lupus anticoagulant, thrombosis, and fetal loss. *N Eng J Med* 1985; **313:** 1348-1350.
5. Sontheimer RD. The anti-cardiolipin syndrome: a new way to slice an old pie or a new pie to slice? *Arch Dermatol* 1987.
6. Wenstein T, Miller AH, Axtens R *et al.* Livedo reticularis associated with raised titres of anti-cardiolipin antibodies in systemic lupus erythematosus. *Arch Dermatol;* In press.
7. Hughes GRV, Harris EN, Gharavi AE. The anti-cardiolipin syndrome. *J Rheumatol* 1986; **13:** 486-489.
8. Chortash EK, Paget SA, Lockshin MD. Lupus anticoagulant associated with aortic and mitral insufficiency. *Arthritis Rheum* 1986; **29:** 595.
9. Buochez B, Arnott G, Hatron PY *et al.* Choréa et lupus erythemateux dissemine avec anticoagulant circulant. *Trols Cas Rev Neurol* 1985; **4:** 571-572.
10. Lubbe WF, Walker EB. Chorea gravidarum associated with circulating lupus anticoagulant: successful outcome of pregnancy with prednisolone and aspirin therapy. Case report. *Br J Obstet Gynaecol* 1983; **90:** 487-490.
11. Asherson RA, Derksen RHWM, Harris EN *et al.* Chorea in systemic lupus and "lupus-like" disease. *Semin Arthritis Rheum* 1987; **16:** 253-259.
12. Harris EN, Chan JKH, Asherson RA *et al.* Thrombosis, recurrent fetal loss and thrombocytopenia: predictive value of the anti-cardiolipin antibody test. *Arch Intern Med* 1986; **146:** 2153-2159.
13. Norberg R, Gardlund B, Thorstensson R, Lidman K. Further immunological studies of sera containing anti-mitochondrial antibodies, type M5. *Clin Exp Immunol* 1984; **58:** 639-644.
14. Meroni P, Harris EN, Brucato A *et al.* Anti-mitochondrial type M5 and anti-cardiolipin antibodies in autoimmune disorders: studies on their association and cross-reactivity. *Clin Exp Immunol* 1987; **67:** 484-491.
15. Harris EN. Syndrome of the black swan. *Br J Rheumatol* 1987; In press.
16. Catterall RD. Biological false positive reactions and systemic disease. In: *Ninth Symposium on Advanced Medicine.* Ed: G Walker, London: Pitman Medical, 1973; pp.91-111.
17. Moore JE, Mohr CF. Biologically false positive serological tests for syphilis: type, incidence and cause. *J Am Med Assoc* 1952; **140:** 467-473.
18. Haserick JR, Long R. Systemic lupus erythematosus preceded by false-positive tests for syphilis: presentation of five cases. *Ann Intern Med* 1951; **37:** 559-565.
19. Moore JE, Lutz WB. The natural history of systemic lupus erythematosus: an approach to its study through chronic biological false positive reactors. *J Chronic Dis* 1955; **1:** 279-316.
20. Harvey AM, Shulman LE. Systemic lupus erythrematosus and chronic biological false positive test for syphilis. In: *Lupus Erythematosus* 2nd Edition, Ed. E Dubois. Los Angeles: University of California Press, 1974; pp.196-209.
21. Pangborn MC. A new serologically active phospholipid from beef heart. *Proc Soc Exp Biol Med* 1941; **48:** 484-486.
22. De Bruijn JH. Chemical structure and serological activity of natural and synthetic cardiolipin and related compounds. *Br J Vener Dis* 1956; **42:** 125-136.
23. Inoue K, Nojima S. Immunochemical studies of phospholipids IV: the reactions of antisera against natural cardiolipin and synthetic cardiolipin analogues containing antigens. *Chem Phys Lipids* 1969; **3:** 70-77.

Anti-phospholipid antibodies 55

24. Conley CL, Hartmann RC. A haemorrhagic disorder caused by circulating anti-coagulant in patients with disseminated lupus erythematosus. *J Clin Invest* 1952; **31:** 621-622.
25. Margolius A, Jackson DP, Ratnoff OD. Circulating anticoagulants: a study of 40 cases and a review of the literature. *Medicine* 1961; **40:** 145-202.
26. Laurell AB, Nilsson IM. Hypergammaglobulinemia, circulating anticoagulant and biological false positive Wasserman reaction: a study of two cases. *J Lab Clin Med* 1957; **49:** 694-707.
27. Feinstein DI, Rapaport SI. Acquired inhibitors of blood coagulation. In: *Prog Haemostas Thromb*. Ed. TN Spael. New York: Grune and Stratton, 1972, pp.75-95.
28. Veltkamp JJ, Kerkhoven P, Loeliger EA. Circulating anticoagulant in disseminated lupus erythematosus: proposed mode of action. *Haemost*. 1974; **2:** 253-259.
29. Shapiro S, Thiagarajan P. Lupus anticoagulant. *Prog Haemostas Thromb*, 1987; **6:** 263-285.
30. Bowie WEJ, Thompson JH, Pascazzi CA, Owen CA. Thrombosis in systemic lupus erythematosus despite circulating lupus anticoagulant. *J Clin Invest* 1963; **62:** 416-430.
31. Johansson EA, Niemi KM, Mustakallio KK. A peripheral vascular syndrome over-lapping with systemic lupus erythematosus. *Dermatologica* 1977; **155:** 257-267.
32. Mueh JR, Herbst KD, Rapaport SI. Thrombosis in patients with the lupus anti-coagulant. *Ann Intern Med* 1980; **92:** 156-159.
33. Nilsson IM, Astedt B, Hedner V, Berezin D. Intrauterine death and circulating anticoagulant ("antithromboplastin"). *Acta Med Scand* 1975; **197:** 153-159.
34. Firkin BG, Howard MA, Radford N. Possible relationship of the lupus inhibitor and recurrent abortion in young women. *Lancet* 1982; **2:** 366.
35. Soulier RP, Boffa MC. Avortements à répétition, thromboses et anticoagulants circulant antithromboplastine. *Nouvelle Presse Médicale* 1982; **9:** 859-864.
36. Carreras LO, Vermylen JG. "Lupus" anticoagulant and thrombosis—possible role of inhibition of prostacyclin formation. *Thromb Haemost* 1982; **48:** 38-40.
37. Lubbe WF, Butler WS, Palmer SJ, Liggins GC. Fetal survival after prednisolone suppression of maternal lupus anticoagulant. *Lancet* 1983; **1:** 1361-1363.
38. Prentice RL, Gatenby PA, Loblay RH, Shearman RP, Kronenberg H, Basten A. Lupus anticoagulant in pregnancy. *Lancet* 1984; **2:** 464.
39. Ros JO, Tarres MV, Baucells MV et al. Prednisone and maternal lupus anticoagulant. *Lancet* 1983; **2:** 576.
40. Jungers P, Liote E, Dautzenberg MD et al. Lupus anticoagulant and thrombosis in systemic lupus erythematosus. *Lancet* 1984; **1:** 574-575.
41. Elias M, Eldor A. Thromboembolism in patients with the 'lupus'-type circulating anticoagulant. *Arch Intern Med* 1984; **144:** 510-515.
42. Gårdlund B. The lupus inhibitor in thromboembolic disease and intrauterine death in the absence of systemic lupus. *Acta Med Scand* 1984; **215:** 293-298.
43. Branch DW, Scott JR, Kochenour NK, Hershgold E. Obstetric complications associated with the lupus anticoagulant. *N Eng J Med* 1985; **313:** 1322-1326.
44. Derue GJ, Englert HJ, Harris EN et al. Fetal loss in systemic lupus: association with anti-cardiolipin antibodies. *J Obstet Gynaecol* 1985; **5:** 207-209.
45. Lockshin MD, Druzin ML, Goei S, Quamar T, Magid MS, Jovanovic L, Ferenc M. Antibody to cardiolipin as a predictor of fetal distress or death in pregnant patients with systemic lupus erythematosus. *N Eng J Med* 1985; **313:** 152-156.
46. Cowchock S, Smith JB, Gocial B. Antibodies to phospholipids and nuclear antigens in patients with repeated abortions. *Am J Obstet Gynecol* 1985; **155:** 1002-1010.
47. Thornton JG, Foote GA, Page CE, Clayden AD, Tovey LAD, Scott JS. False positive results of tests for syphilis and outcome of pregnancy: a retrospective case-control study. *Br Med J* 1987; **295:** 355-356.

48. Harris EN, Gharavi AE, Boey ML *et al.* Anti-cardiolipin antibodies: detection by radioimmunoassay and association with thrombosis in systemic lupus erythematosus. *Lancet* 1983; **2:** 1211-1214.
49. Harris EN, Gharavi AE, Patel SP, Hughes GRV. Evaluation of the anti-cardiolipin antibody test: report of a standardisation workshop held April 4, 1986. *Clin Exp Immunol* 1987; **68:** 215-222.
50. Harris EN, Gharavi AE, Hughes GRV. Anti-cardiolipin antibody testing: the need for standardisation. *Arthritis Rheum* 1987; **30:** 835-837.
51. Colaco CB, Male DL. Anti-phospholipid antibodies in syphilis and thrombotic subset of SLE: distinct profiles of epitope specificity. *Clin Exp Immunol* 1985; **59:** 449-456.
52. Harris EN, Gharavi AE, Wasley GD, Hughes GRV. Use of an enzyme-linked immunosorbent assay and of inhibition studies to distinguish between antibodies to cardiolipin from patients with syphilis or autoimmune disorders. *J Infect Dis;* In press.
53. Gharavi AE, Harris EN, Asherson RA *et al.* Anti-cardiolipin isotypes in autoimmune disorders, syphilis, and chlorpromazine treated patients. *Arthritis Rheum* 1986; **29:** 596.
54. Canoso RT, Zon LI, Groopman JE. Antocardiolipin antibodies associated with HTLV-III infection. *Br J Haematol* 1987; **65:** 495-498.
55. Schleider MA, Nachman RL, Jaffe EA, Coleman M. A clinical study of the lupus anticoagulant. *Blood* 1976; **48:** 499-509.
56. Manoharan A, Gibson L, Rush B, Feery BJ. Recurrent venous thrombosis with a 'lupus' coagulation inhibitor in the absence of systemic lupus. *Aust N Z J Med* 1977; **7:** 422-426.
57. Williams H, Laurent R, Gibson T. The lupus coagulation inhibitor and venous thrombosis: a report of four cases. *Clin Lab Haematol* 1980; **2:** 139-144.
58. Gastineau DA, Kazmier FS, Nichols WL, Bowie EJW. Lupus anticoagulant: an analysis of the clinical and laboratory features of 219 cases. *Am J Hematol* 1985; **19:** 265-275.
59. Lechner K, Pabinger-Fasching I. Lupus anticoagulants and thrombosis. A study of 25 cases and review of the literature. *Haemost* 1985; **15:** 254-262.
60. Derksen RHWM, Kater L. Lupus anticoagulant: revival of an old phenomenon. *Clin Exp Rheumatol* 1985; **3:** 349-357.
61. Boey ML, Colaco CB, Gharavi AE, Elkon KB, Lorizou S, Hughes GRV. Thrombosis in systemic lupus erythematosus: striking association with the presence of circulating lupus anticoagulant. *Br Med J* 1983; **287:** 1021-1023.
62. Glueck HI, Kant KS, Weiss MA *et al.* Thrombosis in systemic lupus erythematosus: relation to the presence of circulating anticoagulants. *Arch Intern Med* 1984; **145:** 1389-1395.
63. Averbuch M, Koifman B, Levo Y. Lupus anticoagulant, thrombosis and thrombocytopenia in systemic lupus erythematosus. *Am J Med Sci* 1987; **293:** 2-5.
64. Petri M, Rheinschmidt M, Whiting-O'Keefe Q *et al.* The frequency of lupus anticoagulant in systemic lupus erythematosus: a study of sixty consecutive patients by activated partial thromboplastin time, Russell Viper Venom Time and Anti-cardiolipin level. *Ann Intern Med* 1987; **106:** 524-531.
65. Asherson RA, Mercey D, Phillips G *et al.* Recurrent stroke and multi-infarct dementia in systemic lupus erythematosus: association with anti-phospholipid antibodies. *Ann Rheum Dis* 1987; **46:** 603-611.
66. Landi G, Calloni MV, Sabbadini MG, Mannuccio P, Candelise L. Recurrent ischemic attacks in two young adults with lupus anticoagulant. *Stroke* 1983; **14:** 377-379.
67   Hart RG, Miller VT, Coull BM, Bril V. Cerebral infarction association with lupus anticoagulants—preliminary report. *Stroke* 1984; **15:** 114-118.
68. Harris EN, Gharavi AE, Asherson RA, Booey ML, Hughes GRV. Cerebral infarction in systemic lupus: association with anticardiolipin antibodies. *Clin Exp Rheumatol* 1984; **2:** 47-51.

69. D'Alton JG, Preston DN, Bormanis J, Green MS, Kraag GR. Multiple transient ischemic attacks, lupus anticoagulant and verrucous endocarditis. *Stroke* 1985; **16:** 512-514.
70. Merchut MP, Brumlik J. Painful tonic spasms caused by putaminal infarction. *Stroke* 1986; **17:** 1319-1321.
71. Levine SR, Welsh KMA. Cerebrovascular ischemia associated with lupus anticoagulant. *Stroke* 1987; **18:** 257-262.
72. Asherson RA, Mackay IR, Harris EN. Myocardial infarction in a young man with systemic lupus erythematosus, deep vein thrombosis and antibodies to phospholipid. *Br Heart J* 1986; **56:** 190-193.
73. Hamsten A, Norberg R, Bjorkholm M *et al.* Antibodies to cardiolipin in young survivors of myocardial infarction: an association with recurrent cardio-vascular events. *Lancet* 1986; **1:** 113-116.
74. Asherson RA, Derkson RHWM, Harris EN *et al.* Large vessel occlusion and gangrene in systemic lupus erythematosus and "lupus-like" disease. A report of 6 cases. *J Rheumatol* 1986; **13:** 740-747.
75. Hall S, Beuttner H, Luthra HS. Occlusive retinal vascular disease in systemic lupus erythematosus. *J Rheumatol* 1984; **11:** 846-850.
76. Peck B, Hoffman GS, Franck WA. Thrombophlebitis in systemic lupus erythematosus. *J A M A* 1978; **240:** 1728-1730.
77. Asherson RA, Lanham JG, Hull RG, Boey ML, Gharavi AE, Hughes GR. Renal vein thrombosis in systemic lupus erythematosus: association with the 'lupus anticoagulant'. *Clin Exp Rheumatol* 1984; **2:** 75-79.
78. Pomeroy C, Knodell RG, Swaim WR, Arneson P, Mahowald ML. Budd-Chiari syndrome in a patient with the lupus anticoagulant. *Gastroenterology* 1984; **86:** 158-161.
79. Bernstein RM, Salusinsty-Sternback M, Belleflour M *et al.* Thrombotic and hemorrhagic complications in children with the lupus anticoagulant. *Am J Dis Child* 1984; **138:** 1132-1235.
80. Levine SR, Kieran S, Puzio K *et al.*Cerebral venous thrombosis with lupus anticoagulants: report of two cases. *Stroke* 1987; **18:** 801-804.
81. Asherson RA, Morgan SH, Harris EN, Gharavi AE, Kraus T, Hughes GR. Arterial occlusion causing large bowel infarction—a reflection of clotting diathesis in SLE? *Clin Rheumatol* 1986; **5:** 102-106.
82. De Wolf F, Carreras LO, Moerman P, Vermylen J, Van Assche A, Renaer M. Decidual vasculopathy and extensive placental infarction in a patient with thromboembolic accidents, recurrent fetal loss, and a lupus anticoagulant. *Am J Obstet Gynecol* 1982; **142:** 829-834.
83. Carreras LO, Defreyn G, Machin SJ, Vermylen J, Demain R, Spitz B, Van Assche A. Arterial thrombosis, intrauterine death and the "lupus" anticoagulant: detection of immunoglobin interfering with prostacyclin formation. *Lancet* 1981; **1:** 244-246.
84. Asherson RA, Mackworth-Young CG, Boey ML, Hull RG, Saunders A, Gharavi AE, Hughes GR. Pulmonary hypertension in systemic lupus erythrematosus. *Br Med J* 1983; **287:** 1024-1025.
85. Schorer AE, Watson KV. The "lupus anticoagulant" induces functional changes in endothelial cells and platelets. (abstract) *Thromb Haemost* 1987; **58:** 232.
86. Rustin MHA, Bull HA, Dowel DA *et al.* Presence of the lupus anticoagulant in patients with systemic lupus erythematosus does not cause inhibition of prostacyclin production. (abstract) *Thromb Haemost* 1987, **58:** 390.
87. Hasselaar P, Blokzijl L, Derksen RHWM, deGroot PhG. The effect of anticardiolipin positive sera from SLE patients on platelet and endothelial prostanoid synthesis. (abstract). *Thromb Haemost* 1987; **58:** 391.
88. Angeles-Caro E, Sultan Y, Clauvel JP. Predisposing factors to thrombosis in systemic lupus erythematosus: possible relation to endothelial cell damage. *J Lab Clin Med* 1979; **94:** 313-323.

89. Sanfellipo MJ, Drayna CJ. Prekallikrein inhibition associated with the lupus anti-coagulant: a mechanism of thrombosis. *Am J Clin Pathol* 1982; **77:** 275-279.
90. Cosgriff TM, Martin BA. Low functional and high antigenic anti-thrombin III level in a patient with the lupus anticoagulant and recurrent thrombosis. *Arthritis Rheum* 1981; **24:** 94-96.
91. Cariou R, Tobelem G, Caen J. Circulating lupus-type anticoagulant, a risk factor for thrombosis by inhibition of protein C activation. *C R Acad Sci* (III) 1986; **303:** 113-118.
92. Comp PC, De Bault LE, Esmon GT. Human thrombomodulin is inhibited by IgG from two patients with non-specific anticoagulants. *Blood* 1983; **62** (suppl 1): 299.
93. Harris EN, Asherson RA, Gharavi AE, Morgan SH, Derue G, Hughes GR. Thrombocytopenia in SLE and related autoimmune disorders: association with anti-cardiolipin antibody. *Br J Haematol* 1985; **59:** 227-230.
94. Asherson RA, Chan JK, Gharavi AE, Hughes GR. Anticardiolipin antibody, recurrent thrombosis, and warfarin withdrawal. *Ann Rheum Dis* 1985; **44:** 823-825.
95. Lockshin MD, Quamar T, Druzin ML, Goei S. Antibody to cardiolipin, lupus anti-coagulant, and fetal death. *J Rheumatol* 1987; **14:** 259-262.
96. Lockwood CJ, Reece EA, Romero R, Hobbins JC. Anti-phospholipid antibody and pregnancy wastage. *Lancet* 1986; **2:** 742-743.
97. Tincani A, Cattaneo M, Martinelli D *et al.* Anti-phospholipid antibodies in recurrent fetal loss: only one side of the coin? *Clin Exp Rheumatol* In press.
98. Petri M, Golbus M, Anderson R *et al.* Anti-nuclear antibody, lupus anticoagulant, and anti-cardiolipin antibody in women with idiopathic habitual abortion: a controlled, prospective study of forty-four women. *Arthritis Rheum* 1987; **30:** 601-606.
99. Lubbe WF, Butler WS, Palmer SJ, Liggins GC. Lupus anticoagulant in pregnancy. *Br J Obstet Gynaecol* 1984; **91:** 357-363.
100. Farquharson RG, Pearson JF, John L. Lupus anticoagulant and pregnancy management. *Lancet* 1984; **2:** 228-229.
101. Lockshin MD, Druzin ML. Anti-phospholipid antibodies and pregnancy (letter). *N Eng J Med* 1985; **313:** 1351.
102. Gregorini G, Setli G, Remuzzi G. Recurrent abortion with lupus anticoagulant and pre-eclampsia: a common final pathway for two different diseases? Case report. *Br J Obstet Gynaecol* 1986; **193:** 194-196.
103. Chan JK. Harris EN, Hughes GRV. Successful pregnancy following suppression of anti-cardiolipin antibody and lupus anticoagulant with azathioprine in systemic lupus erythematosus. *J Obstet Gynaecol* 1986; **7:** 16-17.
104. Valesini G, Carsetti R, Patricelli S *et al.* Autoimmunity and abortion. In: Serono Symposium No. 45, *Immunological factors in human reproduction.* Eds. S Shulman, F Dondero, M Nicotra. London/New York: Academic Press, 1982; pp.235-239.
105. Cowchock S, Dehoratius RD, Wapner RJ, Jackson LG. Subclinical autoimmune disease and unexplained abortion. *Am J Obstet Gynecol* 1984; **150:** 367-371.
106. Clauvel JP, Tchobroutsky C, Danon F, Sultan Y, Intrator L, Brouet JC. Spontaneous recurrent fetal wastage and autoimmune abnormalities: a study of fourteen cases. *Clin Immunol Immunopathol* 1986; **39:** 523-530.
107. Bresnihan B, Grigor RR, Oliver M *et al.* Immunological mechanism for spontaneous abortion in systemic lupus erythematosus. *Lancet* 1977; **2:** 1205-1207.
108. Hull RG, Harris EN, Morgan SH, Hughes GRV. Anti-Ro antibodies and abortions in women with SLE. *Lancet* 1983; **2:** 1138.
109. Harris EN, Gharavi AE, Hedge U, Derue G, Morgan SH, Englert H, Chan JK, Asherson RA, Hughes GR. Anti-cardiolipin antibodies in autoimmune thrombo-cytopenic purpura. *Br J Haematol* 1985; **59:** 231-234.
110. Margolius J. The Kaolin clotting time: a rapid one-stage method for diagnosis of coagulation defects. *J Clin Pathol* 1958; **11:** 406-409.

111. Exner T, Rickard KA, Kronenberg H. A sensitive test demonstrating lupus anticoagulant and its behavioural patterns. *Br J Haematol* 1978; **40:** 143-151.
112. Triplett DA, Brandt JT, Kaczor D, Schaeffer J. Laboratory diagnosis of lupus inhibitors: a comparison of the tissue thromboplastin inhibition procedure. *Am J Clin Pathol* 1983; **79:** 678-682.
113. Rosner E, Pauzner R, Lusky A, Modan M, Many M. Detection and quantitative evaluation of lupus circulating anticoagulant activity. *Thromb Haemost* 1987; **57:** 144-147.
114. Kelsey PR, Stevenson KJ, Poller L. The diagnosis of lupus anticoagulants by the activated partial thromboplastin time—the central role of phosphatidyl serine. *Thromb Haemost* 1984; **52:** 172-174.
115. Howard MA, Firkin BG. Investigations of the lupus-like inhibitor by-passing activity of platelets. *Thromb Haemost* 1983; **50:** 775-779.
116. Firkin BG, Booth P, Hendrix L, Howard MA. Demonstration of a platelet bypass mechanism in the clotting system using an acquired anticoagulant. *Am J Hematol* 1978; **5:** 81-92.
117. Coots MC, Miller MA, Glueck HI. The lupus inhibitor: a study of its heterogeneity. *Thromb Haemost* 1981; **46:** 734-739.
118. Triplett DA, Brandt JT, Maas RL. The laboratory heterogeneity of lupus anticoagulants. *Arch Pathol Lab Med* 1985; **109:** 946-951.
119. Exner T. Similar mechanism of various lupus anticoagulants. *Thromb Haemost* 1985; **53:** 15-18.
120. Brandt JT, Triplett DA, Musgrave K. The sensitivity of different coagulation reagents to the presence of lupus anticoagulants. *Arch Pathol Lab Med* 1987; **111:** 120-124.
121. Green D, Hougie C, Kazmier FJ, Lehner K, Manucci PM, Rizza CR, Sultan Y. Report of the working party on acquired inhibitors of coagulation: studies of the 'lupus' anticoagulant. *Thromb Haemost* 1983; **49:** 144-146.
122. Alving BM, Baldwin PE, Richards AL, Jackson BJ. The dilute phospholipid APTT: a sensitive assay for verification of lupus anticoagulants. *Thromb Haemost* 1985; **54:** 709-712.
123. Yin ET, Gaston LW. Purification and kinetic studies on a circulating anticoagulant in a suspected case of lupus erythematosus. *Thromb Diath Haemorrh* 1965; **14:** 88-115.
124. Lechner K. A new type of coagulation inhibitor. *Thromb Diath Haemorr*, 1969; **21:** 482-499.
125. Lechner K. Acquired inhibitors in nonhemophilic patients. *Haemostasis* 1974; **3:** 65-93.
126. Thiagarajan P, Shapiro SS, de Marco L. Monoclonal immunoglobulin M lambda coagulation inhibitor with phospholipid specificity. Mechanism of a lupus anticoagulant. *J Clin Invest* 1980; **66:** 397-405.
127. Harris EN, Gharavi AE, Loizou S *et al.* Crossreactivity of anti-phospholipid antibodies. *J Clin Lab Immunol* 1985; **16:** 1-6.
128. Harris EN, Gharavi AE, Tincani A, Chan JK, Englert H, Mantelli P, Allegro F, Ballestrieri G, Hughes GR. Affinity purified anticardiolipin and anti-DNA antibodies. *J Clin Lab Immunol* 1985; **17:** 155-162.
129. Violi F, Valesini G, Ferro D *et al*. Anticoagulant activity of anti-cardiolipin antibodies. *Thromb Res* 1986; **44:** 543-547.
130. Pengo V, Thiagarajan P, Shapiro SS, Heine MJ. Immunological specificity and mechanism of action of IgG lupus anticoagulants. *Blood* 1987; **70:** 69-76.
131. Derksen RHWM, Biesma D, Bouma BN *et al*. Discordant effects of prednisone on anti-cardiolipin antibodies and the lupus anticoagulant. *Arthritis Rheum* 1986; **29:** 1295-1296.
132. Koike T, Sueishi M, Funaki H, Tomioka H, Yoshida S. Anti-phospholipid antibodies and biological false positive serological test for syphilis in patients with systemic lupus erythematosus. *Clin Exp Immunol* 1984; **56:** 193-199.

133. Lafer EM, Rauch J, Andrzejewski C, Mudd D, Furie B, Schwartz RS, Stollar BD. Polyspecific monoclonal lupus autoantibodies reactive with both polynucleotides and phospholipids. *J Exp Med* 1981; **153:** 897-909.
134. Koike T, Maruyama N, Funaki H *et al.* Specificity of mouse hybridoma antibodies to DNA II. Phospholipid reactivity and biological false positive serological test for syphilis. *Clin Exp Immunol* 184; **57:** 345-350.
135. Shoenfeld Y, Rauch J, Massicotte H *et al.* Polyspecificity of monoclonal lupus auto-antibodies produced by human-human hybridomas. *N Eng J Med* 1983; **308:** 414-420.
136. Eilat D, Zlotnick AY, Fischell R. Evaluation of the cross-reaction between anti-DNA and anti-cardiolipin antibodies in SLE and experimental animals. *Clin Exp Immunol* 1986; **65:** 269-278.
137. Edberg JC, Taylor RP. Quantitative aspects of lupus anti-DNA autoantibody specificity. *J Immunol* 1986; **136:** 4581-4587.
138. Smeenk RJ, Lucassen WAM, Swaak TJG. Is anti-cardiolipin activity a cross-reaction of anti-DNA or a separate entity? *Arthritis Rheum* 1987; **30:** 607-617.

Discussion

Chairman: Professor R. W. Beard

Professor JOHNSON: A key point is why these women have or may have anti-cardiolipin in the first place. Is there any evidence that a prior pregnancy, or more particularly prior pregnancy failure, can itself sensitise or unmask for anti-cardiolipin antibody? Then a degree of anticardiolipin seropositivity would be an effect of the recurrent early fetal loss rather than a cause.

Dr HARRIS: That question has been raised time and time again. We have looked at enough patients over a long enough period of time to know that many of these patients are antibody positive before their first detected pregnancy. It is a possibility, but as far as we know, and looking at patients before the event, it seems that the antibody has been there and it is not a result of anything.

Secondly, it is frequently within the framework of autoimmune disorders and there are several other autoantibodies that occur with the anticardiolipin antibody. I cannot think that they are all induced that way.

Dr UNANDER: I appreciate very much Dr Harris's presentation but one thing concerns me. He is talking about SLE patients. We were discussing fetal loss and habitual aborters as such, and I have been looking at habitual aborters. I published some results, the first 49, in the *American Journal of Obstetrics and Gynecology* in March 1986;[1] I have now looked at about 300 patients, I have statistics on 254. These 254 were all habitual aborters of unexplained aetiology. Genetic causes, uterine anomalies and infectious diseases were excluded. Fifty-eight of them (23%) were anticardiolipin antibody positive by exactly the same method used by Dr Harris, and of these 15 (26%) had the anticardiolipin antibody as the aetiology for their recurrent abortions.

If we simply screen for anticardiolipin antibody we may find it in many women in whom it is not the explanation for their recurrent fetal loss, and that is one of my concerns when we talk about this antibody. So many people seem to think that if they screen for anticardiolipin antibody and they find it, they have found the explanation, yet it is very rarely the case. Only 6 or 7% of the 254 patients really held that antibody as an explanation as I see it.

Of these 254 habitual aborters only two had had any thrombosis previously. One of them was in the group with the highest levels, about 10, in anticardiolipin antibody, and the other had 4, and we really cannot expect to explain it by a finding of thrombosis together with habitual abortion.

We have not yet published, but we have been looking at 200 women with normal pregnancies from an antenatal clinic. During pregnancy they may be weakly anticardiolipin antibody positive with levels of 3 or 4, but in all those in whom we have completed the blood samples, 170 were negative at the time of delivery. So it seemed to be a weak transient phenomenon in mid-pregnancy, from the 24th to 30th week of pregnancy, which then disappeared.

Those who look at this antibody must clarify exactly what it is that they do.

Dr HARRIS: That is precisely the point that I have made throughout my presentation. We looked at 600 first trimester aborters and we found three positive. Two were low positive and the third, who was really positive, we already knew about. There were 600 taken blind and the one we all knew. We then looked at a later group and found a slightly higher percentage.

I think I have made the point that one cannot blanket-treat everybody. At the same time I am very concerned about levels. If levels are not defined then one is bound to run into trouble. I hope I have emphasised that clearly. I agree with you.

Professor GILL: I cannot even understand the ground rules of this phenomenon but I do understand correctly that a phospholipid is a coagulant by itself. The antibody found in lupus is an antibody to the phospholipid and hence is called an anticoagulant—but it does coagulate. Is that correct?

Dr HARRIS: It is an anticoagulant defined by what it does in the test tube. It cannot be defined on the basis of what happens *in vivo*. And it is not confined to patients with lupus.

Professor GILL: So this antiphospholipid antibody is a test tube phenomenon. It prevents phospholipids from causing coagulation.

Dr HARRIS: It prevents. Phospholipids serve as a catalytic surface. They block the catalytic surface.

Professor GILL: But *in vivo* patients with antiphospholipid antibodies do clot.

Dr HARRIS: Yes. That is the paradox.

Professor GILL: It certainly is. And the relationship between cardiolipin and phospholipid is that they are both lipids but their conformations apparently are different?

Dr HARRIS: No, not quite. The conformational change that I am referring to is when cardiolipin is mixed with other phospholipids which are not negatively charged.

Professor GILL: But then, at least from the point of view of someone who does not work in this field, and I doubt that I ever will, then the phenomenon ought really to be defined in a rational chemical sense before any attempt is made to associate it with any physiological or pathological change. This would seem to be a set of phenomena some of which are *in vivo* and some of which are *in vitro* and they do not correlate.

Dr HARRIS: With due respect, if one was to look at the whole field of medicine and to try to explain many of the events . . .

Professor GILL: I doubt that I am clever enough.

Dr HARRIS: We are discussing immunotherapy and I think that there are several areas in medicine where there is only an association to deal with that cannot be suitably explained. If we were to wait until we found an explanation then we might not treat several people, and we might miss something that potentially had some clinical importance and relevance. It will take a while to find the whole story.

Dr CARP: Can the type of recurrent fetal loss that these patients have be described in any way clinically? I think that has a great deal of bearing on the outcome of treatment. Is there any particular type of pregnancy loss?

Dr HARRIS: I do not know. It is all retrospective data.

Dr CARP: Our impression certainly is that when we treat these patients with steroids and aspirin, or with steroids, aspirin and heparin, that there is a difference in the way different types of patients behave. We have treated patients who have been primary aborters who have had lupus anticoagulant present, as diagnosed by usually the KCT or the APTT. We have also had patients with what I would call a more typical story of mid-trimester fetal loss in which we have seen some form of growth retardation before the death of the fetus—and we find very different results. When they are treated with steroids and aspirin, six patients out of nine have so far succeeded in achieving live births in their subsequent pregnancies—with early caesarean sections, and with other interventions—but have had live births. However, primary missed aborters, of the type that we were speaking about with immunotherapy, when they have even high levels of lupus anticoagulant present seem to have very poor results and so far we have only succeeded with one patient out of 100 in this series.

Dr HARRIS: When did treatment start?

Dr CARP: In most patients as soon as we had diagnosed that they were pregnant.

Dr HARRIS; Was the intention to suppress the placental coagulant activity completely?

Dr CARP: Yes. And we nearly always succeeded in doing that. But what we also found was that the time of the fetal death in mid trimester seemed to have no bearing. There were patients whose fetus died in spite of their having negative levels of lupus anticoagulant. There were patients who went on to caesarean section with very high levels of lupus anticoagulant.

Dr HARRIS: I think that has been a common experience.

Dr CARP: Should we then be treating the first trimester aborters?

Dr HARRIS: I think again a prospective randomised study is needed.

Dr LOKE: I have always understood that the formation of autoantibodies is a result of cellular destruction rather than the cause of any disease. This being the case, I wondered whether the presence of antiphospholipid antibodies is not just a secondary phenomenon and one is therefore measuring the predilection of those patients who will make these antibodies rather than the predilection of thrombotic phenomena.

Dr HARRIS: In autoimmune disorders we do not know what generates those antibodies; in autoimmune thyroiditis for instance. We do not really know what causes those antibodies in SLE. They are antibodies of many specificities without any apparent cause.

Dr LOKE: Right. So those antibodies are not the cause of disease, they are merely a result.

Dr HARRIS: We are not sure that they are not the cause. We are not sure of that. There is evidence for instance that anti-DNA antibodies in SLE certainly have something to do with nephritis, and it certainly looks as if anti-rho may have something to do with congenital heart block in fetuses born to mothers with those autoantibodies. So we cannot dismiss it as not having a cause.

Dr LOKE: But how can an antibody direct an intracellular antigen of any significance *in vivo*?

Dr HARRIS: One of the possibilities that we are playing with—phospholipids exist in all sorts of cell surfaces. One current explanation is that they could bind the platelet membrane, alter platelet function and cause thrombosis. There is no reason to dismiss the possibility that they can cause disease.

Dr PAGE FAULK: Within the context of the statement that there were alterations in the placental vasculature, about the only way that I am aware that this could occur is that the mother had an IgG lupus-like anticoagulant, or IgG AC/A. Could there be any correlation between the isotype of the antiphospholipid antibodies and the coefficient of fetal wastage?

Dr HARRIS: I am not sure what is meant by the coefficient of fetal wastage.

Dr PAGE FAULK: We cannot talk very clearly about whether it is primary or secondary that is being studied. What I am trying to do is to approach the problems of fetal loss. The problem is to decide whether fetal loss is due to placental immunopathology. A very convenient way for this to occur would be for the mother to make an IgG lupus-like anticoagulant which is transported into the placental circulation. Thus we might expect to find a difference between fetal loss when maternal IgM antibody is present, compared with fetal loss when maternal IgG antibody is not present. Have such differences been seen?

Dr HARRIS: We have not looked carefully enough at that data. There are certainly a few women who seem to have IgM alone who are subject to fetal loss, but the trouble with the IgM, and why I have been hesitant even in looking at data with IgM, is that that particularly is the non-specific isotype. We see IgG frequently at low levels. IgM also happens at high levels and I can quote many instances where there is no apparent effect from the IgM being present. But there have been a few women with recorded fetal loss who have only IgM. The majority have IgG, and so we presume that it is the IgG that is doing whatever it is supposed to be doing to the placenta.

Professor JENKINS: I presume somebody has done the obvious experiment and that I may be forgiven for not knowing the answers. Has anticardiolipin antibody been given to pregnant animal models and has someone looked for histological damage in the placenta and in the fetus in the animal model?

Dr HARRIS: No we have not.

Professor JENKINS: Why not?

Dr HARRIS: That is the obvious question to ask. Anticardiolipin was certainly raised in several mouse models in the sixties. We ourselves had not done it. The anticardiolipin test was only developed some three or four years ago. It is an obvious move to make, but there are questions which I would like clarified first.

We need to characterise better what antigen it is that these antibodies bind. It may not be cardiolipin. We do not see phospholipids alone. There are confirmational things involved and so on. So it may be that inducing anti-cardiolipin by injecting cardiolipin into mice and seeing whether they do or they do not abort does not tell us enough until we know more about the immunological characteristics of the antibody. But an obvious direction in which to go is an animal model, yet I feel that we need to tie down more precisely what this antibody is. We have not done so.

Professor BEARD: It seems to me that two things emerge. One is that the epidemiology of miscarriage is pretty sparse and there is a need for prospective observational type population-based studies to determine the natural history of miscarriage, including recurrent miscarriage. We have no good evidence to say as yet that there is any difference between pregnancy outcomes of those having 1, 2 and 3 miscarriages other than some data about outcome of pregnancies.

Apart from these observational studies it seems to me that there is also a need for investigation-type studies. As the study group proceeds we shall be able to determine what sort of investigations are valid and which we shall have to wait for, and it does seem on the immunological side as if we are still in the infancy of investigation-type studies.

As for lupus, anticardiolipin antibody, a history of thrombosis, these are all areas where more work is needed.

The second major point is that there clearly is an association between recurrent miscarriage and serious complications of the babies of these women which really needs to be borne in mind when designing the prospective studies of the future. We are all very interested in aetiology but one should not forget that the outcome indices that we have discussed, of severe growth retardation, pre-term delivery and perinatal death are very serious complications that the women of course, and we are interested in. These are outcome indices that should always be borne in mind whenever studies are done.

REFERENCES
1. Unander AM, Lindholm A. Transfusions of leukocyte-rich erythrocyte concentrates: A successful treatment in selected cases of habitual abortion. *Amer J Obstet Gynecol* 1986; **154:** 516-520.

SECTION 2

EXPERIMENTAL MODELS OF EARLY PREGNANCY FAILURE

Anatomical and immunological aspects of fetal death in the *Mus musculus/Mus caroli* model of pregnancy failure

M. A. Crépeau, S. Yamashiro, B. A. Croy

SUMMARY

M. caroli embryos transferred to the *M. musculus* uterus implant but subse-quently resorb about mid-gestation. Failure is a function of *M. caroli* trophoblast and, in immunocompetent *M. musculus* recipients, is associated with deficient recruitment of intrauterine suppressor cells followed by lymphocytic infiltration of the conceptus and development of cytotoxic lymphocytes (CTL). To determine the events initiating pregnancy failure in this model system, *M. caroli* blastocysts were transferred to severe combined immunodeficient (scid) mice of genotype *scid/scid*. C.B.-17 *scid/scid* mice were unresponsive to *M. caroli* xenoantigens in immunological assays but *M. caroli* embryos transferred to them failed to survive and were resorbed efficiently. These results indicated that CTL, antibody, delayed-type hypersensitivity (DTH) and T-cell activated macrophages neither initiated *M. caroli* failure nor were essential for resorption of embryos in the murine uterus.

To investigate further the events initiating failure of *M. caroli* embryos in *M. musculus* recipients, semi-thin serial sections of Day 8.5 pregnancies were studied. Evidence was obtained that supports a primary failure of *M. caroli* trophoblast giant cells which is unlikely to have an immunological basis.

THE M. caroli-M. musculus PREGNANCY MODEL

A large number of complex but physiologically normal interactions contribute to the success of the mammalian fetus.[1,2] Alterations to the mother's immune system resulting from pregnancy are well characterised in many species[3-8] but the role of the immune system during pregnancy remains unclear. It has been proposed that maternal immune recognition of the fetus is immunotrophic and directly promotes fetal growth.[9-12] Alternatively, the maternal immune system has been regarded as aggressive, aware of the fetal allograft, but in some extraordinary way, prevented from destroying it.[13,14] Many mechanisms have been proposed that could protect the fetus from maternal immune-mediated destruction.[15-20] However, the demonstration of an obligatory biological requirement for specific immunological events to ensure pregnancy success remains elusive, since the fetus usually succeeds despite experimental manipulation.[11,21,22] To advance understanding of the immunological events critical to the success of pregnancy we have sought an animal model system of consistent pregnancy failure, initiated by immunological events and reversible by immunological manipulations, in a species suitable for extensive immunological and genetic analysis. The system we have selected involves embryo manipulation and embryo transfer between two distinct species of mice, *Mus musculus* and *Mus caroli*.[23]

M. caroli blastocysts transferred to pseudopregnant *M. musculus* recipients implant and develop to mid-gestation, then resorb.[24] Prior to resorption, a deficiency of intrauterine suppressor cell activity can be demonstrated at the *M. caroli* implantation sites.[17] Subsequently, the *M. caroli* embryos become infiltrated by lymphocytes, including maternal cytotoxic T lymphocytes (CTL).[24] Major experimental observations made in this model system are summarised in Table 1. Rescue of *M. caroli* embryonic cells in *M. musculus* recipients (ie. survival to term) has only been achieved by producing *M. caroli* <-> *M. musculus* chimeras that have trophoblast of *M. musculus* genotype.

Table 1

Observations on *M. caroli* embryos transferred to the *M. musculus* uterus

First Pregnancy

0-72 hr.	Cleavage of *M. caroli* embryos is much faster than cleavage of *M. musculus* embryos.[25]
Day 4.5-5.5	*M. caroli* embryos successfully implant in *M. musculus*.[24,25]
Day 9.5	Intrauterine suppressor cells of the small granulated null lymphocyte phenotype are deficient at *M. caroli* implantation sites but are present at normal levels at *M. musculus* implantation sites within the same uterus.[17]
Days 10.5-15.5	*M. caroli* embryos all die in normal immunocompetent recipients with histological evidence of lymphocyte infiltration.[24,26]
Days 11.5-13.5	Maternal T lymphocytes cytotoxic for *M. caroli* target cells *in vitro*, can be isolated from resorbing embryos.[24]

Second Pregnancy

Day 10.5	All *M. caroli* embryos are dead and in an advanced state of resorption.[26]

Failure to Rescue

	M. caroli embryos die but resorption is blocked in *M. musculus* recipients treated with Cyclosporin A or anti-IL-2 receptor.[21]
	M. caroli embryos die and are efficiently resorbed in immunodeficient *nu/nu*, *scid/scid*, and *bg/bg* recipients; in recipients immunosuppressed with anti-L3T4 or anti-Ia antibodies; and in putatively tolerant *M. musculus* <-> *M. caroli* chimeras.[21,26]
	M. caroli embryos die in *M. musculus* vaccinated with *M. caroli* lymphocytes or receiving serum from normally pregnant *M. musculus*.

Rescue

	M. caroli are born to *M. musculus* as chimeras or fully xenogeneic offspring if enveloped by *M. musculus* trophoblast.[27,28]

The data collected to date suggest that embryo failure and embryo resorption are two distinct and separable events,[26] that fetal trophoblast is the tissue accounting for *M. caroli* death, and that lymphocytes are associated with *M. caroli* embryos dying in immunocompetent recipients.[24] None of the data demonstrate conclusively, however, whether maternal anti-fetal immune responses do, or do not, initiate failure of *M. caroli* embryos.

To characterise the events responsible for initiation of *M. caroli* failure we selected *M. musculus* with severe combined immunodeficiency syndrome (scid) as the most appropriate embryo transfer recipient because of its stringent immune deficiency. It has been reported that lymphocytes from C.B.-17 *scid/scid* mice fail to respond *in vitro* to B cell or T cell mitogens or to alloantigens.[29,30] They fail to reject allogeneic skin grafts[29] and have no detectable level of circulating immunoglobulins.[29] Furthermore, neither xenografted hybridoma cell lines,[31] nor human tumours, are rejected (R.A. Phillips, personal communication). The *scid* gene is believed to be a mutation in the recombinase enzyme system that, when expressed in homozygotes, results in defective rearrangement of immunoglobulin and T cell receptor genes.[32] It has also been reported that mice, homozygous for the *scid* gene have functional NK cells,[33] antigen presenting cells[34] and pre-B cells.[35] T-lymphocyte independent macrophage function has been observed in C.B.-17 *scid/scid* mice, but at levels insufficient to eliminate a bacterial challenge.[36] Myelopoiesis appears normal.[30] Therefore, we predicted that *M. caroli* embryos transferred to C.B.-17 *scid/scid* mice would escape immune-mediated destruction attributable to CTL, antibody, (DTH) and T-cell activated macrophages. Prolongation of *M. caroli* embryos in *scid/scid* recipients would implicate one or several of these effector pathways in initiating the failure. Alternatively, death and resorption of *M. caroli* embryos in *scid/scid* recipients would eliminate all of these effectors as initiators of the fetal loss.

C.B.-17 *SCID/SCID* MICE RESPONSE TO *M. CAROLI* ANTIGENS

To establish that C.B.-17 *scid/scid* mice were unresponsive to *M. caroli* antigens a series of *in vivo* and *in vitro* studies were performed (Table 2).[37] *M. caroli* skin grafted to C.B.-17 +/+ mice was rejected in 8-12 days (mean = 10.5 days for 5 animals), while that grafted to C.B.-17 *scid/scid* recipients was not observed to fail (C.B.-17 *scid/scid* carrying successful *M. caroli* skin grafts were killed 42, 52, 52 and 88 days after transplantation). Primary and secondary foot pad challenges of C.B.-17 *scid/scid* mice with 10^7 *M. caroli* splenocytes failed to induce a significant DTH response and C.B.-17 *scid/scid* splenocytes failed to respond to irradiated *M. caroli* splenocytes in the mixed leucocyte reaction. These results suggested that C.B.-17-*scid/scid* mice were unable to respond, in an antigen specific manner, to xenoantigens of *M. caroli*.

FATE OF *M. CAROLI* EMBRYOS IN C.B.-17 *SCID/SCID* RECIPIENTS

Bilateral transfers of *M. caroli* and *M. musculus* (CD1) blastocysts were successful in three C.B.-17 *scid/scid* recipients, thereby providing a total of 10 *M. caroli* and 8 *M. musculus* implantation sites for study. Since most *M. caroli* embryos, in immunocompetent recipients have died by Day 13.5 of gestation,[24-26] this time point was selected for study of the pregnancies in *scid/scid* recipients. In the present experiment 9 of the 10 *M. caroli* embryos were dead and in an advanced state of resorption and the remaining embryo was dying but had not begun to resorb (Figure I). Conversely, 7 of the 8 *M. musculus* embryos were viable. The rate of resorption and the gross appearance of the resorption sites in C.B.-17 *scid/scid* recipients were not different to those measured previously for

Figure I

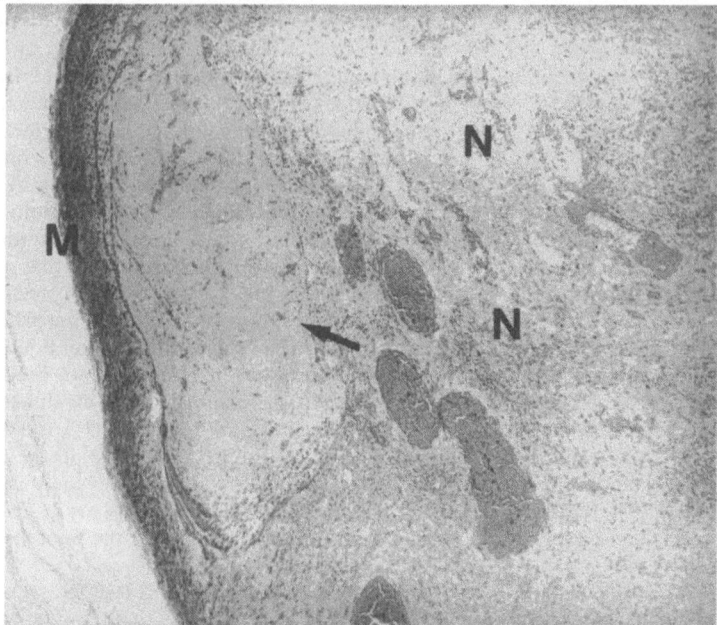

Placental lesion in a Day 13.5 *M. caroli* implantation site in a C.B.-17 *scid/scid* uterus. A large thrombus (arrow) and surrounding necrotic tissue (N) are seen. M = myometrium (× 64).

M. caroli embryos transferred to immunocompetent *M. musculus* recipients.[24-26] These results suggest that specific immune responses involving CTL, antibody, DTH and T-lymphocyte activated macrophages are unlikely to initiate *M. caroli* failure in the *M. musculus* uterus. Furthermore, these effector cell populations do not appear to be essential for efficient resorption of embryos in the murine uterus.

The identity of potential effector cells in mice of *scid/scid* genotype was examined histologically since the number of cells that could be recovered from implantation sites in advanced stages of resorption was too low for functional studies. Most *M. caroli* resorption sites showed extensive haemolysis, dead embryonic and trophoblastic cells and acellular deposits.[37] Granulocytes were prominent and macrophages, as well as large granular lymphocytes, were common. Examination of 1.4 μm methacrylate sections only rarely revealed cells that were morphologically similar to lymphocytes. In the single large *M. caroli* conceptus, a thick layer of extravascular amorphous material separated maternal uterine and fetal trophoblast tissues and a large number of granulocytes surrounded the fetoplacental unit. Thus, efficient embryo resorption appears to involve either phagocytes and/or non-specific immune effector cells such as NK cells, and to be T cell and B cell independent. The lymphoid-like cells at the resorption sites are probably pre-B or pre-T cells,[35] that have little or no

Table 2

Failure of C.B.-17 *SCID/SCID* to respond to *M. caroli* splenocytes

Assay	Response induced by	
	M. caroli cells	*Control cells*
Primary footpad challenge[a]	0.11 ± 0.04[b]	0.24 ± 0.05[b]
Secondary footpad challenge[a,c]	0.26 ± 0.11[c]	0.14 ± 0.04[c]
MLR: C.B.-17 *scid/scid* responders	3.0 ± 0.2[d]	3.0 ± 0.4[d]
MLR: C.B.-17 +/+ responders	21.1 ± 3.6[d,e]	3.4 ± 0.6[d]

[a] 10^7 *M. caroli* splenocytes or control cells injected in a volume of 20 μl into opposite footpads. Swelling measured 24 hr following injection.

[b] Mean net swelling calculated in mm by subtracting the preinjection footpad thickness from the 24 hr post injection thickness for 11 animals.

[c] Secondary challenge of 10^7 *M. caroli* splenocytes given 6 days after the primary challenge. Data presented as mean net swelling (mm) for 7 animals.

[d] Mean cpm ^{3}H-TdR incorporation in 84 hr MLR's consisting of 2.5×10^5 responser cells and 2×10^5 irradiated *M. caroli* or syngeneic control cells.

[e] $p < 0.05$ using Student's t-test.

functional importance (Table 2).[32] To address the role of NK cells in initiating the death of *M. caroli* embryos and in their intrauterine resorption we are preparing stocks of double mutant mice homozygous for both *scid* and *bg* genes for use as embryo transfer recipients. Greatly reduced NK cell activity has been reported in mice homozygous for both *nu* and *bg* genes, compared to mice homozygous for *nu* alone.[38]

It is possible that non-immunological events initiate the failure of *M. caroli* embryos in the *M. musculus* uterus. These events could be of a developmental nature, such as differential molecular imprinting of genes.[39-41] Alternatively, they could be physiological, involving dysfunction in the transport or signalling of molecules or cells. In any non-immunological hypothesis, however, the role of the trophoblast must remain central. The event initiating *M. caroli* embryonic failure has been sought through a careful histological investigation of serially sectioned *M. caroli* embryos collected from uteri of normal, immunocompetent *M. musculus* recipients on Day 8.5 of gestation.

PATHOLOGICAL FINDINGS IN TRANSFERRED DAY 8.5 *M. CAROLI* EMBRYOS

The earliest known abnormalities associated with gestation of *M. caroli* embryos in the *M. musculis* uterus occur at Day 9.5 (deficiency of intrauterine suppressor cells and lymphocyte infiltration). Consequently, Day 8.5 of gestation was selected for detailed morphological study. From two embryo transfer recipients (CD1) 4 *M. caroli* and 2 *M. musculus* control embryos were studied. Embryos were embedded in methacrylate and examined as 2.8 μm serial sections stained with toluidine blue, haemotoxylin and eosin or periodic acid-schiff (PAS).

Both *M. musculus* embryos had developed normally to the midsomite stage,[42] whereas the development of the *M. caroli* embryos was not uniform. One *M. caroli* embryo was at the presomite stage with emerging allantois (Figure IIa), another was at the early somite stage with fused allantois (Figure IIb) and two other mid-somite stage embryos were undergoing rotation (Figures IIc, d).

Figure II

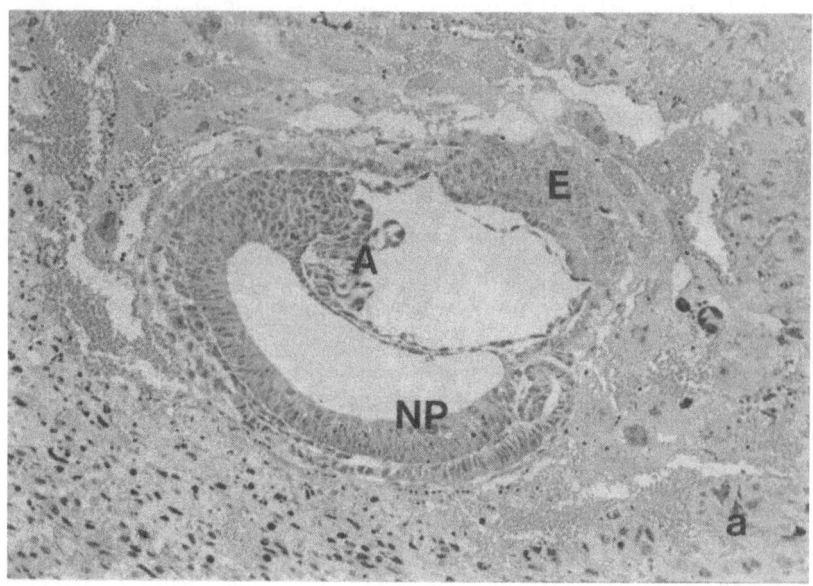

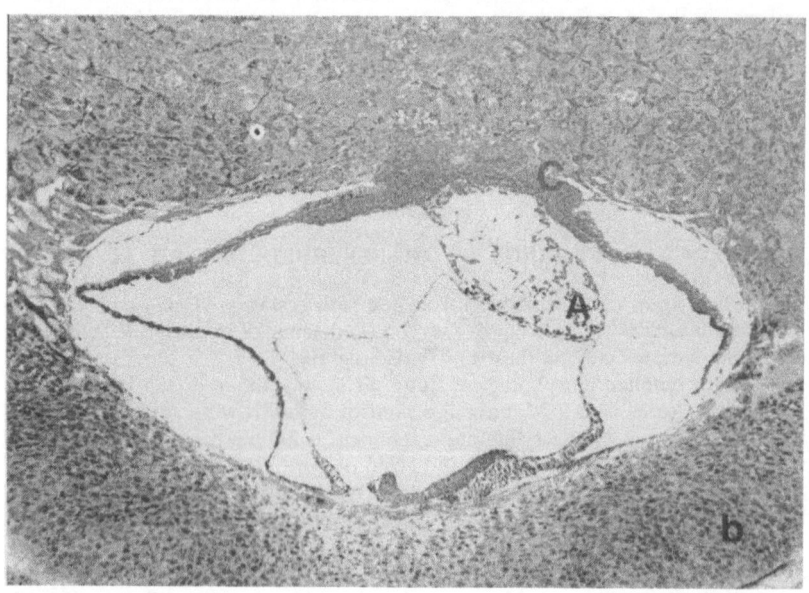

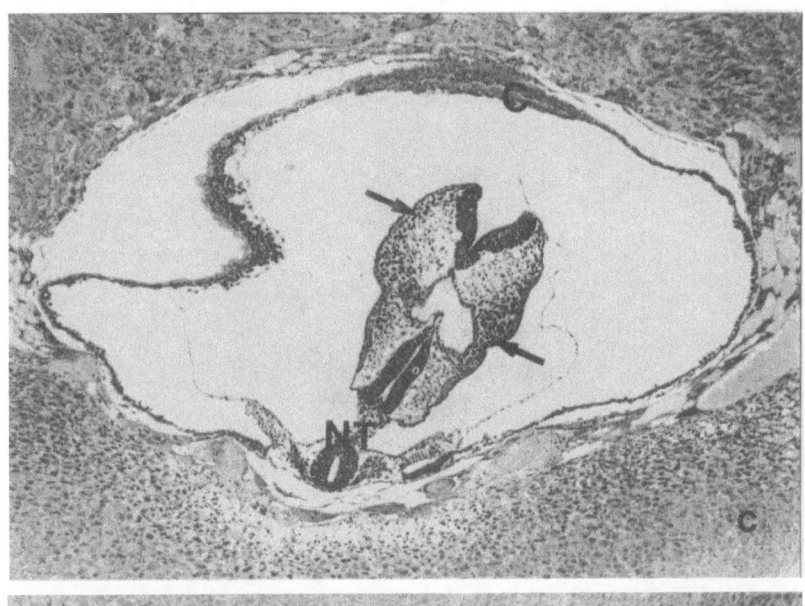

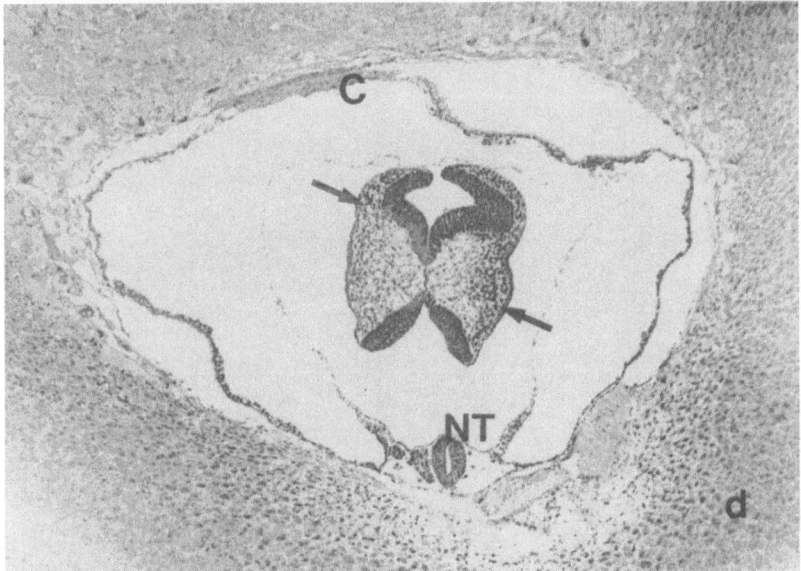

Saggittal sections of Day 8.5 *M. caroli* embryos in *M. musculus* uteri. a) presomite stage with neural plate (NP), budding allantois (A) and ectoplacental cone (E) (× 160). b) early somite stage with allantois (A) fused to chorion (C) (× 64). c, d) midsomite stage with closed posterior neural tube (NT), head region (arrows) and fused chorion (C) (× 64).

Figure III

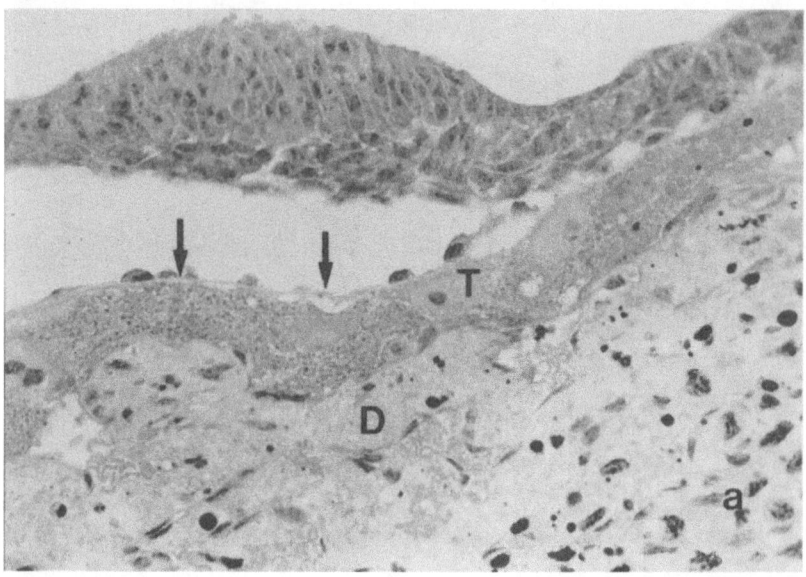

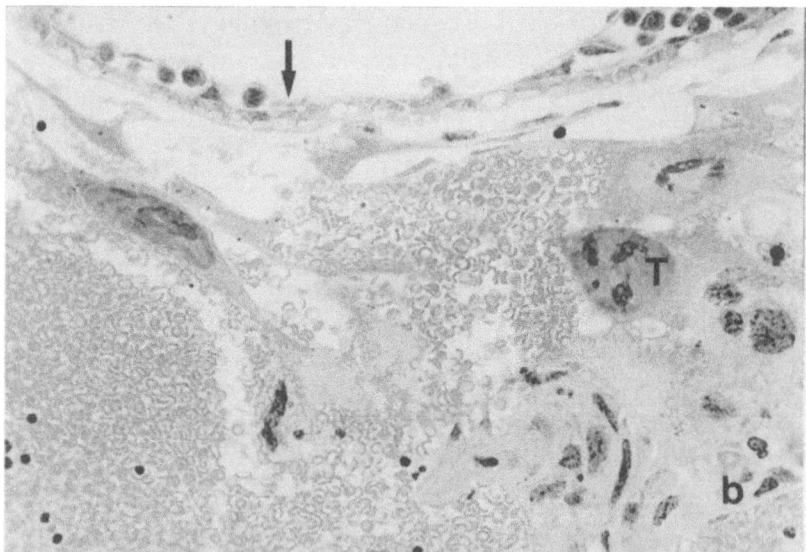

a) continuous barrier of Day 8.5 mural trophoblast giant cells (T) from a *M. musculus* embryo in a *M. musculus* uterus between necrotic decidual cells (D) and Reichert's membrane (arrow) (× 390). b) discontinuous barrier of Day 8.5 mural trophoblast giant cells (T) from a *M. caroli* embryo in a *M. musculus* uterus with erythrocytes infiltrating the area near the yolk sac (arrow) (× 390).

Figure IV

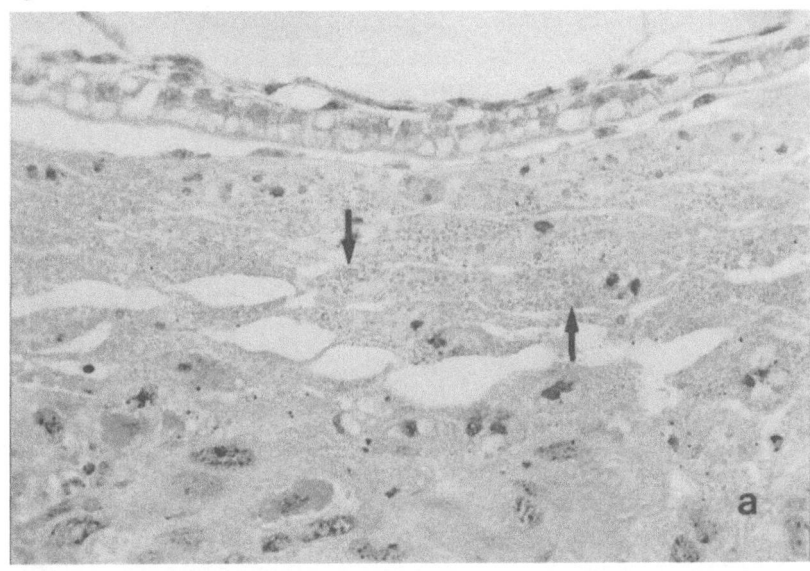

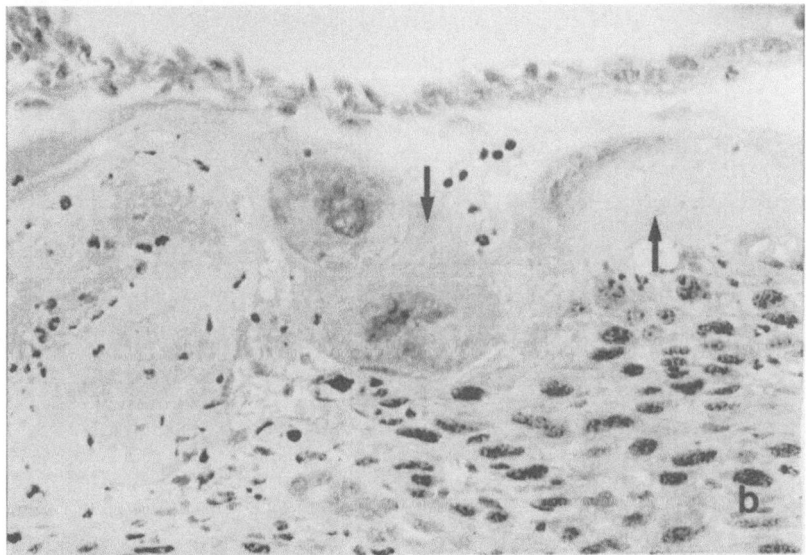

a) mural trophoblast giant cells from a Day 8.5 *M. musculus* embryo in a *M. musculus* uterus with numerous cytoplasmic granules (arrows) (× 390). b) mural trophoblast giant cells from a Day 8.5 *M. caroli* embryo in a *M. musculus* uterus with ill-defined cytoplasm, absence of granules, and nuclei undergoing karyolysis (× 390).

Figure V

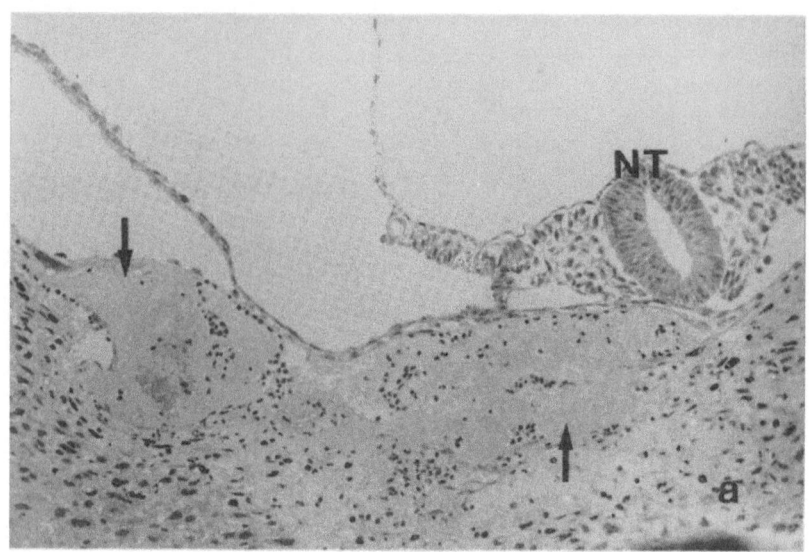

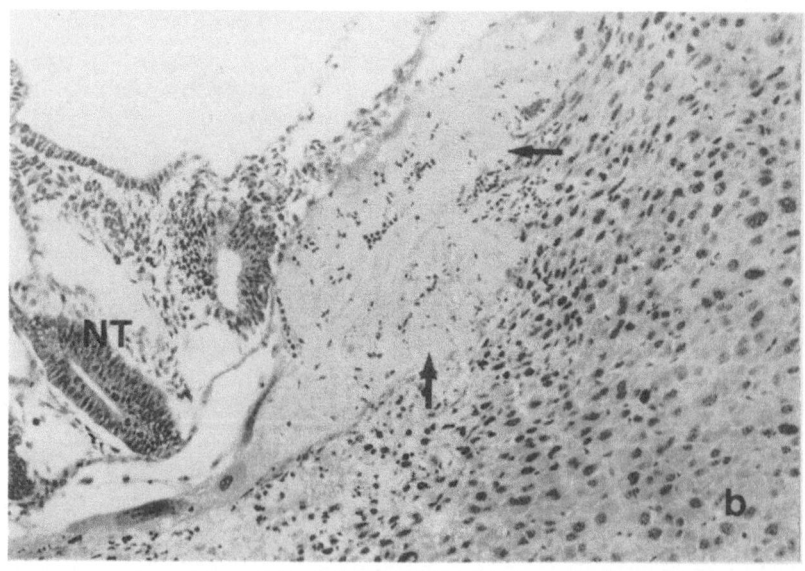

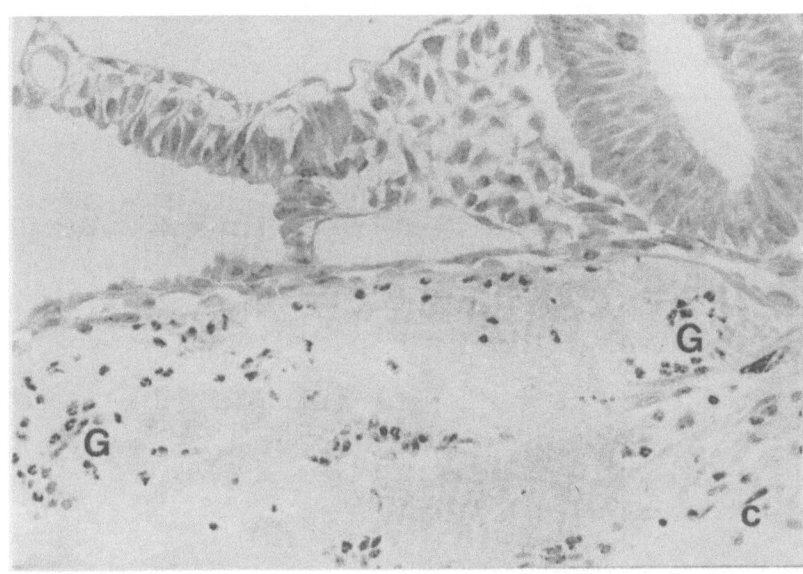

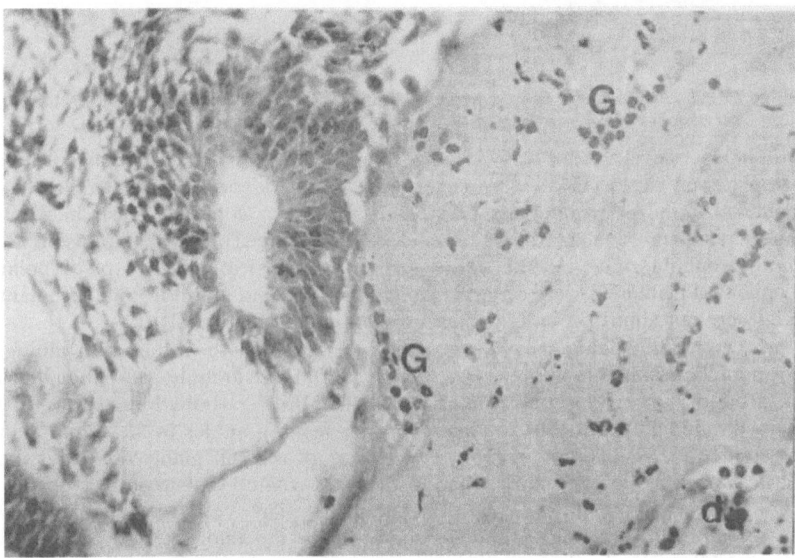

a, b) foci of exudate (arrows) near the neural tube (NT) in Day 8.5 *M. caroli* embryos in a *M. musculus* uterus (× 160). c, d) higher magnification of the exudates showing granulocytes (G) (× 390).

Figure VI

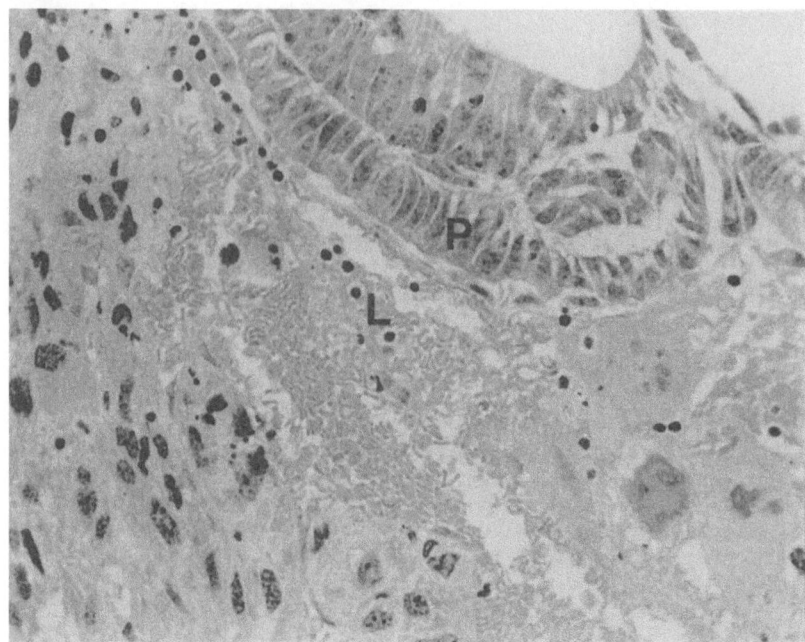

A Day 8.5 *M. caroli* embryo in a *M. musculus* uterus. An engorged blood vessel containing erythrocytes and lymphocytes (L) is near the primitive streak (P) (× 390).

Trophoblast development was extensive around *M. musculus* embryos and their ectoplacental cones (EPC) were covered by several layers of polar trophoblast giant cells; mural trophoblast giant cells formed a cohesive mesh between Reichert's membrane and the maternal decidua (Figure IIIa). By comparison, *M. caroli* trophoblast development was sparse. A few irregular layers of polar trophoblast giant cells were observed above the EPC and mural trophoblast giant cells were not abundant and appeared discontinuous (Figure IIIb).

M. musculus giant cells were densely packed with intensely staining, eosinophilic granules of variable size (Figure IVa); these granules were thought to be secretory inclusions of proteins containing little carbohydrate since they stained only lightly with PAS. There were far fewer granules in *M. caroli* giant cells (Figure IVb), although more granules were seen in giant cells from the earliest stage *M. caroli* embryo than in the later rotated embryos. This observation suggests that the *M. caroli* trophoblast giant cells were functioning abnormally or were undergoing degeneration in the enogeneic *M. musculus* uterus. Alternatively, however, the paucity of granules in Day 8.5 *M. caroli* embryos gestating in *M. musculus* could be due to species differences, and the question needs to be resolved by carrying out similar studies on successful *M. caroli* gestating in the *M. caroli* uterus.

Numerous *M. caroli* giant cells had ill-defined cellular outlines, vacuolated cytoplasm, pyknotic and/or karyorrhexic nuclei (Figure IVb). Foci of mildly eosinophilic exudate were evident near the neural tube region of two *M. caroli* embryos (Figure V). These exudates formed in areas that appeared to be devoid of trophoblast giant cells and those giant cells that were adjacent to the areas appeared to be dying. The exudative foci were infiltrated by granulocytes and they abutted Reichert's membrane (Figure V). In one *M. caroli* embryo, the Reichert's membrane cells had vacuolated cytoplasm suggestive of degeneration. An engorged blood vessel containing erythrocytes and leucocytes appeared to disrupt the giant cell barrier of the earliest stage *M. caroli* embryo and to contact Reichert's membrane (Figure VI). In this implantation site, lymphocytes were present but they were usually within vessels and were not in embryonic tissues. This observation, and the finding of lymphocytes around control *M. musculus* feto-placental units in the same recipient, suggest that on Day 8.5 of gestation, lymphocytes may not yet be directly involved in *M. caroli* death in immunocompetent recipients.

The results of this histological study suggest that *M. caroli* and trophoblast giant cells are the first cells of the *M. caroli* fetoplacental unit to undergo degenerative changes and die in a *M. musculus* mother. Trophoblast cells, particularly trophoblast giant cells, have been shown to be highly resistant to immunologically mediated destruction[15] and *M. caroli* trophoblast giant cells are resistant to immune destruction in the *M. musculus* kidney.[43] Thus, it seems unlikely that the necrosis of *M. caroli* trophoblast giant cells in the *M. musculus* uterus is immunologically mediated.

Localised necrosis of trophoblast giant cells appears to be associated with increased vascular permeability and plasma seepage from maternal blood vessels. Expansion of the exudate against fetal membranes could lead to pressure-induced embryonic cell death with eventual disruption of development. Or it could cause displacement of the embryo from maternal tissue and subsequent nutritional failure. Further morphological studies of *M. caroli* gestation in *M. musculus* and *M. caroli* using electron microscopy and autoradiography are in progress.

ACKNOWLEDGEMENTS

This work is supported by grants from the Ontario Ministry of Agriculture and Food and the Natural Sciences and Engineering Council of Canada. M.A. Crépeau is a recipient of a research training studentship from the Province of Ontario.
The assistance of Mr. T. Bast and Ms. C. Chapeau is gratefully acknowledged.

REFERENCES
1. Finn CA, Ed. *Oxford Review of Reproductive Biology.* Vol. 8. New York: Oxford University Press, 1986.
2. Costantini F, Jaenisch R, Eds. *Genetic Manipulation of the Early Mammalian Embryo.* Banbury Report 20. Cold Spring Harbor: Cold Spring Harbor Laboratory, 1985.

3. Chatterjee-Hasrouni S, Parhar R, Lala PK. An evaluation of the maternal natural killer cell population during the course of murine pregnancy. *Cell Immunol* 1984; **84:** 264-275.
4. Antczak DF, Miller JM, Remick LH. Lymphocyte alloantigens of the horse. II. Antibodies to ELA antigens produced during equine pregnancy. *J Reprod Immunol* 1984; **6:** 283-297.
5. Nymand G, Heron I, Jensen KG *et al.* Cytotoxic antibodies in serum of pregnant women at delivery. *Acta Pathol Microbiol Scand* (B)1971; **79:** 595-598.
6. Bell SC, Billington WD. Major anti-paternal alloantibody induced by murine pregnancy is non-complement-fixing IgG. *Nature* 1980; **288:** 387-388.
7. Smith RN, Amsden A, Sudiolovsky O, Coleman N, Margolies R. The alloantibody response in the allogeneically pregnant rat. In: *Immunoregulation and Fetal Survival.* Eds. TJ Gill III, TG Wegmann, E Nisbet Brown. New York: Oxford University Press, 1987; pp.27-36.
8. Jones WR. Hawes CS, Kemp AS. Studies on cell-mediated immunity in human pregnancy. In: *Immunology of Reproduction.* Eds. TG Wegmann, TJ Gill III. New York: Oxford University Press, 1983; pp.365-380.
9. Clarke B, Kirby DRS. Maintenance of histocompatibility polymorphisms. *Nature* 1966; **211:** 999-1000.
10. Croy BA, Gambel P, Rossant J, Wegmann TG. Characterization of murine decidual natural killer (NK) cells and their relevance to the success of pregnancy. *Cell Immunol* 1985; **93:** 315-326.
11. Athanassakis I, Wegmann TG. The immunotrophic interaction between maternal T cells and fetal trophoblast macrophages during gestation. In: *Reproductive Immunology 1986.* Eds. DA Clark, BA Croy. Amsterdam: Elsevier, 1986; pp.99-105.
12. Athanassakis I, Bleackley RC, Paetkau V, Guilbert L, Barr PJ, Wegmann TG. The immunostimulatory effect of T cells and T cell lymphokines on murine fetally derived placental cells. *J Immunol* 1987; **138:** 37-44.
13. Medwar PB. Some immunological and endocrinological problems raised by the evolution of viviparity in vertebrates. *Soc Exp Biology: Evolution* 1954; **7:** 320-338.
14. Chaouat G. Ed. The riddle of the fetal allograft. *Ann Immunol* 1984; **135D:** 301-351.
15. Simmons RL, Russell PS. The antigenicity of mouse trophoblast. *Ann NY Acad Sci* 1962; **99:** 717-732.
16. Slapsys RM, Clark DA. Active suppression of host-vs-graft reaction in pregnant mice. IV. Local suppressor cells in decidua and uterine blood. *J Reprod Immunol* 1982; **4:** 355-364.
17. Clark DA, Slapsys RM, Croy BA, Rossant J. Suppressor cell activity in uterine decidua correlates with success or failure of murine pregnancy. *J Immunol* 1983; **131:** 540-542.
18. Stiles DP, Siiteri PK. Steroids as immunosuppressants in pregnancy. *Immunol Rev* 1983; **75:** 117-138.
19. Chaouat G, Kolb JP, Wegmann TG. The murine placenta as an immunological barrier between the mother and the fetus. *Immunol Rev* 1984; **75:** 31-60.
20. Rocklin RE, Kitzmiller JL, Carpenter CB, Garovoy MR, David JR. Maternal-fetal relation: absence of an immunologic blocking factor from the serum of women with chronic abortions. *New Eng J Med* 1976; **295:** 1209-1213.
21. Croy BA, Crepeau MA, Yamashiro S, Clark DA. Further studies on the transfer of *Mus caroli* embryos to immunodeficient *Mus musculus.* In: *Reproductive immunology: materno-fetal relationship.* Ed. G Chaouat. Paris: INSERM, 1987; pp.101-111.
22. Gronvik K-O, Hoskin DW, Murgita RA. Monoclonal antibodies against murine neonatal and pregnancy-associated natural suppressor cells induce resorption of the fetus. *Scand J Immunol* 1987; **25:** 533-540.

23. Marshall JT. Taxonomy of Thailand Sinda species of *Mus* (*Rodentia, Muridea*). *Mammal Chrom Newsl* 1972; **13**: 13-16.
24. Croy BA, Rossant J, Clark DA. Histological and immunological studies of post-implantation death of *Mus caroli* embryos in the *Mus musculus* uterus. *J Reprod Immunol* 1982; **4**: 277-293.
25. Frels WI, Rossant J, Chapman VM. Intrinsic and extrinsic factors affecting the viability of *Mus caroli-Mus musculus* hybrid embryos. *J Reprod Fert* 1980; **59**: 387-392.
26. Croy BA, Rossant J, Clark DA. Effects of alterations in the immunocompetent status of *Mus musculus* females on the survival of transferred *Mus caroli* embryos. *J Reprod Fert* 1985; **74**: 479-489.
27. Rossant J, Mauro VM, Croy BA. Importance of trophoblast genotype for survival of interspecific murine chimeras. *J Embryol Exp Morphol* 1982; **69**: 141-149.
28. Rossant J, Croy BA, Clark DA, Chapman VM. Interspecific hybrids and chimeras in mice. *J Exp Zool* 1983; **228**: 223-233.
29. Bosma GC, Custer RP, Bosma MJ. A severe combined immuno-deficiency mutation in the mouse. *Nature* 1983; **301**: 527-530.
30. Dorshkind K, Keller GM, Phillips RA, Miller RG, Bosma GC, O'Toole M, Bosma MJ. Functional status of cells from lymphoid and myeloid tissues in mice with severe combined immunodeficiency disease. *J Immunol* 1984; **132**: 1804-1808.
31. Ware CF, Donato NJ, Dorshkind K. Human, rat or mouse hybridomas secrete high levels of monoclonal antibodies following transplantation into mice with severe combined immunodeficiency disease (SCID). *J Immunol Meth* 1985; **85**: 353-361.
32. Schuler W, Weiler IJ, Schuler A, Philips RA, Rosenburg N, Mak TW, Kearney JF, Perry RP, Bosma MJ. Rearrangements of antigen receptor genes is defective in mice with severe combined immune deficiency. *Cell* 1986; **46**: 963-972.
33. Dorshkind K, Pollack SB, Bosma MJ, Phillips RA. Natural killer (NK) cells are present in mice with severe combined immunodeficiency (*scid*). *J Immunol* 1985; **134**: 3798-3801.
34. Czitrom AA, Edwards S, Phillips RA, Bosma MJ, Marrack P, Kappler JW. The function of antigen-presenting cells in mice with severe combine immunodeficiency. *J Immunol* 1985; **134**: 2276-2280.
35. Fulop GM, Bosma GC, Bosma MJ, Phillips RA. Evidence for normal numbers of early B cell precursors in *scid* mice. Submitted.
36. Bancroft GJ, Bosma MJ, Bosma GC, Unanue ER. Regulation of macrophage Ia expression in mice with severe combined immunodeficiency: induction of Ia expression by a T cell independent mechanism. *J Immunol* 1986; **137**: 4-9.
37. Crepeau MA, Croy BA. Specific cellular immunity cannot account for death of *Mus caroli* embryos transferred to *Mus musculus* with severe combined immune deficiency disease (SCID). Submitted.
38. Hioki K, Maruo K, Susuki S, Kato H, Shimamura K, Saito M, Nomura T. Studies on beige-nude mice with low natural killer cell activity. I Introduction of the *bg* gene into nude mice and the characteristics of the beige-nude mice. *Lab Anim* 1987; **21**: 72-77.
39. Surani MAH, Barton SC, Norris ML. Development of reconstituted mouse eggs suggests imprinting of the genome during gametogenesis. *Nature* 1984; **308**: 548-550.
40. Sapienza C, Peterson AC, Rossant J, Balling R. Degree of methylation of transgenes is dependent on gamete of origin. *Nature* 1987; **328**: 251-254.
41. Reik W, Collick A, Norris ML, Barton SC, Surani MA. Genomic imprinting determines methylation of parental alleles in transgenic mice. *Nature* 1987; **328**: 248-251.
42. Theiler K. *The House Mouse.* New York: Springer-Verlag, 1972.
43. Croy BA, Rossant J, Clark DA. Recruitment of cytotoxic cells by ectopic grafts of xenogeneic, but not allogeneic, trophoblast. *Transplantation* 1984; **37**: 84-90.

Discussion

Chairman: Dr. W.R. Allen

Professor GILL: Perhaps some sort of discourse is required between mother and the developing embryo in order to turn on the appropriate sequences in embryonic development. This need not be immunological but will require interaction of the maternal tissues.

Dr. CROY: Very definitely.

Dr. BILLINGTON: It appears that *Mus caroli* may possess a slow preimplantation development gene (PID) whereas *Mus musculus* has the fast equivalent. In Dr. Croy's model, a slow embryo was being put into a fast mother. That in itself may confound the signal and result in embryonic failure.

Dr CROY: The fact that we can get viable chimeras would tend to dispute that possibility. One cell population would dominate in chimeras if the genes were incompatible.

Dr BILLINGTON: I don't think I would conclude that from the data. The chimeras would be both PID gene-fast and PID gene-slow producers.

Dr CROY: But why should they interact within the single animal?

Dr BILLINGTON: Because in the F1 hybrid, a fast and a slow gene gives us a fast-developing embryo.

Dr CROY: But these are not hybrids. In the chimera there is a population of slow growing and a population of fast growing cells and so we get coordinated regulation within the animal.

Dr BILLINGTON: I cannot accept that as proof of the hypothesis without first looking at a recipient domestic mouse which is also PID gene-slow. And not to use just *M. caroli* but something like the C-57-Black 6 strain as well.

Dr. CROY: We have transferred *M. caroli* into Black 6.

Dr. BILLINGTON: Then it is the same.

Dr. REDMAN: Do the *scid* mice have small granulocytes in their decidua?

Dr. CROY: I think that is a question for Professor Clark. We have been trying to get the *scid* mice pregnant for histological examination but have been unsuccessful so far.

Professor CLARK: I can confirm our lack of success in achieving pregnancies in scid mice during the past several months. Their fecundity is not as good as *M. musculus* for some reason. Those we have looked at have had *M. musculus* transplants and we have found in the spleens of these animals cells that will kill a *M. musculus* trophoblast cell line *in vitro*. We don't know what these cells are but it is established that *scid* mice can reject certain types of grafts, notably bone marrow grafts, by a mechanism that is thought to be dependent on natural killer (NK) cells.

What is going on in the sites of trophoblast failure is still an open question. We would very much like to have a pregnant *scid* mouse to answer the question asked—perhaps by the next meeting.

Dr. BELL: This is fascinating and it highlights the possibility that pregnancy failure is due to factors other than immunological ones. Interactions between the mother and the embryo come into the picture. May I ask, have any endocrine parameters been looked at in these animals, particularly in terms of mouse chorionic gonadotrophins? Perhaps there is species variation in the ability of chorionic gonadotrophin to bind to new receptors?

Dr. CROY: We did try to supplement with progesterone early in pregnancy but it would take too long to explain why this failed. I think Dr. Bell is quite right. Even though we can associate a larger and larger phenomenon with an event, this does not mean it is cause and effect. Many things still point towards the antigenicity of *M. caroli* trophoblast stimulating an immunological event. But I rather doubt that and tend to think that a hormonal deficiency exerting its effect either as a functional failure, or perhaps through gene imprinting, is a likely solution. In all species it is trophoblast which fails in nuclear gene transplantation experiments. The paternal genome is preferentially expressed in the placenta.

Dr. BELL: There is, in fact, a recognition between systems which is not entirely immunological. Is there any histological evidence of differences in the pattern of endometrial decidualisation between the successful and unsuccessful pregnancies?

Dr. CROY: Not that we could find.

Dr. ALLEN: Are those trophoblast cell granules that you mentioned as being absent in the *M. caroli* in *M. musculus* uterus present in the normal intraspecies *M. caroli* in *M. caroli* pregnancy?

Dr. CROY: We are looking at this question at the moment. I believe they are. I must point out that all our early histological studies were done with haematoxylin and eosin (H & E) staining and these granules do not stain with H & E. Many people describe the presence of these granules in trophoblast cells in the literature around 1957 to 1960.

Dr. ALLEN: They are very like steroid hormone granules in appearance.

Dr. CROY: Yes, but we think it is definitely a polypeptide product.

Dr. BILLINGTON: Was any attempt made to manipulate the NK and macrophage activity, either positively or negatively, in these models; or in the scid model?

Dr. CROY: The scid model inherently has some deficiency of macrophage function. Namely, the whole of the T-dependent macrophage system is absent. Their level of NK cells is normal but because they have no T-cells or B-cells, the NK cells appear functionally elevated. It is merely a problem of cell numbers.

A report from Japan which looked at nude mice crossed to beige mice showed an 85% reduction of NK activity compared to the situation in straight nude mice. This gave us the idea to cross our mice to get double mutant scid x beige offspring. We expect these to be NK efficient.

Dr. RUSHTON: I am a little concerned about the interpretation that the granulocytes are involved in the actual process of cell killing. I suspect they might have arrived on the scene because dead material is present. In our studies in ferrets many of the granules seen in trophoblast cells were, in fact, phagocytosed fragments of maternal red cells. I am wondering whether any of Dr. Croy's granules are phagocytosed maternal material which might be missing from inappropriate trophoblast.

Dr. CROY: We really have not gone deeply into the granules. It is the next thing on the agenda. At the moment I am only prepared to say that the absence of this material probably represents a dysfunction of the cells. In the very early stage *M. caroli* embryo we examined the giant cells had more granules than those in the embryos that had begun to rotate. Thus, we do think their absence is associated with degeneration.

Dr. Janet Rossant has been using the *M. caroli* hybridisation model to look at Day 5½ and Day 6½ ectoplacental cone formation in chimeras (Personal Communication). On both these days the giant cells are a mixed population. But we know at Day 9½ they become totally *M. musculus* in origin, indicating that those from *M. caroli* have died off.

Dr. CHAOUAT: Can one lyse placental cells from *M. caroli* by NK cells coming from a nude mouse or from a normal *M. musculus* mouse? Secondly, is anything known about the level of histamine in the placentae of *M. caroli* versus *M. musculus*?

Dr. CROY: The answer to both questions is no.

Dr. PAGE FAULK: One product of allogeneic recognition, even though immunologists do not like to talk about it, is the release of tissue thromboplastin from endothelium. This thromboplastin activates Factor VII which, in turn, causes fibrinoid areas like those shown in Dr. Croy's histological sections. Other evidence for tissue thromboplastin derives from alterations in the endothelium. Did you look for abnormalities in the endothelial cells in any of your preparations?

Dr. CROY: Not directly. We are soon to have an opportunity to examine sections under the electron microscope but there was nothing obvious at the light level.

Dr. PAGE FAULK: It would be very hard to see these changes under normal light microscopy although one can sometimes see marked endothelial proliferation in the release of tissue thromboplastin following allogeneic recognitiion.

Genetic aspects of the CBA × DBA/2 and B10 × B10.A models of murine pregnancy failure and its prevention by lymphocyte immunisation

G. Chaouat, D. A. Clark, T. G. Wegmann

THE CBA × DBA/2 SYSTEM

Dr. David Clark first highlighted the research value of the CBA × DBA/2 model of murine pregnancy failure when he recorded an increased rate of spontaneous resorption in CBA/J females (H-2k) mated to DBA/2 males (H-2d), which did not occur in another H-2k × H-2d mating, namely C3H females mated to DBA/2 males.[1] Soon afterwards it was discovered that CBA/J females mated to another H-2d male (Balb/c) also had a normal resorption rate.

Subsequent investigations have shown that resorption rates, whether they be the "background" or control rates such as those exhibited by CBA × CBA, DBA/2 × DBA/2, DBA/2 females mated to CBA males and CBA/J females mated to Balb/c males, or whether they are the higher rate in the CBA/J × DBA/ 2 mating model, all vary considerably between breeding centres. For example, control versus CBA/J × DBA/2 resorption rates range from 5-7% vs 24-30% in a laboratory in Villejuif, to 5% vs. 13-16% in one in Nice.[2] Further marked variations in rates include 8-11% vs 28-42% in another breeding room at the same institute in Villejuif[3] and 9-15% vs 35-45% at The Institut Curie in Paris, but with the values falling to a low of 4% vs 28.4% during the spring of 1986.[1] Other published comparisons include 9% vs 48-50% at a laboratory in Cochin[4,6] and 5-14% vs 30% at The Pasteur Institute, Paris.[5] As discussed elsewhere,[7,8] these differences between laboratories may reflect environmental influences on the immunotrophic loop.

The next important step in the overall story was the finding that immunisation of DBA/J females with Balb/c male spleen cells 7 days before mating to DBA/2 males, reduced the resorption rate from 16-22% down to 5% (p < 0.001).[2]

Both the increased resorption rate and the immunisation effects are specific for the CBA/J female × DBA/2 male mating combination. Furthermore, the increased resorption rate is seen only in certified strains of CBA mice originating from the Jackson Laboratory's line (CBA/J). For example, the resorption rate of

28.4% obtained in the Institut Curie when mating CBA/J females to DBA/2 males, drops to 5.6% when using CBA/Ca females, 8.3% when using CBA/J.Han females and 4.2% when using CBA/N females. Other H-2k strain females mated to DBA/2 males give equally low resorption rates; for example C3H/HeJ females show a resorption rate of only 2.8%, B10.Br females exhibit a rate of 3.6% and Balb/K females a rate of 4.6%.

In view of the "normal" (low) resorption rates shown by CBA/J females mated to H-2d strain males other than DBA/2, the effects of immunising CBA/J females with either spleen cells or placental cells obtained from other H-2d congenic strains, or Balb/c background congenic strains, was investigated. The results of these immunisations are summarised in Table 1. Of considerable interest was the finding that systemic immunisation with placental cell preparations of the correct strain type were equally effective as splenic leucocytes in lowering the resorption rate.

Table 1

Conceptus resorption rates in CBA × DBA/2 matings following immunisation of the CBA mothers

Immunising Strain	% Resorptions
CONTROL (Sham immunised)	31.7
10^7 SPLENOCYTES I.P. from:	
Balb/c (H-2d, Mls b)	7.4
Balb/b (H-2b)	28.4
Balb/k (H-2k)	33.6
B10.D2 (H-2d, Mls b)	27.8
NZB (H-2d, Mls a)	35.9
C57B1/6-H-2d (Mls b)	25.7
Balb/b × Balb/c (F1)	5.3
Balb/k × Balb/c (F1)	8.7
B10.D2 × DBA/2 (F1)	37.8
NZB × DBA/2 (F1)	35.4
B10.D2 × Balb/c (F1)	9.1
DBA/2 × Balb/c (F1)	6.3
DBA/2 × Balb/b (F1)	9.5
DBA/2 × Balb/k (F1)	15.8
10^4 PLACENTAL CELLS I.P. from:	
Balb/c × Balb/c matings	13.6
Balb/b × Balb/c matings	35.8
Balb/k × Balb/k matings	33.4

Prior immunisation with cells from MHC-identical strains that differ at the Mls locus can lead to strong inhibition of some immune reactions *in vivo* and *in vitro*. It is known that, in some cases, the inhibition is due to Mls induction of suppressor cells. However, the use of B10.D2 and NZB strains in the present immunisation experiments does not rule out Mls locus involvement as claimed previously,[9] since these strains do differ from Balb/c by a large number of minor antigens which could contribute to negative allogeneic effects. Although the restriction still applies,[10] it would be preferable to use the Balb.D2-Mls a

Table 2
Lysis of YAC-1 and L 1210 cells by cells from resorbing embryos

Origin of cells	Day of pregnancy	YAC-1 (% lysis)	L 1210 (% lysis)
FETUS	10-11	65.3	3.2
	11-12	51.4	1.8
	12-13	75.3	28.7
PLACENTA	10-11	8.5	4.2
	11-12	37.8	5.9
	12-13	65.3	32.8

congenic as the immunising strain. This strain has, unfortunately, been unavailable to us up to now. Nevertheless, we still believe that the Mls locus is probably not involved in the phenomenon since B10.D2 × DBA/2 F1 hybrids, which carry the Mls b gene, are as ineffective as NZB × DBA/2 F1 hybrids which carry Mls a. Both these strains behave like DBA/2.

Further evidence that the increased rate of resorption in the CBA/J × DBA/2 model is immunologically mediated comes from the finding that Ficoll isolation of lymphocytes from fetuses or placentas unveils anti-Yac-1 activity (Natural Killer Cells, NKs), followed by anti-L210 activity (Cytotoxic T-lymphocytes; Table 2). The anti-L-1210 specific activity is expandable in medium containing Interleukin-2 (IL-2) and it remains specific for H-2d, with minor crossreactivity to H-2b. In conjunction with the abrogation of the effect by anti LyT 2.1 + C' treatment (Table 3), this evidence proves that the cells are CTLS.

Table 3
Lytic activity of lymphocytes infiltrating embryos after expansion by Interleukin-2

Cell type	YAC-1	L1210	BW5147	MBL2
H-2 haplotype	a	d	k	b
NK sensitivity	+	−	−	−
% Lysis untreated	53.8%	24.3%	4.4%	8.9%
% Lysis after treatment with anti LyT 2.1 + complement	11.3%	2.0%	1.5%	1.8%

Another argument in favour of an immunological basis to the increased resorption rate phenomenon in the CBA/J × DBA/2 model, is its display of memory. So-called "good" and "bad" mothers have been identified in CBA/J colonies, with the latter showing increasing resorption rates with successive pregnancies.[11] In a similar vein, recurrent pre-immunisation with DBA/2 lymphocytes causes an increase in resorption rates with the effect being difficult to reverse by vaccination (Table 4).

Of equal importance in establishing the immunological basis of the CBA/J × DBA/2 pregnancy losses, are the immunological concomitants which accompany vaccination. For example, vaccination correlates with the induction of anti H-2d antibodies and the triggering of MLR and CML suppressor activities,[12] and with

Table 4

Resorption rates in CBA × DBA/2 matings following immunisation of CBA mothers

Treatment	% Resorption (p <)	
Untreated age-matched controls	31.8	(0.001)
Immunised females	18.3	
1 injection of 10^7 DBA/2 lymphocytes I.P.	35.6	(0.01)
2 injections of 10^7 DBA/2 lymphocytes I.P.	41.3	
3 injections of DBA/2 lymphocytes followed by Balb/c vaccination	37.6	(0.001)
4 injections with DBA/2 splenocytes	53.8	

Table 5

Resorption rates in the CBA × DBA/2 pregnancy model following immunisation of the CBA mothers on Day 0 of pregnancy

i/v injection of	% Resorptions (p < c.f. control)
Nil (control)	31.3
Saline	35.3
Virgin CBA/J serum	34.5
CBA/J anti DBA/2 serum	37.2
CBA/J anti DBA/2 splenocytes	34.4
CBA/J anti Balb/c serum	12.6 (0.01)
CBJ/J anti Balb/c serum absorbed with Balb/k spleen cells	16.8 (0.01)
CBJ/J anti Balb/c serum absorbed with DBA/2 spleen cells	29.7
CBJ/J anti Balb/c serum absorbed with B10.D2 spleen cells	34.2
CBA/J anti Balb/c splenocytes	18.3 (0.02)
CBA/J anti Balb/c B cells*	15.4 (0.01)
CBA/J anti Balb/c T cells*	19.6 (0.05)
CBJ/J anti Balb/c T cells LyT 2−*	14.7 (0.001)
CBJ/J anti Balb/c T cells LyT 2+*	18.7 (0.02)

*Separated by Mage plate panning.

Table 6

Effect of anti-idiotype immunisation on resorption rates in the CBA × DBA/2 pregnancy model

Treatment	No. of viable conceptuses	No. of resorbing conceptuses	% resorptions
Nil (control)	95	40	29.4
Mating control (CBA♀ × Balb/c ♂)	104	8	7.1
Anti-Balb/c vaccination	88	6	5.7
Anti-Balb/c serum	112	14	11.1
Anti-(anti-CBA anti-Balb/c) serum	101	8	7.3

the local recruitment accumulation of decidual suppressor cells.[13,14] But perhaps the most conclusive evidence is that protection against increased resorption can be adoptively transferred to virgin CBA/J females by antibodies or sensitised T cells. As shown in Table 5, the antibodies in serum are clearly directed towards an MHC determinant, since the protective effect can be ablated if the serum is first absorbed with H-2d cells, but not if it is absorbed with Balb/k cells.[12] The anti DBA/2/J serum which, unlike anti Balb/c serum, contains few, if any, anti H-2d antibodies at the immunising dose used, is ineffective (Table 5). Similarly, as shown in Table 6, resorption can also be prevented by anti-idiotypic immunisation.[15]

It is of interest to find that local intrauterine immunisation is also effective in lowering resorption rates and that placental cells from Balb/c × Balb/c conceptuses are a good immunogen. As summarised in Table 7, these placental cells showed themselves to be slightly more efficient than spleen cells in a dose-response experiment.

Table 7

Effects of intra-uterine vaccination with low doses of spleen cells or placental cells

No. of cells injected	Type of cells	% Resorptions
Nil	DBA/2 splenocytes	37.3
1,000	DBA/2 splenocytes	39.4
10,000	DBA/2 splenocytes	45.7
100,000	DBA/2 splenocytes	48.5
1,000,000	DBA/2 splenocytes	44.3
1,000	DBA/2 placental cells*	41.4
10,000	DBA/2 placental cells*	43.5
1,000	Balb/c splenocytes	28.5
10,000	Balb/c splenocytes	18.3
100,000	Balb/c splenocytes	12.8
1,000,000	Balb/c splenotypes	21.6
1,000	Balb/c placental cells*	25.1
10,000	Balb/c placental cells*	19.4
10,000,000	DBA/2 splenocytes (I.P.)	42.3
10,000,000	Balb/c splenocytes (I.P.)	8.9

*Placental cells prepared by collagenase digestion of placentae from Day 14 conceptuses.

Finally, although overall resorption rates increase with increasing age of the CBA/J females, previous pregnancies sired by a Balb/c male provide protection from the ageing effect (Table 8), in a similar manner to immunisation with Balb/c spleen cells.[16] As shown in Table 9, the protective effect of previous pregnancies is also transferable by immunising with the lymphoid components of the pregnant mice although, in keeping with the immunoabsorbent role of the placenta during pregnancy, only postpartum serum is effective. Interestingly, only Lyt2+ T cells seem to carry the protective effect (Table 9).

Table 8

Effect of previous pregnancies sired by Balb/c males on resorption rates in CBA/J females mated to DBA/2 males

Type of pregnancy	% Resorptions
Maiden CBA/J (8 weeks of age)	28.3
Maiden CBA/J (vaccination control at 8 weeks of age)	11.5
1 prior Balb/c pregnancy	19.3
1 prior Balb/k pregnancy	38.3
1 prior Balb/b pregnancy	31.6
1 prior B10.D2 pregnancy	35.2
Age control	34.5
Vaccination control (equivalent age)	8.5
1 prior DBA/2 pregnancy	39.5
2 prior Balb/c pregnancies	15.6
Age control	43.8
Vaccination control (equivalent age)	14.1
2 prior DBA/2 pregnancies	45.8
3 prior Balb/c pregnancies	17.3
Age control	41.2
Vaccination control (equivalent age)	16.5
3 prior DBA/2 pregnancies	61.8

Table 9

Effects of passive transfer of serum and immune cells on resorption rate in the CBA/J × DBA /2 pregnancy model

Transferred material	% Resorptions
Nil (control)	34.3
Serum from CBA/J × Balb/c D.16 pregnancy	28.4
Serum from CBA/J × Balb/c D.7 post partum	16.8
10^8 spleen cells (after 1 pregnancy)	31.3
10^8 spleen cells Day 7 p.p. (after 2 pregnancies)	19.8
10^8 spleen cells Day 7 p.p. (after 3 pregnancies)	16.7
B cell equivalent (after 2 pregnancies)	20.3
T cell equivalent (after 2 pregnancies)	36.5
B cell equivalent (after 3 pregnancies)	18.3
T cell equivalent (after 3 pregnancies)	21.8
LyT2− equivalent (after 3 pregnancies)	35.9
LyT2+ equivalent (after 3 pregnancies)	20.4

Thus, the increased resorption rate phenomenon seems to depend on an anti-MHC response that is itself dependent on the correct allogeneic environment furnished by minor antigens. It could be termed "MHC restricted, minor loci dependent".[17,18] By using recombinants between DBA/2 and Balb/c, Kiger was able to show that, during immunisation of 9 such mice, 6 behaved like Balb/c and 3 like DBA/2. This finding strongly suggests that the genes coding for the immunising effect are either a closely linked cluster, or a single Mendelian gene.[19,20] On Day 10 in that system, immunisation with protective strains produced an increase in decidual suppressor activity. This contrasts with the fact that the NK suppressor activity of the placenta is sometimes decreased on Day 10. In fact, some protective strains produce an increase in NK activity after incubation with placental cells on Day 10, although on Day 14, NK suppressor activity of the hybrid placenta has always returned to the level of the CBA/J × Balb/c mating.[14,21] None of the systemic correlants follow the segregation of the protective effects of the recombinants.[19,22] However, this should be re-examined using samples from individual animals.[23]

THE B10 × B10.A SYSTEM

This other model of murine pregnancy failure stems from the original observation by Melnick of an abnormally high resorption rate in B10 females mated to B10.A males.[24] Melnick and his colleagues examined every parameter in the model, including ovulation and implantation rates. We confirmed their observations with our first batch of B10 congenic mice and we found that the increased resorption rate was lowered only after immunisation with B10.A cells, not by third party cells (Table 10). Furthermore, we observed a marked increase in resorption rate with increasing age of the B10 females (Table 11). And, as in the CBA/J × DBA/2 model, the protective effects of outcross matings can be passively transferred in serum. The protection can be removed from serum by absorption with B10.A, A/J cells, but not by absorption with B10.S cells (Table 12). This too suggests an anti-MHC component in the immune serum.

Table 10

Effect of immunisation on resorption rate in the
B10 × B10.A pregnancy model

Matings	% Resorptions*
B10 × B10.A (H-2b × H-2a)	13.5
B10.A × B10 (H-2a × H-2b)	5.6
B10 × B10.D2 (H-2b × H-2d)	3.2
B10.D2 × B10 (H-2d × H-2b)	3.8
B10 × B10.D2 after:	
immunisation with B10.A	6.3
immunisation with B10.D2	15.6
immunisation with B10.BR	12.9

*Resorptions counted on Days 13 and 14 of pregnancy.

Table 11

Effect of maternal age on resorption rate in the B10 × B10.A
pregnancy model

Age of B10 mothers	% Resorptions
2 months	14.7
3 months	32.5
5 months	48.3

Table 12

Effect of various treatments on resorption rate in the B10 × B10.A
pregnancy model

Treatment Group	% Resorptions
Nil-control (3 month old B10 females)	31.7
B10 anti-B10.A spleen cell transfer	14.4
B10 anti-B10.A serum transfer	7.6
B10 anti-B10.A serum (absorbed with B10.A cells)	35.6
B10 anti-B10.A serum (absorbed with A/J cells)	29.4
B10 anti-B10.A serum (absorbed with B10.S cells)	4.3

Thus, the B10 × B10.A model of pregnancy failure provides us with an MHC-dependent model with the same genetic background. It is therefore important to examine in detail which of the many similar congenic strains will provide immunisation protection and which will absorb the protective effects from immune serum. Our findings to date in both models of pregnancy loss lead us to believe that an anti-MHC response in the proper allogeneic context is involved. This is likely to be a monomorphic determinant.

ASPECTS OF THE MECHANISMS INVOLVED

Expansion of existing CBA × DBA/2 recombinant mice, the segregation of new recombinants and mapping the genes in the CBA × DBA/2 system are just some of the problems yet to be solved before we may learn the true nature of the mechanisms involved in this most interesting model of pregnancy failure.

One unexpected finding in our study was that both aggregated human gamma globulin and heat aggregated normal mouse serum confer protection when administered to CBA females mated to DBA/2 males. In a similar manner, deaggregation of CBA anti-Balb/c serum causes it to lose some of its protective activity, with the residual activity again being removed by absorption with cells bearing the appropriate MHC antigens (Table 13).

Table 13

Effects of injected serum and gamma globulin on resorption rates in the
CBA/J × DBA/2 pregnancy model

Material injected i/v on Day 0 of pregnancy	% Resorptions
Nil (control)	37.5
Normal CBA/J serum	35.1
Heat aggregated CBA/J serum*	18.4
Heat aggregated, then deaggregated, CBA/J serum*	42.3
Heat aggregated human gamma globulins*	12.4
Deaggregated human gamma globulins*	38.2
CBA/J anti Balb/c serum	8.3
CBA/J anti Balb/c serum, deaggreagated*	17.3
CBA/J anti Balb/c serum (absorbed with Balb/c thymocytes)	45.8
CBA/J anti Balb/c serum (absorbed with Balb/k thymocytes)	19.8
CBA/J anti Balb/c serum (absorbed with DBA/2 thymocytes)	41.2

*Protocols as described in Reference 26.

Hamilton and Hamilton[25] made a second important discovery when they noted differential resorption rates in CBA/J × DBA/2 matings between one breeding room of their colony and another. Resorption rate was low (normal) in one room and was not altered by anti Balb/c immunisation. In the other room, however, the resorption rate was characteristically high and was significantly lowered by immunisation.

Table 14

Prevention of the anti-abortive effects of anti-Balb/c immunisation of CBA/J females mated to DBA/2 males and the induction of abnormal abortion rates in CBA/J × Balb/c matings by injection of anti-L3T4 plus anti Lyt 2.1 monoclonal antibodies (M/Abs) purified by HPLC

Mice	Treatment 1	Treatment 2	% Resorptions (p<)	Placental weight (mg) (p<)	Placenta/ phagocytosis index* (Units) (p<)
Mating Experiment 1					
CBA/J × Balb/c	—	Control	10.4	148.75	277
			(0.001)	(0.01)	(0.01)
CBA/J × Balb/c	—	M/Abs	43.7	85.3	117
CBA × DBA/2	—	Control	37.0	77.3	286
			(0.05)	(0.01)	(0.01)
CBA/J × DBA/2	—	M/Abs	42.5	94.2	207
Mating Experiment 2					
CBA/J × Balb/c	—	Control	8.7	139.9	321
			(0.001)	(0.01)	(0.001)
CBA/J × Balb/c	—	M/Abs	51.3	81.3	169
CBA × DBA/2	—	Control	33.5	79.1	198
			(0.01)	N.S.	N.S.
CBA/J × DBA/2	—	M/Abs	46.1	85.6	157
Immunisation Experiment 1					
CBA × DBA/2	—	—	46.4	51.4	81
			(0.001)	(0.01)	(0.001)
CBA × DBA/2	Balb/c	—	7.9	88.8	232
CBA × DBA/2	Balb/c	Control	7.4	97.1	235
			(0.001)	(0.001)	N.S.
CBA × DBA/2	Balb/c	M/Abs	45.6	68.1	202
Immunisation Experiment 2					
CBA × DBA/2	—	—	42.1	67.3	185
			(0.001)	(0.01)	(0.05)
CBA × DBA/2	Balb/c	—	9.9	124.8	274
CBA × DBA/2	Balb/c	Control	6.3	118.7	246
			(0.001)	(0.001)	(0.05)
CBA × DBA/2	Balb/c	M/Abs	51.3	62.4	162

For Mating Experiment 1, immunisation carried out on Day −7, injections given on Days 8, 10 and 13 and conceptuses checked on Day 15. For all the other experiments, injections given on Days 8, 10 and 12, and conceptuses checked on Day 14.

*Placenta/phagocytosis index: This reflects the mean phagocytosis of fluorescent latex beads as described in Reference 28.

Table 15

Correction of placental hypertrophy in MRL/Mp 1pr/1pr (CSEA1 MRL/L) mice* and reduction of placental weight in normal MRL (CSEA1 MRL/mp) mice* by injection of anti L3T4 (GK.15) plus anti LyT 2.1 purified monoclonal antibodies on Days 8, 10 and 12 of pregnancy.

Strain	Treatment	Mean placental weight in mg (p<)		Mean placenta/ phagocytosis index** (units) (∞)	
Experiment 1					
Conceptuses examined on Day 14					
Normal MRL	IgG Control	133.6	(0.001)	76.1	N.S.
Normal MRL	M/Abs	103.3		71.3	
MRL Mp 1pr/1pr	IgG Control	166.2	(0.001)	97.6	(0.01)
MRL Mp 1pr/1pr	M/Abs	93.7		73.3	
C3H controls		109.3		N.T.	
Conceptuses examined on Day 15					
Normal MRL	IgG Control	112.3	(0.001)	312.6	(0.001)
Normal MRL	M/Abs	69.7		238.0	
MRL Mp 1pr/1pr	IgG Control	152.5	(0.001)	490.6	(0.001)
MRL Mp 1pr/1pr	M/Abs	91.5		271.8	
Experiment 2					
Conceptuses examined on Day 14					
Normal MRL	IgG Control	124.0	(0.001)	433.7	(0.001)
Normal MRL	M/Abs	67.0		327.0	
MRL Mp 1pr/1pr	IgG Control	165.3	(0.001)	535.2	(0.001)
MRL Mp 1pr/1pr	M/Abs	89.2		297.3	
Experiment 3					
Conceptuses examined on Day 14					
Normal MRL	IgG Control	131.0	(0.001)	357.7	(0.001)
Normal MRL	M/Abs	59.0		243.0	
MRL Mp 1pr/1pr	IgG Control	171.3	(0.001)	642.6	(0.001)
MRL Mp 1pr/1pr	M/Abs	93.7		319.6	

*CSEA1 Orleans MRL/L is Lpr/Lpr++, while CSEA1 Orleans MRL/mp is LPR 1pr negative and corresponds to "Normal MRL". This strain was termed Mrl/l in Reference 30, while Mrl/MP 1 pr/pr in Reference 30 is the CSEA1 Orleans MRL/L strain referred to in this table.
**Mean placenta/phagiocytosis index: This reflects the mean phagocytosis of fluorescent latex beads as described in Reference 28.

A third key observation in the overall picture came from weighing the placentae of immunised and non-immunised CBA/J × DBA/2 newborn mice. This showed a definite increase in mean placental weight in actively immunised mice (0.144 mg) and in mice passively immunised with serum (0.162 mg) and immune cells (0.146 mg), compared to non-immunised controls (0.132 mg).[12,26]

Table 16

Effects of intraperitoneal injections of 10^7 splenocytes and purified monoclonal antibodies on resorption rate and placental weight

Mice	Treatment 1 (10^7 splenocytes)	Treatment 2	% Resorption	Placental weight in mg (p<)
CBA/J × Balb/c	—	—	8.9	137.9
CBA/J × Balb/c	NL MRL	—	7.8	142.7
CBA/J × Balb/c	MRL lpr/lpr	—	6.3	165.4 (0.05)
CBA/J × Balb/c	—	Control	9.7	145.3
CBA/J × Balb/c	MRL lpr/lpr	Control	6.9	170.9
CBA/J × Balb/c	MRL lpr/lpr	M/Abs	38.9	93.2 (0.01)
CBA/J × DBA/2	—	Control	41.7	85.7 (0.01)
CBA/J × DBA/2	anti Balb/c	—	10.2	146.2 (0.05)
CBA/J × DBA/2	MRL	—	33.1	101.6 (0.01)
CBA/J × DBA/2	MRL lpr/lpr	—	13.7	172.4 N.S.
CBA/J × DBA/2	MRL lpr/lpr	Control	15.5	168.9 (0.01)
CBA/J × DBA/2	MRL lpr/lpr	M/Abs	28.4	110.6

One further set of recent observations has led to an "immunotrophic theory" to explain the CBA/J × DBA phenomenon.[27] Namely, placental cells cultivated *in vitro* show enhanced growth in the presence of the lymphokines, IL-3, GM-CSF and CSF-1.[26,28] In a similar vein, we have observed that the teratocarcinomas, Terc/b and A6B91C5, both grow better *in vitro* in synergy with a monoclonal anti H-2b antibody of the IgG1 subclass. Also consistent with this immunotrophic theory is Armstrong's observation that C3H × DBA/2 placental cells grow better on an irradiated C3H anti Balb/c feeder layer than on an irradiated C3H anti-C3H layer.[29]

In the light of the finding that placental growth and phagocytosis *in vivo* are diminished by treatment with a mixture of anti-LyT-2 and anti-L3T4, we tested whether such treatment could: a) increase resorption rate in the CBA × Balb/c matings and, b) prevent the anti-abortive effect of anti-Balb/c immunisation on the CBA × DBA/2 mating. As shown in Table 14, the answer is affirmative for both questions. Injection of anti-LyT 2.1 plus anti-L3T4 hybridoma antibodies on Days 8, 10 and 12 of pregnancy did reduce fetal survival rate and placental weights in CBA × Balb/c pregnancies and in CBA × DBA/2 matings in which the CBA mothers had been immunised against Balb/c. The same treatment also reduced placental weights in pregnant H-2k MR1/1 (MRL.mp/1pr/1pr) mice in which their autoimmunity leads to severe lymphoproliferative disorders and greatly increased placental weight without harming fetal survival (Table 15). This result is important since MRL/mp 1pr/1pr T cells have been shown to secrete high levels of IL-3 and possibly IL-2 and other lymphokines.[30] Since they are H-2k, it is possible to inject these mice intraperitoneally 2 days before mating with 10^7 splenocytes from either MRL/L +/+ (Mrl Mp, or normal MRL) or Lpr +/+ (MRL mp 1pr/1pr, alias MRL/L) animals. These cells have never seen the H-2d antigen, nor the placental antigen involved, but are hyper-secreting IL-3. Yet, as shown in Table 16, they do reduce the resorption rate when injected alone into CBA/J mice mated to DBA/2 males. Since the cells differ from CBA/J cells by minor background antigens, they could either be cleared from the circulation after injection or they could induce graft versus host (GVH) disease. Of 10 mice injected with 1pr/1pr spleen cells as non-pregnant viability controls to date, 9 have survived normally for 3 weeks and the other died in a manner suggestive of GVH.

This experiment obviously needs to be repeated and the time-lapse ratio of LyT 1.2 (MRL) cells to 1.1 (CBA) cells measured by FACS, and the outcome of pregnancies beyond Day 14 will also need to be tested. We will also need to examine the system for the possible involvement of the claimed aberrant H-2d, 1a-d monocyte subset in the MRL 1pr+ 1pr+ mouse.[30] But despite these isolated findings, we nevertheless believe that the immunotrophic loop theory, as proposed originally by Wegmann, plays an important part in placental survival. Thus, anti-MHC recognition or homing, or the degradation of immune complexes to provide chemotactic signals, would attract sensitised T cells and reinforce placental growth and functions. Amongst these functions are placental neutralisation of killer cells and placental recruitment of decidual suppressor cells whose factors suppress killer cell expansion and their lytic functions, while at the same time acting as a placental growth factor. In this manner, immunotrophism would set up a paracrine loop, the intricacy of which we are just now beginning to tackle.

ACKNOWLEDGEMENTS

The close co-operation of N. Kiger, J. P. Kolb, D. Lankar, M. Riviere and J. L. Guennet in these studies is gratefully acknowledged.

ADDENDUM

Recent experiments show that the trophic effects of immunised T-cells in preventing abortion can be replaced by injections of granulocyte macrophage colony stimulating factor (GMCSF) which lowers the abortion rate from 47% to 8.3% following 3 i.v. injections of 600 units on Days 8, 10 and 12. The trophic effect seems to affect lysis-resistant spongiotrophoblast cells. Recombinant IL-2 does not affect the abortion rate in normal pregnancies, but it slightly increases the resorption rate in CBA/J × DBA/2 pregnancies.

REFERENCES
1. Clark DA, McDermott MR, Szewczuk MR. Impairment of host-versus-graft reaction in pregnant mice: II) Selective suppression of cytotoxic cell generation correlates with soluble suppressor activity and with successful allogeneic pregnancy. *Cell Immunol* 1980; **52**: 106-118.
2. Chaouat G, Kiger N, Wegmann TG. Vaccination against spontaneous abortion in mice. *J Reprod Immunol* 1983; **5**: 389-392.

3. Chaouat G, Kolb JP, Kiger N, Stanislawski M, Wegmann TG. Immunologic sequences of vaccination against abortion in mice. *J Immunol* 1985; **134:** 1594-1598.
4. Chaouat G, Lankar D, Kolb JP, Clark DA. 2 modules d'avortements d'origine immunitaire chez la souris de laboratoire: mécanismes abortifs, modalités et mécanismes du traitement par l'immunisation contre un mâle relié ou non relié suivant les différences antigéniques père ere. In: *Immunologie de la relation féto-maternelle.* Ed: G Chaouat. Paris: Editions INSERM. J Libbey. Colloque INSERM 154, 1987. pp.243.
5. Kiger N, Chaouat G, Kolb JP, Wegmann TG, Guennet JL. Immunogenetic studies of spontaneous abortion in mice. Preimmunization of females with alloantigenic spleen cells. *J Immunol* 1985; **134:** 2966-2970.
6. Bobé P, Kiger N. Role of minor histocompatibility antigens in fetal tolerance. In: *Reproductive Immunology 1986.* Eds: DA Clark, BA Croy. Amsterdam: Elsevier, 1987; pp.246.
7. Clark DA, Croy BA, Wegmann TG, Chaouat G. Immunological and para-immunological mechanisms in spontaneous abortion: Recent insights and future directions (opinion). *J Reprod Immunol* 1987; In press.
8. Wegmann TG, Athanassakis I, Mogil R, Chaouat G. Placental immunotrophism: maternal T cells contribute to the growth and survival of the fetal allograft. Submitted.
9. Bobé P, Kiger N. Immunogenetic aspects of spontaneous abortion in mice: Role of non-MHC antigens in the induction of semi-allogeneic fetus tolerance. *J Reprod Immunol* 1986. (Abstract). p.24.
10. Klein J. *Natural history of the H-2 complex.* Chichester: John Wiley, 1986; pp.320.
11. Clark DA, Chaput A, Tutton D. Active suppression of host-versus-allograft reaction in pregnant mice. VII. Spontaneous abortion of allogeneic CBA × DBA/2 fetuses in the uterus of CBA/J mice correlates with deficient non-T suppressor cell activity. *J Immunol* 1986. **136:** 1668-1675.
12. Chaouat G, Kolb JP, Riviere M, Chaffaux S. Local and systemic regulation of maternal antifetal cytotoxicity during murine pregnancy. In: *Gynaecology and Obstetrics.* Eds: V Toder, AE Beer. Basel: S Karger, 1985; pp.55-65.
13. Clark DA. Local suppressor cells and the success or failure of the foetal allograft. *Ann Immunol* 1984; **135:(D):** 321-324.
14. Clark DA, Chaouat G, Guennet JL, Kiger N. Local active suppression and successful vaccination against spontaneous abortion in CBA/J mice. *J Reprod Immunol* 1987; **10:** 79-85.
15. Chaouat G, Lankar D. Vaccination against spontaneous abortions in mice by preimmunisation with an anti-idiotypic antibody. *Amer J Reprod Immunol Microbiol*; In press.
16. Bobé P, Kiger N. Immunogenetic aspects of feto-maternal tolerance. In: *Immunologie de la relation féto-maternelle.* Ed. G Chaouat. Paris: Editions INSERM, 1987; Colloque INSERM 154. pp.235.
17. Chaouat G, Kolb JP, Wegmann TG. Studies on a murine model of immunologically mediated abortion and its treatment. 7th European Immunology Meeting, Jerusalem, 1985. *Int Arch Allergy Appl Immunol* 1985; **Suppl:** 1.
18. Chaouat G, Kolb JP, Wegmann T. The CBA/J × DBA/2 murine abortion model. *J Reprod Immunol* 1986; **Suppl:** 135.
19. Bobé P, Stanislawski M, Kiger N. Immunogenetic studies of spontaneous abortions in mice. In: *Immunoregulation and fetal survival.* Eds: TJ Gill 3rd, TG Wegmann. Oxford: Oxford University Press, 1987; pp.252.
20. Bobé P, Kiger N. Immunogenetic studies of spontaneous abortion in mice: role of non-MHC antigens in the induction of semi-allogeneic fetus tolerance. *6th Intl Congress of Immunology.* Abstract 6.22.4.

21. Chaouat G, Kolb JP. Effet protecteur d'anticorps dans un modèle murin des avortements immunitaires et de leur traitement. *Proceedings of May 1985 meeting of the S.F.I. (Société Française d'Immunologie)*, Grenoble, 1985. Paris: Institut Pasteur, 1985.
22. Bobé P, Chaouat G, Stanislawski M, Kiger N. Immunogenetics of spontaneous abortion in mice. II) anti-abortive effects are independent of systemic regulatory mechanisms. *Cell Immunol* 1986; **98:** 2.
23. Chaouat G. Modèles animaux d'immunopathologie de la gestation. In: *Immunologie de la grossesse*. Eds. C Sureau, JF Bach, P Edelmann, GA Voisin. Paris: Flammarion; In press.
24. Melnick M, Jaskoll T, Slavkin HC. The association of H-2 haplotype with implantation, survival and growth of murine embryos. *Immunogenetics* 1981; **14:** 303-308.
25. Hamilton MS and Hamilton BL. Examination on immunologically associated recurrent spontaneous abortion in CBA/J mice. *J Reprod Immunol*; In press.
26. Chaouat G, Kolb JP. Studies on a murine abortion model, and its immunological treatment. *British Society for Immunology* 1985. Liverpool, July 1985.
27. Wegmann TG. Fetal protection against abortion: is it immunosuppression or immunostimulation? *Ann Immunol* 1984; **135D:** 309-312.
28. Athanassakis I, Bleackley RC, Paetkau V, Guilbert L, Barr PJ, Wegmann TG. The immunostimulatory effects of T cells and T cell lymphokines on murine fetally derived placental cells. *J Immunol* 1987; **138:** 37.
29. Armstrong DTA, Chaouat G. Effects of lymphokines and immune complexes on murine placental cell growth *in vitro*. Submitted.
30. Weston KM, Yeh ETH, Man-Sun SY. Autoreactivity accelerates the development of autoimmunity and lymphoproliferation in MRL/Mp 1pr/1pr mice. *J Immunol* 1987; **139:** 734.

Discussion

Chairman: Dr. W.R. Allen

Professor GILL: Could Dr. Chaouat test his hypothesis by giving the animals with the high resorption rate just the purified growth factor, or by trying to elicit the production of growth factor by an unrelated immune combination?

Dr. CHAOUAT: We have been purifying the growth factor and now have it ready for GLC assessment. We are also making an *in vitro* calibration of lymphokines in the growth factor and are injecting these into mice to see whether or not they influence placental growth. The growth factor we have purified contains small amounts of IA-1 and IA-3 so it is not totally pure. Monoclonal antibodies against both recombinant lymphokines are available and I hope to use these to neutralise the activities of the lymphokines *in vivo* and *in vitro*. We plan to use these in the CBA/DBA$_2$ mating combinations.

Dr. BELL: Could there be two phenomena? The results achieved from the transfer of serum could be an antihistamine-type antibody stimulating growth factor receptors on the placenta.

Dr. CHAOUAT: I am doubtful. Since the antibody has to be directed against MHC antigen, we first need to know if the spongiotrophoblast is MHC positive. On the other hand, the antibodies could act simply by being targeted locally and producing chemical signals that are chemotactic and attract T-cells to produce more lymphokines. We don't know this yet but we do know that purified antibodies are not as good as the immune serum. However, immune serum apparently loses some of its activity when absorbed so it is a question of targeting.

When we look at the CBA/BALB C immunisation, the antibodies by themselves may be absent so that the protective effect cannot be seen. We are presently trying to see if the immunised animals have T-cells in the decidua. And whether the decidua is producing growth factor for placental cells *in vitro*.

Dr. BELL: Have you actually selected for these inbred strains to show this phenomenon?

Dr. CHAOUAT: No. We are using a number of inbred strains of which 6 do not protect and 3 do protect when they are used to immunise the CBA females. Thus, if our hypothesis is right, the decidual cells of the CBA females immunised with the appropriate protective recombinant strain should correlate positively for both the decidual growth factor and the T-cell growth factor activities. If they do not correlate it simply means there is something else that we do not understand about lymphokines.

Dr. BELL: Before we see the data from the scid strain, I wonder if, in natural outbred animals, we may be seeing another growth factor. In the normal physiological process of pregnancy there is a growth factor which stimulates placental growth (e.g. IGF) which we know has Type 1 receptors. In the defective pregnancies perhaps Dr. Chaouat is seeing a situation where lymphokines are another type of growth factor which substitutes for the natural growth factor.

Dr. CHAOUAT: The placenta has been shown to have receptors for IL-3 which could act as a growth factor by itself. I don't know whether or not this could bypass the effect of growth but it may well stimulate the production of other growth factors.

Dr BILLINGTON: Dr. Chaouat described the protective effect of passively transferred serum as being protective only in the postpartum situation and not when given during pregnancy. I was not clear if he had an explanation for this.

Dr. CHAOUAT: Yes, I do have an explanation for this finding. During pregnancy the antibody level in blood drops below a certain value due to absorption of the antibodies onto the placenta. In the postpartum period, on the other hand, as seen by using an ELISA assay, there is a slight rise in antibody production. Thus, my explanation is quite simple, although I have not tested it; during pregnancy there is not enough antibody to achieve the effect.

Dr. BILLINGTON: So it is purely a quantitative effect?

Dr. CHAOUAT: It could be many things, but most likely it is a question of amounts of antibody.

Dr. PAGE FAULK: In the light of this, could one get the same kind of protection by passively transferring placental eluate?

Dr. CHAOUAT: I would like to do that and we have begun working on placental eluates. I think it is a strong possibility that anti-MHC antibody eluded from the placenta would be protective.

Professor MOWBRAY: Associated with that, the immunoglobulin that is on placenta is almost exclusively IgG, although it was shown some years ago that it is a rather odd distribution of subclasses. But is there any direct evidence from serum transfer that IgG is effective?

Dr CHAOUAT: The immunoglobulins that can be eluded from the placenta are mostly IgG-1, but not exclusively.

Effects of feto-maternal major histocompatibility differences on litter size in pigs

C. Renard

INTRODUCTION

In mammalian reproduction the role of immunogenetic incompatibility between parents has been widely discussed.[1] The Major Histocompatibility Complex (MHC) of mammalian species is known to play a crucial role, both in self-recognition and in the recognition and response to antigens presented by an allograft. As the fetus can be considered a semi-allograft, the MHC has been a prime candidate for investigation as an influencing factor in reproduction.[2,3]

The role of the MHC in pregnancy has been studied chiefly in the human,[4] in mice[5] and rats.[6] These species all have a haemochorial placentation that allows intimate contact between the maternal and fetal circulations. By contrast, pigs have the least intimate type of feto-maternal contact, the non-invasive epitheliochorial placenta.[7] It is therefore of interest to compare the influence of the porcine MHC in pregnancy with observations made in other species.

In this paper the characteristics of pregnancy in the pig, the immunological developments during pregnancy and the characteristics of the swine MHC (swine leucocyte antigen; SLA) will be outlined. The findings of my own laboratory, and those of others, on the influence of SLA on reproduction in the pig will also be described.

GESTATION

Gestation in sows lasts 114 days. Initial morula formation is followed by blastocyst hatching at Day 6, and the fetus begins to elongate by Day 11. This is followed by migration and positioning in the uterine horns which is a critical stage for successful implantation.[8] Protrusions from the uterine epithelium immobilise the blastocyst between Days 13 and 14, and implantation is achieved between Days 13 and 18. Contact between the uterine epithelium and the trophoblast is increased during Days 15 to 20 by the formation of apical domes from the uterus and interdigital microvilli from the fetus. Placentation continues in the peripheral zone of the placenta to about Day 26,[9] corresponding to the first quarter of gestation. Beyond this time, growth occurs exponentially from Day 28 to Days 60 to 80[10] (Figure I).

Figure I

PIG GESTATION TIMING

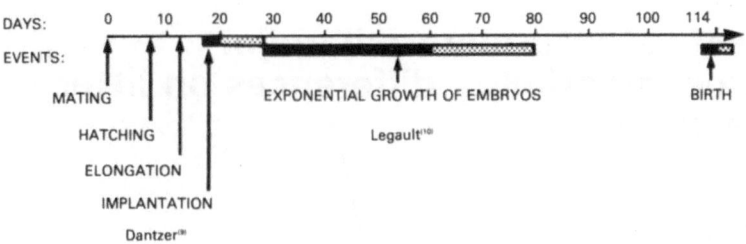

THE IMMUNE RESPONSE DURING PREGNANCY

This subject has been extensively reviewed by Koch[11] so only the major points are summarised here. Histologically, the epitheliochorial placenta of the pig is similar to that of the horse and although this form of placentation presents the most substantial anatomical barrier to contact between fetal and maternal circulations, some degree of contact does occur. For example, chromosome analyses carried out in pregnant gilts has demonstrated that male karyotypes regularly constitute 1-4% of metaphases from peripheral blood leucocytes.[12]

Antigen expression

The question arises as to whether, for the pregnancy to be successful, the "foreign" antigens of the fetus are either not expressed, or are subject to some masking mechanism that reduces the immunogenicity of fetal cells which come into contact with the maternal lymphoid system. Concerning non-expression, Meziou *et al*[13] investigated the expression of SLA antigens on the embryo before and after implantation. Whereas classical polyclonal SLA antibodies pre-absorbed by maternal cells gave inconclusive results, the use of monoclonal anti-bodies to beta 2 microglobulin (which forms part of the Class 1 MHC molecule) showed that antigen is expressed on pig trophoblast between elongation and implantation, but not after implantation. Regarding possible reduction of immunogenicity, the reproductive tract of the sow is equipped with an effective mucosal immune system.[14] Thus, a mucopolysaccharide layer may cover the surface of trophoblast cells.

Maternal humoral response

As in the horse, no maternal antibodies have been observed in the pig embryo before birth, even in 2nd pregnancies.[15,16] Immunoglobulin secretion occurs

Figure II

EMBRYONIC MORTALITY RATE IN THE PIG DURING PREGNANCY

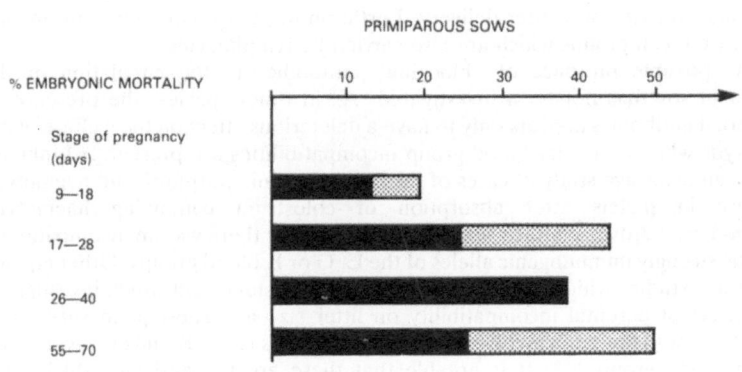

PRIMIPAROUS SOWS

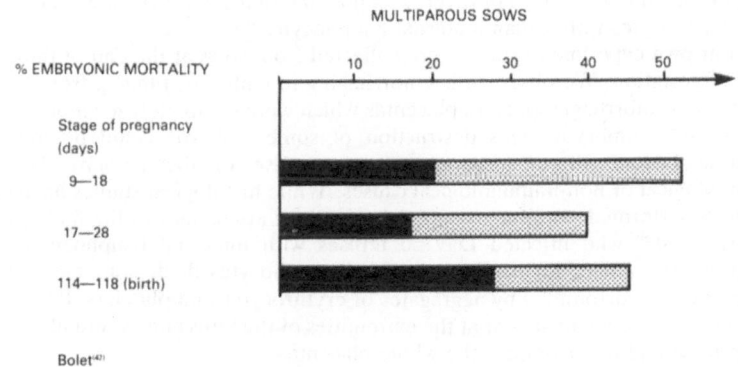

MULTIPAROUS SOWS

Bolet[42]

locally in the uterus,[14] but immunoglobulins do not appear to cross the placental barrier in either the pig or the horse.[15] Active immunisation of sows by boar spermatozoa does increase the number of stillborn, but only after the second pregnancy in which reimmunisation is carried out.[17] Unlike mares which do produce cytotoxic anti-MHC antibodies during pregnancy,[15] sows produce lymphocytotoxins only after delivery. Furthermore, these antibodies are mainly against red cell groups which are also carried by lymphocytes.[18]

The possible presence of "blocking" antibodies in the circulation of the pregnant sow has not been investigated. As in other species, the presence of maternal antibodies appears only to have a deleterious effect on the welfare of pig embryos when particular blood group incompatibilities are present.[19] Linklater made an extensive study of cases of thrombocytopenia purpurea and haemolytic disease in piglets after absorption of colostrum containing haemolytic antibodies.[20] Adverse effects were noted only where there was an incompatibility for the strongly immunogenic alleles of the E, G or K blood groups. Other equally extensive studies which included 12 blood group systems and which investigated the effect of parental incompatibility on litter size and subsequent survival of piglets showed the same involvement of blood groups E, G, K and also A, but not other blood groups.[21-24] It is notable that these are the antigens which most readily induce the production of lymphocytoxic antibodies by skin grafting.[25] An association between "biological fitness" of the conceptus due to heterosis and the H blood group system, and a possible pre-zygotic selection linked to the B blood group system, was also described.[24,26]

Maternal cellular response

The histological studies of Marrable and Flood[27,28] indicated the presence of lymphoid cells in the necrotic tips of the allantochorion of the pig placenta, and a large number of "lymphocytes" was observed in the placenta and interlocular zone of the endometrium. However, it is possible that these cells were nuleated fetal erythrocytes rather than maternal lymphocytes.[28]

In our own experiments, uteri were collected from sows at the end of the first third of gestation. We observed haemorrhaging in embryos, ranging from small petechial haemorrhagic spots, to placentas which were completely haemorrhagic, with necrotic embryos. This destruction of some embryos could be due to maternal factors, or to a spontaneous response of the embryo due to immunological or non-immunological causes. While histological studies have not yet been performed, our macroscopic observations are similar to the findings of Gerard et al[29] who injected Day 50 fetuses with maternal lymphocytes. In Gerard's experiment, many of the injected lymphocytes died, apparently as a result of being surrounded by aggregates of erythrocytes and platelets. Petechial haemorrhages began to appear at the extremities of the fetus and eventually these began to spread to encompass the whole placenta.

THE SWINE MHC

The swine lymphocyte alloantigen system (SLA) has been studied since 1970[30] and is now well characterised. It resembles closely the equivalent systems found in other species, whether studied by serological[30] or cellular techniques,[32] or at the molecular DNA level.[33]

Three Class I and two Class II loci, all closely linked,[34] have been identified by observation of recombinants and from biochemical studies.[35] Polymorphism for the genes which control the level of haemolytic complement activity (a Class III determinant) has also been mapped to the same region by segregation studies.[36] The gene coding for the 21-hydroxylase enzyme has also been investigated in our laboratory using molecular biological techniques. We have shown this to be on the same chromosome (Number 7) as the SLA Class I genes, which were identified by chromosome sorting and spot hybridisation.[37] 21-hydroxylase is known to be involved in steroid metabolism, and it will be interesting to study the activity of this enzyme, or its DNA sequence modification, in conjunction with reproductive traits.

The polymorphism of SLA has so far been studied mainly with regard to Class I antigens, although at the Class II region 10 alleles at the D locus, and 5 at the Dr locus, have also been described.[38] The First International Workshop was held in 1986 in Helsinki, when Class I antisera from 6 laboratories in Europe and USA, were shown to define clearly 18 of the 35 local specificities previously described by the different laboratories. Table 1 shows the internationally agreed nomenclature for the more frequent SLA haplotypes, and the corresponding local nomenclature used in previous publications. In order to simplify reference to specificities of the 3 Class I loci which segregate together in families, a coded name has been assigned to these haplotypes.[39] Thus, previously reported results concerning associations between SLA and proliferacy can now be compared.

Table 1

EQUIVALENCE BETWEEN INTERNATIONAL NOMENCLATURE OF CODED SLA HAPLOTYPES AND LOCALLY USED NAMES

SLA Haplotype Workshop-coded name	Bern Haplotype	French and Danish nomenclature
H 1	HBe 2	SLA 15.1.18
H 2	—	SLA 10.14
H 4	HBe 1	SLA 13.9
H 5	HBe 11	SLA 5.21
H 7	HBe 13	SLA 20.8.2.11
H 14	HBe 18	SLA 16.11
H 16	HBe 9	SLA 13.19
H 19	HBe 3	SLA 6
H 21	HBe 6	SLA 20.2.11
H 23	HBe 19	SLA 26

Polymorphism for SLA is high and 61 Class I haplotypes have been observed in segregation studies.[38,40] Within a given breed, however, the variation may be much more restricted, with only 3 or 4 haplotypes having a frequency greater than 0.10.[38] Consequently, only a few haplotypes were common enough to be studied extensively in relation to reproductive traits.

SLA MATING TYPE AND REPRODUCTION

In the four laboratory studies to be described, Class I antigens were identified by serological methods, and formed the basis of the SLA analysis. In addition, Class II antigens were also identified in certain cases by the mixed lymphocyte reaction (MLR) or by serology. And in a few instances, RFLP was used to compare apparently identical haplotypes.

The animals studied came chiefly from the Yorkshire and Landrace breeds of pig. Two mating types were studied; those in which the boar and sow shared an SLA haplotype, when a proportion of SLA homozygous offspring which would be compatible with the mother could be expected, and those in which the boar and sow differed for both SLA haplotypes and could thus produce only heterozygous offspring. In the majority of matings only the parents were SLA-typed, but in some cases the piglets, including stillborn animals, were also tested.

Litter size depends on fertilisation rate and on embryonic loss at various stages of gestation. We have looked at these factors in relation to SLA at different stages of gestation.

The fertilisation rate

In pigs the fertilisation rate is generally considered to be very high. Failure of fertilisation is indicated by a return to oestrus at around 21 days after mating. A delayed return to oestrus may indicate failure of fertilised ova to implant rather than failed fertilisation, but the two phenomena are difficult to distinguish.

We looked at the percentage of sows returning to oestrus after mating in a herd selected for prolificacy over 14 generations. Sows were mated with boars from the same breed for their first litter, and with boars from another breed for their second litter. From three generations this gave 370 within-breed/first parity matings and 212 cross-breed/second-parity matings. An SLA haplotype was shared in one-third of matings in each group. There was no significant difference in fertilisation rate between any of the groups, although the highest failure rate was noted for cross-breed matings that shared an SLA haplotype (Table 2). Numbers were insufficient to make the same comparison by any of the 3 individual SLA haplotypes in the study which could be identified. However, an Australian group using different haplotypes,[41] also found no SLA related differences in fertilisation rates.

Table 2

PERCENTAGE RETURN TO OESTRUS

SLA MATING TYPE	PURE BREED	CROSS BREED	
A/− × A/−	14%	16%	NS
A/− × −/−	15%	13%	
Number of sows	370	212	

Embryonic mortality

The rate of embryonic mortality in pigs has been reviewed by Bolet,[42] and the values are shown in Figure I. The period prior to implantation seems to be the most critical stage for embryonic loss and, as estimated by return to oestrus, a 20% loss occurs at this stage in first pregnancies, with the rate rising to 20-50% in subsequent pregnancies. A second peak in fetal loss occurs at around Day 50 as a result of overcrowding in the uterine horns.

To study embryonic loss prior to implantation we looked at 64 sows which were slaughtered between Days 30 and 35 of gestation. The number of *corpora lutea* on the ovaries, and the number of allantochorionic sacs were counted and the viability of each was assessed. Two values for percentage of embryonic loss were calculated; the first based on the difference between *corpus luteum* (CL) and chorionic sac (CS) numbers, and the second, reflecting a later mortality, by the difference between (CL) and live embryo (LE) numbers. These observations were made on three generations of sows of first or third parity in cross-breed matings. No effect of either generation or parity was observed. Sire effect was corrected for by comparing figures between sows served by the same boar when sharing of an SLA haplotype did or did not exist.

For the offspring of two boars in which the haplotype SLA-H1 was the shared haplotype, no difference in embryonic loss rate was observed which could be attributed to SLA. However, in two sire families when the haplotype SLA-H2 was shared, the embryonic loss was far greater in the shared-haplotype matings when measured by the second criterion of embryo viability. This embryonic loss rate was, of course, calculated without prior knowledge of the SLA type of mating. In this particular herd, sows carrying the SLA-H2 haplotype had inherited it from one or other of two different boars two generations previously. When the litters of these two groups of sows were considered separately, the higher embryonic loss rate was marked in the SLA-matched matings of one group, whereas the loss rate was similar in SLA compatible and incompatible matings in the other group. The identity of these two maternal SLA-H2 haplotypes was confirmed by RFLP analysis using probes for both Class I and Class II regions. Consequently, this effect on embryonic loss of a shared SLA haplotype appears to be mediated by genes *linked* to SLA, rather than to SLA directly. When sows were slaughtered between Days 30 and 35, early embryonic loss could have occurred already due to SLA homozygosity, or the situation could have been affecting the subsequent development and viability of embryos still *in utero* at that time. This could explain the high standard variation seen in Table 3.

642 embryos sired by 4 different boars were weighed and measured. Variance analysis, using a model which allowed for sire and dam effect, showed an influence of mating type, a relation between mating type and day of gestation at harvesting, and an influence of SLA shared by the boar and sow.

Progressive analysis showed no mating type effect in the case of boars that shared SLA-H1 with the sows (Table 4). However, mating type clearly influenced embryonic and placental growth in the case of boars that shared SLA H2 with the sows ($p < 0.05$), although only at Days 31-32; this result is not apparent when sows were slaughtered at Day 30. Thus, at Days 31-32, SLA homozygosity, or SLA compatibility between embryo and sow, was beginning to influence fetal development.

Table 3

EMBRYONIC LOSS IN RELATION TO SLA STATUS
AT DAYS 30-35

SLA sire	dam	PERCENTAGE OF LOSS $\dfrac{\text{CL-CS} \times 100}{\text{CL}}$		PERCENTAGE OF LOSS $\dfrac{\text{CL-LE} \times 100}{\text{CL}}$	
		n	M%	n	M%
2a/−	2a/−	(17)	21.2 ± 4.8	(17)	35.5 ± 6.1
2a/−	2b/−	(11)	14.8 ± 3.3	(11)	20.4 ± 3.3
2a/−	−/−	(16)	15.7 ± 2.9	(16)	19.8 ± 4.3
2/a−	2/b−				
	−/−	(27)	14.5 ± 2.0	(27)	19.8 ± 2.6

*

Pooled results from 3 generations
a : haplotype derived from boar 1586 in the 13th generation
b : haplotype derived from boar 1460 in the 13th generation
CL : corpora lutea
CS : chorionic sacs
LE : live embryos
n : number of litters
m : mean percentage of embryonic loss

Table 4

EMBRYONIC DEVELOPMENT AT 31 AND 32 DAYS OF PREGNANCY
(263 EMBRYOS)

SLA mating type sire	dam	Placental Weight g	Fluid Volume ml	Embryonic Weight g	Length of Embryo mm
2/−	2/−	27.8	171	1.76	25.9
2/−	−/−	43.5	208	2.69	29.2
1/−	1/−	37.3	241	2.61	29.1
1/−	−/−	43.9	228	2.41	28.1

At 30 days of gestation, H2 SLA mating type does not decrease the growth of embryos and placenta (150 embryos).

SLA and litter size at birth

When litter size at birth was considered, the number of SLA-homozygous offspring was found to be lower than expected in some cases. An earlier study in 1980[43] looked at 47 litters from matings where SLA haplotypes were shared, and found that in one of 4 haplotypes investigated, SLA H1, there was a significantly lower incidence of homozygous piglets at birth. However, no general effect on litter size was obvious some days after birth in relation to SLA matching, and this lower proportion of SLA H1 homozygous piglets was lost in the following generation. Similarly, Kristensen[44] who was working with a different breed in Switzerland, found a deficit of piglets homozygous for the SLA H14 haplotype in the first generation, but not the second. More recently the same author found no influence of homozygosity for 12 SLA haplotypes in piglets born live and weaned from 217 Danish litters.[44]

In 1985 an Australian investigator examined the question of whether mating between MHC compatible individuals can lead to improved reproductive success in terms of litter size and birth weight.[41] In a large series of 424 matings between 47 boars and 123 sows no significant difference in litter size could be attributed to SLA. One antigen, locally named SU6, was associated with increased birth weight, but this was not significant after correction for the number of tests performed. Again, in Switzerland in 1986, Gautschi[45] found a trend towards reduced litter size with SLA compatible matings for 4 of 7 haplotypes studied, although this was significant for only one haplotype, H19.[45] For one other haplotype, H7, litter size at birth increased with homozygosity, but was also associated with a significantly higher stillbirth rate.

We have also looked for effect of SLA on litter size in two Yorkshire herds, one unselected and the other selected over 14 generations for large litter size at birth.[46] In the selected herd, litters were studied over two generations, with around 100 sows in each. For each generation the sows had litters first by a boar (1 of 8) of the same breed, and secondly by a boar (1 of 5) of another breed. Parity and cross-breed effects could not be independently assessed. Two thousand piglets, including stillborns and their parents, were typed for SLA in the following groups: a) first-parity/within breed; b) second-parity/cross-breed combinations. In the pure breed matings there was no effect on litter size in shared haplotype

Table 5

COMPARISON BETWEEN LITTER TRAITS FOR BOARS HAVING SLA-LINKED
GENES WHICH INFLUENCE HOMOZYGOUS PIGLET PROPORTIONS

Herd selected for prolificacy

Mating type sire	dam	Number of litters	Percentage of homozygous piglets	Mean litter size	Mean live births	Mean offspring weaned
1/−	1/−	6	17	9.5 ⎫ ₒ	9.3	8.4
1/−	−/−	13	—	10.6 ⎭	9.7	6.7
2/−	2/−	7	9	9.8 ⎫ **	9.3	5.3
2/−	−/−	12	—	12.7 ⎭	11.9	7.1

Unselected herd

Mating type sire	dam	Number of litters	Percentage of homozygous piglets	Mean live births	Mean offspring weaned
1/6	1/−	3	15	12.3	8.6
1/6	−/6	4	25	11	8.7
1/3	1/−	3	14	10.6	10
1/3	−/3	6	21	10.8	10.1
1^{d1}/1^{d6}	1^{d1}/−	5 ⟨ d1/d1 / d1/d6	16 / 29	11.2	11

matings, but in cross-breed matings litter size was significantly lower for SLA haploidentity; and this was the case for all 4 SLA haplotypes if they were compared to the heterozygous mating type. However, intra-boar comparison showed this effect on litter size was only due to one boar used in cross-breeding, and his sharing SLA H2 with some sows (Table 5). In the pure-breed combinations we were unable to observe any effect of SLA H2 homozygosity, because mating was always performed between boar and sows from different paternal lineages, of which only one showed an effect of SLA H2 homozygosity on embryonic loss. When the actual types of the offspring were examined the proportion of homozygous piglets at birth, including stillborns, was lower than expected only for the SLA H2 haplotype in cross-breed combinations. Some results showed striking intra-boar effects in both herds. For example, in the unselected herd with pure-breed mating, SLA H1 homozygosity had no greater effect on litter size than other homozygous haplotypes, and reduced numbers of homozygous piglets were noted only when there was complete homozygosity for both Class I and Class II determinants; this suggested that recessive deleterious genes were more likely to remain in linkage with SLA when the whole SLA haplotype was the same in both parents. When observations were pooled for haplotype or breed mating, the homozygous deficit was less significant. Consequently, litter size appears to be independent of feto-maternal SLA compatibility, except in cases when recessive deleterious genes linked to SLA may be homozygous in the embryo or piglet, as we observed for some SLA H2 haplotypes.

With regard to birth and weaning weights, in litters in which homozygotes were expected, the average birth weight was lowered for SLA H16 in one study,[45] but no such general effect was noted in our study in which all SLA haplotypes were pooled and subjected to complete model variance analysis.[47] Results from simplified models which ignored sire and dam effects suggested that SLA Class I homozygosity lowered birth weights, but at weaning the effect of homozygosity on weight could be either positive or negative, depending on the haplotype concerned. The same SLA haplotype was shown to be advantageous for birth weight in one herd,[48] thereby suggesting an effect of a particular SLA haplotype, rather than of homozygosity *per se*.[47]

CONCLUSIONS

In conclusion, these observations indicate that compatibility or incompatibility for SLA as such, does not affect litter size, although certain SLA haplotypes may have an effect, one way or another, which is more marked in homozygotes. The existence of SLA-linked genes affecting embryo growth or development would also be consistent with our observations regarding the SLA H2 haplotype and early embryonic loss. Furthermore, the haplotype which seems to have some effect also has the highest frequency in the breed studied. A parallel situation was noted in the mouse in relation to the T complex, but segregation distortion has not been observed for SLA H2 in pigs, as it has been described in man[49] and mice.[50] However, to explain the viability of some homozygotes, and the loss of this effect with generation, either SLA linkage cannot be very close, penetrance must be low, or recombination events must be postulated between SLA and any linked deleterious genes. A further similarity with the mouse T complex is the segregation distortion of SLA H7 which was clearly observed in Danish pigs,[51] and an increased stillborn rate associated with the same haplotype in Switzerland.[45] In previous studies no deficit of SLA H7 homozygotes was observed.

Thus it seems likely that the porcine MHC does play some part, directly or indirectly, in reproductive success. However, we cannot be sure by which of several possible mechanisms this may occur, and our observations could have been caused by a number of different phenomena. We wish to continue our investigations in experimental herds, with more planned matings and with a statistical model that is better adapted to the analysis of porcine reproductive traits and SLA markers.

In the present study we had to take into account the possible epistatic effects of other genes which seem to influence litter size or piglet survival, such as certain blood group incompatibilities and fertilisation failure related to transferrin types.[52] The model of interaction between HLA and transferrin genes developed by Weitkamp showed that such an epistatic effect is possible.[53] For future studies, histological examination of neural development in SLA homozygous embryos must be performed to see if a T-like system might exist. And to determine if there is any non-classical Class I gene effect, such as that observed in the rat,[54,55] we would like to analyse sow sera which lack blood group antibodies in order to look for public determinants of Class I on the trophoblast. Haemorrhagic embryos must be studied in more detail and RFLP techniques will make more precise analyses of genes in embryos possible.

ACKNOWLEDGEMENTS

I am most grateful to Dr P. Cullen, M. Vaiman and P. Chardon for their advice in the preparation of this manuscript. I thank J. P. Bidanel for his statistical analysis of results and P. Rombauts, P. Dando, N. Bourgeaux and J. J. Leplat for their collaboration throughout the experiments. I am also grateful to Isabelle Chifflet for excellent secretarial assistance.

REFERENCES
1. Gill TJ. Immunological and genetic factors influencing pregnancy and development. *Am J Reprod Immunol Microbiol* 1986; **10:** 116-120.
2. Beer AE, Billingham RE. Histocompatibility gene polymorphisms and maternal-fetal interactions. *Trans Proc* 1977; **9:** 1393-1401.
3. Giphart MJ, D'Amaro J. HLA and reproduction? *J Immunogenet* 1983; **10:** 25-29.
4. Coulam CB, Moore SB, O'Fallon WM. Association between major histocompatibility antigens and reproductive performance. *Am J Reprod Immunol Microbiol* 1987; **14:** 54-58.
5. Voisin JE, Monnot P, Voisin GA. Maternal alloimmune reactions towards the murine conceptus and graft-versus-host reaction (GVHR) I. Priming for anti-paternal GVHR by gestation. *J Reprod Immunol* 1986; **9:** 73-83.
6. Günther E. Genetic control of anti-male immune responsiveness in rat. *Trans Proc* 1985; **17:** 1840-1841.

7. Steven DH. Biology of trophoblast. In: *Interspecies differencies in the structure and function of trophoblast.* Eds. YW Loke, A Whyte. Amsterdam: Elsevier, 1983; pp.114-119.

8. Anderson LL. Early embryonic development in the pig. *J Anim Sci* 1974; **39:** 986 (Abstract).

9. Dantzer V. Electron microscopy of the initial stages of placentation in the pig. *Anat Embryol* 1985; **172:** 281-293.

10. Legault C, Leuillet M. Etude de quelques facteurs de variation du poids de l'embryon et du placenta chez la truie primipare au trentiène jour de la gestation. *Ann Bio Anim Bioch Biophys* 1973; **13:** 25-36.

11. Koch E. Establishment of pregnancy and its immunological implications in the pig. *J Reprod Fertil* 1985; **Suppl. 33:** 65-81.

12. Rudek Z, Kwiatkowska L. The possibility of detecting fetal lymphocytes in the maternal blood of the domestic pig, *sus scrofula. Cytogenet Cell Genet* 1983; **36:** 580-583.

13. Meziou W, Chardon P, Flechon JE, Kalil J, Vaiman M. Expression of beta 2-microglobulin on preimplantation pig embryos. *J Reprod Immunol* 1983; **5:** 73-80.

14. Hussein AM, Newby TJ, Bourne FJ. Immunohistochemical studies of the local immune system in the reproductive tract of the sow. *J Reprod Immunol* 1983; **5:** 1-15.

15. Antczak DF, Miller JM, Remick LH. Lymphocyte alloantigens of the horse: II. Antibodies to ELA antigens produced during pregnancy. *J Reprod Immunol* 1984; **6:** 283-297.

16. Linklater KA. Iso-antibodies to red cell antigens in pigs' sera. 1-Isoimmunisation of pregnancy in sows. *Anim Blood Grps Biochem Genet* 1971; **2:** 201-214.

17. Veselsky L, Stanek R, Hradecky J. Effect of antibodies to boar spermatazoa on fertility in sows and rabbits. *Arch Androl* 1981; **7:** 337-342.

18. Schmid DO, Cwik S, Krausslich H, Meyer J, Graf zu Dohna R. Uber lymphocyto-toxische antikorper bei weiblichen zuchtschweinen. *Zbl Vet Med B* 1978; **25:** 517-523.

19. Linklater KA. Iso-antibodies to red cell antigens in pigs' sera. 2. The incidence of iso-antibodies to red cell antigens in the sera of adult pigs. *Anim Blood Grps Biochem Genet* 1971; **2:** 215-220.

20. Linklater KA, McTaggart, Imlah T. Haemolytic disease of the newborn, thrombo-cytopenic purpurea and neutropenia occurring concurrently in a litter of piglets. *Br Vet J* 1973; **129:** 36-40.

21. Jensen EL, Smith C, Baker IN, Cox DF. Quantitative studies on blood group and serum protein systems in pigs: II. effects on production and reproduction. *J Anim Sci* 1968; **27:** 856-862.

22. Rasmusen BA, Hagen KL. The H blood group system and reproduction in pigs. *J Anim Sci* 1973; **37:** 568-573.

23. Rasmusen BA. A and O blood types and reproduction in pigs. 67th annual meeting of the American Society of Animal Science. *J Anim Sci* 1975; **41:** 256 (abstr).

24. Yau FD. Association of polymorphic blood group systems and relative fitness in pigs. *Dissertation abstracts international, B (sciences and engineering)* 1982; **43:** 629.

25. Hruban V, Simon M, Hradecky J. Alloantigens common to erythrocytes and leucocytes in pigs. *Anim Blood Grps Biochem Genet* 1972; **3:** 157-161.

26. Rasmusen BA, Yau FD. Association of H blood types with heterosis for reproductive fitness in pigs. *18th International Conference on Animal Blood Groups and Biochemical Polymorphisms.* Ottawa, Canada 1982; 112 (Abstract).

27. Marrable AW. The ischaemic extremities of the allantochorion of the pig and their relation to the endometrium. *Res Vet Sci* 1968; **9:** 578-582.

28. Flood PF. Endometrial differentiation in the pregnant sow and the necrotic tips of the allantochorion. *J Reprod Fert* 1973; **32:** 539-543.

29. Gerard H, Salmon H, Rombauts P. Les organes cibles potentiels de l'alloreactivité maternelle antifoetale, étude chez le porc. In: *Reproductive Immunology: materno-fetal relationships*. Ed. G. Chaouat, Paris: Colloques INSERM, 1987; **154:** pp.141-150.

30. Vaiman M, Renard C, Lafage P, Amateau J, Nizza P. Evidence for a histocompatibility system in swine (SLA). *Transplantation* 1970; **10:** 155-164.

31. Renard C, Chardon P, Vaiman M. The pig histocompatibility system SLA: serological study on a group of antigenic specificities. *Anim Blood Grps Biochem Genet* 1982; **13:** 161-177.

32. Chardon P, Renard C, Vaiman M. Characterization of class II histocompatibility antigens in pigs. *Anim Blood Grps Biochem Genet* 1981; **12:** 59-65.

33. Vaiman M, Chardon P, Cohen D. DNA polymorphism in the major histocompatibility complex of man and various farm animals. *Anim Genet* 1986; **17:** 113-133.

34. Geffrotin C, Popescu CP, Cribiu EP, Boscher J, Renard C, Chardon P, Vaiman M. Assignment of MHC in swine to chromosome 7 by *in situ* hybridization and serological typing. *Anim Genet* 1984; **27:** 213-219.

35. Vaiman M, Chardon P, Renard C. Genetic organization of the pig SLA complex. Studies on nine recombinants and biochemical and lysostrip analysis. *Immunogenetics* 1979; **9:** 353-361.

36. Vaiman M, Hauptmann G, Mayer S. Influence of the major histocompatibility complex in the pig (SLA) on serum haemolytic complement levels. *J Immunogenet* 1978; **5:** 59-65.

37. Geffrontin C, Grunwald D, Chardon P, Vaiman M. Swine MHC: mapping by chromosome flow sorting and spot hybridization. *Anim Genet* 1987; **18:** 118 (Abstract).

38. Renard C, Luquet M, Gouillieux P, Vaiman M. Le polymorphisme du systeme majeur d'histocompatibilité SLA dans plusieurs races porcines en France. In: *18ème Journées de la recherche porcine en France*. Paris: Institut Technique du Porc, 1986; pp.285-298.

39. Renard C, Kristensen B, Gautschi C, Hruban V, Fredholm N, Vaiman M. Joint report on the first international comparison test on swine lymphocyte alloantigens (SLA). *Anim Genet* 1987; In press.

40. Kristensen B, Philipsen M, Lazary S, Renard C, de Weck AL. The swine histocompatibility system SLA: serological studies in the common Swiss and Danish swine breeds. *Anim Blood Grps Bioch Genet* 1985; **16:** 109-124.

41. Willis GL, Baglin MJ, Love RJ, Brown SC, Nicholas FW. A study of histoincompatibility and reproductive performance in pigs. *Vet Rec* 1985; p.601.

42. Bolet G. Timing and extent of embryonic mortality in pigs, sheep and goats: genetic variability. In: *Embryonic mortality in farm animals*. Program of coordination of research on livestock production and management. Ed. JM Sreenan, MG Diskin. Dordrecht: Martinus Nijhoff, 1986; pp.12-45.

43. Vaimann M, Renard C. Deficit of piglets homozygous for the SLA histocompatibility complex in families. *Anim Blood Grps Biochem Genet* 1980; **11:** 57 (Abstract).

44. Kristensen B, Waflet P, de Weck AL. Histocompatibility antigens (SLA) in swine. Possible correlation between SLA haplotype and performance of piglets. *Anim Blood Grps Biochem Genet* 1980; **11:** 58-59.

45. Gautschi C, Gaillard C, Schwander B, Lazary S. Studies on possible associations between the major histocompatibility complex and reproduction traits in swine. In: *3rd world congress on genetics applied to livestock production. Lincoln, 1986*; **12:** 70-75.

46. Renard C, Bolet G, Dando P, Vaiman M. Effect of SLA haplotypes on birth and weaning weight and on deficit of homozygotes in Meishan pigs. *17ème Journée de la recherche porcine en France*. Institut Technique du Porc, 1985; pp.105-112.

47. Rothschild MF, Renard C, Legault C, Vaimann M. Effect of SLA haplotypes on birth and weaning weight and on deficit of homozygotes in Meishan pigs. *Anim Genet* 1987; **18:** 33-34 (Abstract).

48. Rothschild MF, Renard C, Bolet G, Dando P, Vaiman M. Effect of swine lymphocyte antigen haplotypes on birth and weaning weights in pigs. *Anim Genet* 1986; **17:** 267-272.
49. Awdeh ZL, Raum D, Yunis EJ, Alper CA. Extended HLA/complement allele haplotypes: evidence for T/t-like complex in man. *Proc Natl Acad Sci USA* 1983; **80:** 259-263.
50. Seitz AW, Bennett D. Transmission distortion of t-haplotypes is due to interactions between meiotic partners. *Nature* 1985; **313:** 143-144.
51. Philipsen M, Kristensen B. Preliminary evidence of segregation distortion in the SLA system. *Anim Blood Grps Biochem Genet* 1985; **16:** 125-133.
52. Kristjanson FK. Transferrin types and reproductive performance in the pig. *J Reprod Fertil* 1964; **8:** 311-317.
53. Weitkamp LR, Schacter BZ. Transferrin and HLA: spontaneous abortion, neural tube defects, and natural selection. *N Eng J Med* 1985; **313:** 925-932.
54. Ghani AM, Gill TJ III, Kunz HW, Misra DN. Elicitation of the maternal antibody response to the fetus by a broadly shared MHC class I antigenic determinant. *Transplantation* 1984; **37:** 187-194.
55. Macpherson TA, Ho HN, Kunz HW, Gill TJ III. Localization of the Pa antigen on the placenta of the rat. *Transplantation* 1986; **41:** 392-394.

Discussion

Chairman: Dr. W.R. Allen

Professor GILL: There is a critical point in talking about the lethals that Dr. Renard suspects might exist in the pig. There is a difference between MHC-linked lethals and the effect of segregation and distortion. The two do not necessarily have to come together. There are MHC-linked lethals in the mouse and rat and there is some evidence that they may exist in the human too. Segregation distortion is unique to the mouse and unique to the T complex. There is an inversion of the DNA which locks that set of genes together and this is a separate phenomenon to the existence of the lethals. If one looks for lethals in the pig system one should concentrate on that and not use segregation distortion as the criterion, because they are two separate phenomena.

Dr. RENARD: Thank you.

Dr. ANTCZAK: For many years David Sachs at The National Institutes of Health has maintained inbred lines of homozygous pigs. They are homozygous only for the MHC and are outbred for other genes. What is known of their reproductive performance?

Dr. RENARD: I do not know about their reproduction, but I do know about their haplotype and that they are not involved in the two cases where we found some inherited deleterious genes. I have observed in many herds the haplotype that is common to David Sachs' pigs and they have never shown homozygote tendencies.

Dr. CROY: We established a minipig herd 5 years ago from David Sachs' herd and we have recently submitted a paper on reproductive performance. The differences do not affect ovulation rate, and they do not affect the litter size except in one combination which Sachs refers to as AA. We think this is probably an embryonic loss.

Professor GILL: In an extensive study we did with various combinations of inbred rat strains and using all different kinds of crosses, there was no correlation between the MHC haplotype of the mating pairs and litter size. Nor was there any correlation between the development of an antibody response and litter size. From Dr. Renard's work, and from other studies, I find the idea that it is just MHC compatibility alone which affects litter size is not tenable. I think attention should focus on the possibility of MHC linked with recessive lethals. By using RFLP techniques one can measure this in the rat because there are specific and very clear RFLP markers for the GLC and wild type genes.

Dr. RENARD: We anticipated that and are just beginning to refine DNA from the embryos we are collecting. It is quite a lot of work.

Dr. CROY: One of the things Dr. Renard pointed out, and which we also found in our pigs, was a deficit of one particular genotype of offspring from particular matings. I wonder if this has been observed in some of the human pregnancy studies? That is, the embryos that go to term do not represent the full span of haplotypes available in the mating couple.

Professor GILL: There was one report of an HLA A2 linkage in this regard, although it has never been shown in any other system. However, HLA deficit may be a reflection of a linkage of recessive lethals to that haplotype and it need not primarily concern the haplotype itself.

Dr. ALLEN: I keep hearing that inbred strains of mice mate satisfactorily and produce good litters despite complete matching at the MHC barrier. Is this the case or are litter sizes lower?

Dr. CHAOUAT: Even the possibility that litter size is smaller in inbred matings has been challenged. There are several studies showing minimal and largely insignificant differences between many strains. There is little doubt that certain inbred strains of mice are perfectly MHC identical and can breed without any problem. I want to refer to this in some detail in a later session but suffice to say at this point that the influence of feto-maternal histocompatibility on litter size and newborn weight is inconclusive.

Professor GILL: It may come up in the session on Genetic Causes, but what Dr. Chaouat says is true in the rat as well as the mouse. When we inbreed strains from the wild, using say 10 mating pairs from the wild, we end up with two inbred strains. Whatever we inbreed for, we automatically inbreed for reproductive capacity. Once this has been done, however, the inbred strains can reproduce with litter sizes that are larger than those of intercrossed strains. Thus, what we are dealing with when we inbreed from the wild is a lot of homozygous recessive lethals that come together. And we pass through an inbreeding recession in the 7th generation that is reduced in the 14th and is even less in the 21st. This phenomenon has been noted by people who inbred both mice and rats and it is what prevented rabbits from being inbred.

Eventually, when we come down to the kinds of recessive lethals we are now discussing, we have weeded out a great number of lethals from the rest of the genome and we see only the few that are left. And in many cases these are semi-lethal.

Dr. ANTCZAK: The question here is not exactly of homozygosity, but of identity between mother and fetus.

Dr. CHAOUAT: The question is simply whether differences in the MHC haplotype between sire and dam lead to an increase in feto-placental weight.

Again, one study says no and there has not been another study to confirm whether or not it is true.

Professor BEER: Even in a totally inbred model there are truncated antigens, or embryonic antigens, presented to the mother and which direct a new response that can be assayed almost with greater facility than in an allogeneic mating. So I think we can understand the 80% of inbred lines which are lost. It is the 20% that continue to produce, and in which a new response can be assayed, that constitute the puzzle. But whether this responsiveness is related to their success remains an open question.

Dr. CHAOUAT: My comment about this is, if we look at the CBA/DBA$_2$ system we find differences in reproductive performance between one breeding room and another, even within the same breeding centre. Given what we now know about factors that influence this system, I would be even more careful now to say that we are looking at MHC difference.

Dr. RENARD: It is why we work by herd and try to compare within herds.

Professor BEER: If one looks at human isolates that have been tissue-typed for Class I and Class II antigens, and then looks at the offspring in that society, there is always an over representation of heterozygotes. If the predicted frequency is a particular figure, the actual value is usually 2-3 times higher in terms of representation by heterozygotes.

Professor GILL: Although they were not tissue-typed at the time, there is the interesting archeological evidence that the 18th Ptolemaic dynasty of Egypt propagated the dynasty by brother-sister matings. The dynasty showed all the characteristics of achievement and produced viable and apparently intelligent offspring during 17 generations of inbreeding. It comes back to the statement that those who start with a good gene pool and inbreed will end up with a good gene pool. However, most of the time there is a lot of recessive linkage that can kill off the gene pool very quickly.

Dr. ANTCZAK: It is important that we understand the difference between heterozygosity maintained by genetic factors and having nothing to do with maternal immunological recognition of the fetus. That is the point I was really trying to make.

A non-genetic development defect in trophoblast formation in the horse: immunological aspects of a model of early abortion

D. F. Antczak, W. R. Allen

INTRODUCTION

Embryogenesis and placentation in the horse family (Genus *equus*) is unusual and interesting for several reasons. For example: a) the chorion of the equine conceptus is composed of two morphologically and functionally distinct forms of trophoblast which can be studied *in situ* and *in vitro*;[1,2] b) there is evidence for strong humoral[3] and cell-mediated maternal[4] anti-fetal immune responses in normal intraspecies equine pregnancy; c) member species of the genus have the capacity to interbreed to produce viable, but usually infertile, hybrid offspring;[5] d) embryo transfer can be performed successfully between many member species of the genus with the birth of live foals.[6]

The defect in placentation which occurs when the donkey (*E. assinus*) embryo is placed in the uterus of the domestic horse (*E. caballus*), and the immunological and pathological consequences which usually result in abortion, are the subjects of the present paper.

EQUINE PLACENTATION

The equine conceptus retains a spherical, fluid-filled outline until as late as Day 45-50 of gestation. At Day 21 it measures 6-7 cm in diameter and is covered externally by a single layer of trophoblast cells which constitutes the chorion; the splanchnic layer of mesoderm forms the outer layer of the yolk sac and rests on the inner surface of the chorion. The embryo is just visible to the naked eye and is situated at one pole of the conceptus. It is already enveloped by the amnion and the allantois is just beginning to develop into the coelomic cavity.[7,8,9] During the next 15 days vascularised mesoderm develops between the chorion and yolk sac endoderm. The allantois enlarges rapidly at the embryonic pole while, at the same time, the yolk sac regresses steadily. This means that the embryo, attached by the yolk stalk (umbilicus), appears to move across the conceptus from one pole to the other. Fusion of the allantoic and chorionic layers gives rise to the allantochorion which will eventually become the definitive placenta.

On the outer surface of the chorion, in the region where the enlarging allantoic and regressing yolk sac membranes abut, a discrete portion of the trophoblast is thrown into a series of simple folds. This ridge formation commences at Day 25 and progresses steadily during the next 10 days. The trophoblast cells at the apices of the ridges multiply rapidly with the result that each ridge increasingly assumes the appearance of an elongated villus of hyperplastic cells. This specialised area of trophoblast is termed the chorionic girdle. By Day 36 it is clearly visible as a pale, thickened band of tissue, some 20-40mm in width, that passes around the circumference of the conceptus (Figure I).[1,4]

Figure I

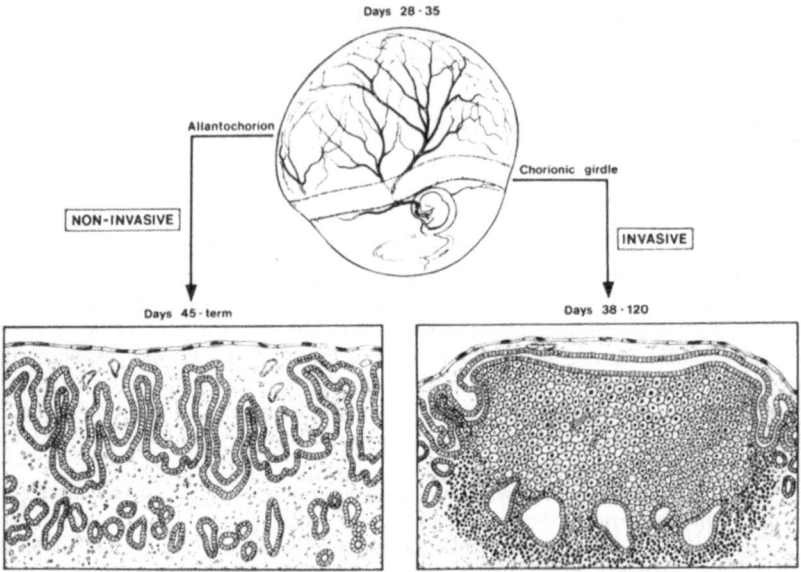

Diagrammatic representation of the major steps in the differentiation of equine trophoblast. *Top*: intact conceptus at Day 33-35, showing the annulate band of invasive trophoblast, the chorionic girdle, at the junction of the allantoic and yolk sac membranes. *Lower right*: section of a mature endometrial cup (Day 60) which originates from invasion of the endometrium by chorionic girdle cells. *Lower left*: section of the allantochorion-endometrium interface (Day 60) where the trophoblast is non-invasive.

Between Days 36 and 38, the entire chorionic girdle separates from the placenta and becomes attached to the overlying endometrial surface. The girdle cells vigorously invade and destroy the lumenal endometrial epithelium and they pass down the endometrial glands beneath the glandular epithelium. Within a few hours they penetrate the basement membrane to enter the endometrial stroma. Here, however, they undergo a series of striking morphological and functional changes; they become sessile, enlarge greatly, acquire a second, large enchromatic nucleus and cease to divide.[10] The hypertrophy of the invading cells causes them to become tightly packed together in discrete clusters within the endometrial stroma. As such they form a series of raised endometrial protruberances, known as endometrial cups, which are arranged in a circle around the developing conceptus in the gravid uterine horn (Figure IIa).[10]

Figure II

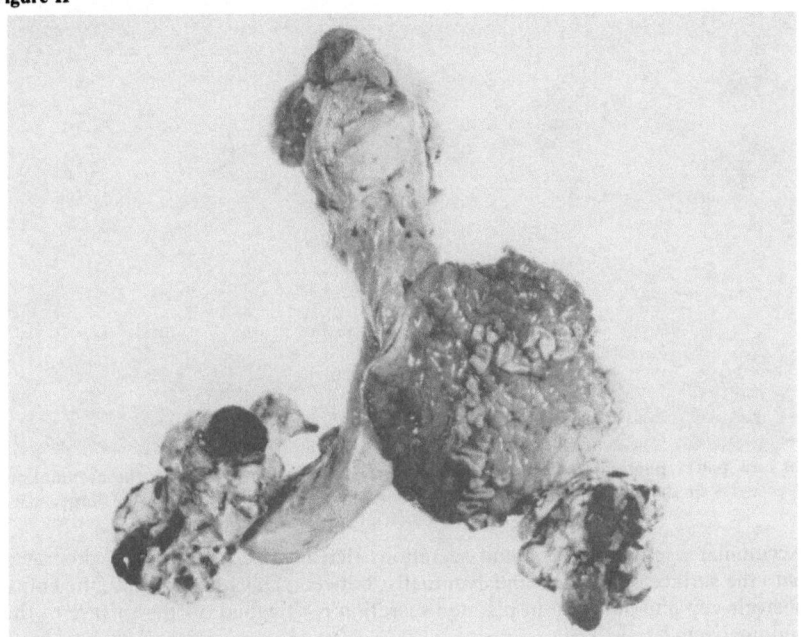

a) Horse uterus at Day 65 of gestation with the conceptus removed. The eCG-secreting fetal endometrial cups form a circle of raised, ulcer-like protruberances in the endometrium of the gravid horn.

Endometrial cups are unique to *Equidae* and they are the source of the high concentrations of equine Chorionic Gonadotrophin (eCG) found in the serum of pregnant mares between Days 40 and 120 of gestation.[11,12] The hormone is secreted by the large, fetal endometrial cup cells[2] and it reaches the maternal bloodstream via a complex network of lymph sinuses which develop in the endometrial stroma beneath each cup.[13] Few blood vessels remain intact within the cup tissue and the apical portions of most endometrial glands are destroyed by the initial invasion of chorionic girdle cells at Day 36. The distal portions of the glands remain intact, however, and become increasingly distended due to hypertrophy and accumulation of their exocrine secretory products (Figure IIb).[14]

The endometrial cups reach their maximum size and secretory activity by Day 55-65 after ovulation but thereafter they become increasingly pale and cheesy in appearance due to degeneration and necrosis of cup cells at the lumenal surface.

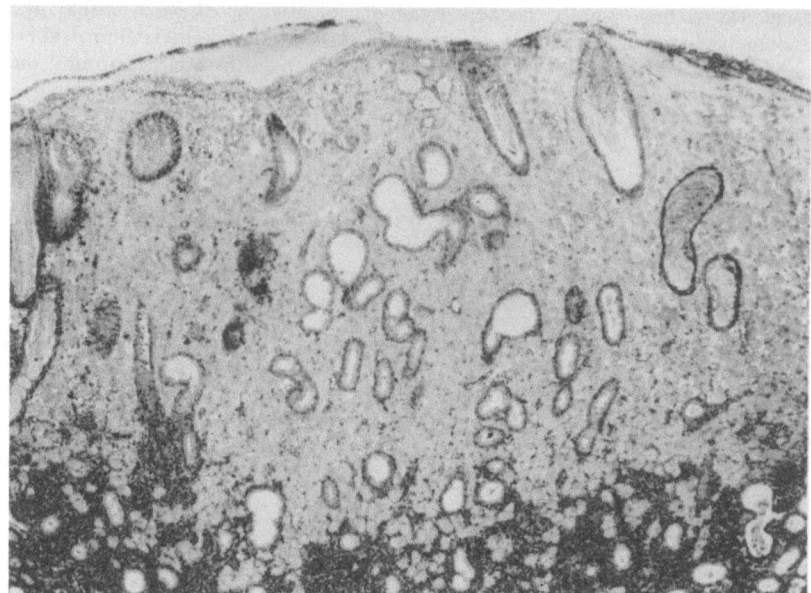

b) **Low power photomicrograph of an endometrial cup at Day 65. Note the accumulated leucocytes in the maternal stroma surrounding the densely packed mass of large, eCG-secreting fetal endometrial cup cells (× 45).**

Accumulated endometrial gland secretion, rich in eCG activity,[12] is liberated onto the surface of the cups and eventually, between Days 100 and 140, the entire necrotic cup and admixed inspissated secretion is sloughed off the surface of the endometrium.[13]

The non-invasive trophoblast of the normal allantochorion constitutes the great majority of the feto-maternal interface in pregnant equids. Beginning around Day 40-45 after ovulation, simple finger-like villi of allantochorion begin to inter-digitate with corresponding crypts or sulci in the endometrial surface and the trophoblast cells establish a stable, microvillous contact with the endometrial epithelium. The whole conceptus expands and elongates slowly during the next 6-8 weeks so that, by Day 90-100, allantochorion becomes attached to the endometrium over the entire internal surface of the uterus. The allantochorionic villi become increasingly branched and complex during this expansion period (Figure IIIa), thereby giving rise to the definitive microcotyledonary placenta which greatly increases the total area for placental interchange between mother and fetus.[15]

Thus, the equine endometrial cups represent a unique form of trophoblast development. They have a short lifespan of only 60-80 days within the total gestation period of 340 ± 30 days and they possess an endocrinological function that is well recognised.[16] However, their immunological role in the maintenance of pregnancy is much less clear and it forms the basis of our investigation.

Figure III

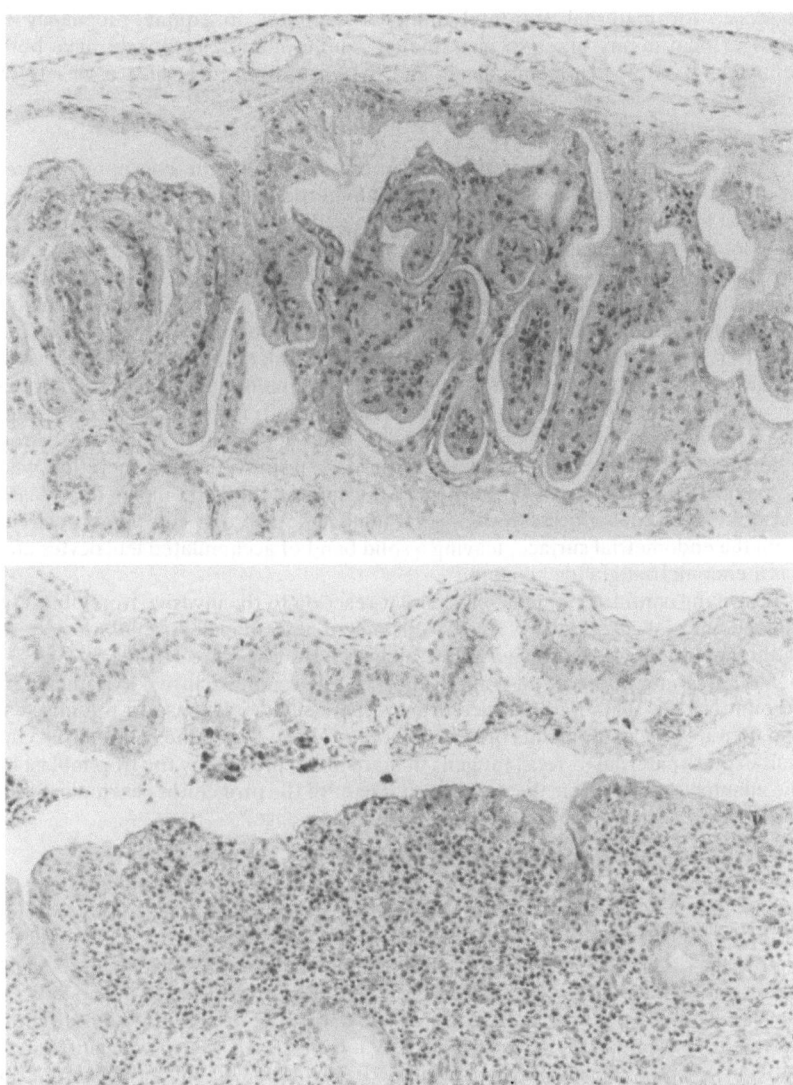

Low power photomicrograph of a section of the allantochorion-endometrium interface in a) a mare carrying a normal intraspecies horse conceptus at Day 85 of gestation; b) a mare carrying a transferred donkey conceptus at Day 85. Note the intense accumulation of maternal leucocytes in the endometrium in b) and the accumulation of exocrine secretion between fetal and maternal epithelial surfaces (× 120).

IMMUNE RESPONSES TO THE EQUINE CONCEPTUS

Evidence for maternal anti-fetal immune responses in equine pregnancy is stronger than in any other species studied. These immune responses have both cellular and serological components and they are directed against a variety of antigens.

Cell-mediated response

The evidence for cellular immune responses to the equine conceptus derives from observations on the kinetics of the endometrial cup reaction. Commencing from the time of the invasion of the chorionic girdle cells into the endometrium at Day 36, maternal leucocytes accumulate in the endometrial stroma around each cup. These invading cells are composed mainly of lymphocytes, with small clusters of macrophages recognisable by their endogenous peroxidase activity. Few neutrophils are observed in the leucocytic infiltrate but, with advancing gestation, increasing numbers of plasma cells and macrophages become visible (Figure IIb).[4,13] At first the leucocytes tend to remain clustered in the stroma around the cup, appearing to wall off the fetal cup cells from the maternal tissue. But beyond Day 70-80 they can be seen to invade the cup and appear to destroy individual cup cells. This coincides with the start of the degeneration and desquamation of cells from the surface of the cups and the accompanying release of accumulated exocrine secretion. Eventually, the necrotic cup tissue dehisces from the endometrial surface, leaving a solid band of accumulated leucocytes and basal endometrial glands beneath.[4]

In striking contrast to this strong cellular reaction to the invasive trophoblast of the endometrial cups, there is a complete lack of any equivalent cellular response to the non-invasive trophoblast of the allantochorion (Figure IIIa).

The foregoing observations suggested one of two non-exclusive hypotheses to account for the striking difference in maternal cellular response to the invasive and non-invasive components of the trophoblast. Namely, do the endometrial cup cells express paternal or fetal antigens that are not expressed by the trophoblast of the allantochorion? Or, is the invasive character of the progenitor chorionic girdle sufficient to account for the maternal cellular response?

Humoral response to fetal antigens

Evidence for maternal sensitisation to paternally inherited tissue alloantigens was first established by studies of the Major Histocompatibility Complex (MHC) of the horse. This is termed the Equine Lymphocyte Antigen (ELA) system[17,18] and it was observed that virtually all mares that had produced foals harboured serum antibodies which were cytotoxic for lymphocyte antigens of the stallion to which they had been mated. Later studies demonstrated that antibodies are first detected at around Day 60 of pregnancy and most are directed against ELA antigens.[3,19] However, antibodies to non-ELA lymphocyte alloantigens are also produced during early pregnancy.[20]

The temporal correlation between the formation of the endometrial cups and the appearance of cytotoxic anti-ELA antibody in the serum of pregnant mares suggested that the endometrial cups might express ELA antigens. However, the demonstration of paternal ELA antigens on cup cells proved difficult. Absorption with endometrial cup tissue of alloantisera recognising paternal ELA antigens, elution of antibody from cup tissue using low pH, and immunisation of horses with isolated endometrial cup tissue, all gave inconclusive results which suggested that, if the endometrial cups do exhibit ELA antigens, they express them at very low levels.[21,22]

Recent experiments using indirect immunoperoxidase labelling of snap-frozen sections of Day 32-36 fetal membranes with a high titred alloantiserum to paternal ELA antigens demonstrated that the chorionic girdle cells do indeed express high levels of paternal ELA antigens. The adjacent non-invasive trophoblast of the allantochorion, on the other hand, expresses either very low levels of paternal ELA, or none at all.[22] Thus, it seems likely that the invasive chorionic girdle provides the antigenic stimulus which results in maternal sensitisation of mares to paternal ELA antigens. The leucocyte reaction could, therefore, be explained as the maternal cell-mediated response to the same foreign Class I antigens. Furthermore, the apparently low rate of expression of these antigens on mature endometrial cup cells could account for the relatively long lifespan of the cups (2-3 months) compared to the survival (2-3 weeks) of skin allografts made across MHC Class I barriers.

Problems with this hypothesis arise with the finding that the leucocyte reactions against the endometrial cups in MHC-compatible intraspecies horse pregnancies are as strong, or stronger, than those in MHC-incompatible matings.[21] Thus, if the leucocyte accumulation around the cups is indeed an immunological phenomenon, the reaction observed in MHC-compatible pregnancies must be directed against minor histocompatibility antigens or against molecules that are unique to the trophoblast. Furthermore, in view of the absence of very low expression of ELA antigens on cup cells, the effector cells in the leucocyte reaction are probably not classical MHC-restricted cytotoxic T lymphocytes.

The composition of the leucocyte population that surrounds the endometrial cups has not yet been accurately determined. However, preliminary findings in a study of the *in vitro* functional activities of these cells[23] indicate that the population includes non-T, non-B cell suppressor and/or cytotoxic lymphocytes of the types that have been described in mice.[24] The lack of specific markers for lymphocyte subsets in the horse has hampered the characterisation of equine uterine lymphocyte populations thus far.

TROPHOBLAST-RESTRICTED MOLECULES OF THE EQUINE PLACENTA

The strong leucocyte reaction against the endometrial cups in MHC-compatible pregnancies suggests a maternal immune response towards non-ELA trophoblast-specific antigens. Monoclonal antibodies were raised by immunising rats with equine endometrial cup tissue and fusing their immune spleen cells with mouse myeloma cells. Thirteen hybrid cell lines secreting trophoblast-reactive antibodies were identified by indirect immunoperoxidase staining of cryostat sections of endometrial cups, allantochorion and chorionic girdle.[25] These antibodies appear to identify at least 6 different molecules expressed by equine trophoblast. However, the only one of the panel that did not cross-react with another adult tissue was found to be directed against the principal hormonal product of the cups, eCG. No antibody unique to the trophoblast was identified, even though 500 hybrid cell lines were screened.

This failure to detect trophoblast-specific molecules in the horse is consistent with reports of others who have likewise encountered difficulty in identifying unique molecules on human trophoblast.[26] The reactivity pattern of the horse monoclonal antibodies does nevertheless provide a means of identifying different forms of equine trophoblast, both *in situ* and *in vitro*. Furthermore, some of the trophoblast-restricted molecules are regulated developmentally in early pregnancy.[27] However, it has not yet been possible to detect a trophoblast-unique molecule that could serve as an antigenic target for either humoral or cell-mediated maternal immune responses.

INTER- AND EXTRASPECIES PREGNANCY IN EQUIDS

Equidae are unusual in respect to the ease with which mating between all the member species produces viable hybrid offspring despite considerable karyotypic and phenotypic parental differences.[5] The most commonly produced and intensively studied of these man-made equine hybrids are the mule and hinny, produced reciprocally by crossing, respectively, the female horse with the male donkey and *vice versa*. In mares carrying mule fetuses there is an accelerated maternal response to the endometrial cups, marked by an intense infiltration of leucocytes that brings about their early destruction.[4] If the same mares carry a second consecutive mule pregnancy of the same antigenic character, the lifespan of the cups is reduced even further, as estimated by the duration of secretion of eCG.[28] But despite the severity of this maternal anti-fetal immunological response against the endometrial cups in both mule and hinny pregnancies, the fetus is not compromised and it continues safely to term. It is likely that the hybrid conceptus presents a wider range of foreign molecules to the maternal immune system than does a normal, intraspecies conceptus.

Extraspecies pregnancy established by embryo transfer

Even bigger antigenic differences between mother and fetus can be produced by embryo transfer. Once again, equids appear to be unique with respect to the great degree of feto-maternal disparity that can be tolerated. Horse-in-donkey[6], zebra-in-horse (Figure IV) and Przewalski's horse-in-horse[29] pregnancies have now been created and in all three types of extraspecific gestation, some degree of endometrial cup development occurred (as determined by maternal serum eCG measurements), placental development was apparently normal and live offspring were born.

DONKEY-IN-HORSE PREGNANCY: A MODEL OF SPONTANEOUS ABORTION

Transfer of donkey embryos to horse mares provides a striking contrast to the above-mentioned successful extraspecific pregnancies. Some 75% of donkey-in-horse pregnancies end in abortion between Days 80 and 95 of gestation.[6] This failure appears to be the result of a non-genetic defect in trophoblast function. The donkey chorionic girdle develops normally within the surrogate mare but it fails completely to invade the maternal endometrium at Day 36, thereby resulting in an absence of endometrial cup tissue and a lack of eCG in maternal blood. But despite this early defect, the donkey conceptus continues to develop for a further 35-50 days before it is expelled.

Certain aspects of the later degeneration and final abortion of the donkey-in-horse conceptus suggest a complex pathological process. Following the failure of chorionic girdle invasion at Day 36, the trophoblast of the allantochorion also fails to form the characteristic non-invasive interdigitating villous connection with the endometrium. Fetal and maternal epithelial surfaces lie apposed but unattached and increasing numbers of leucocytes accumulate in the endometrial stroma along the whole length of the endometrium-allantochorion border (Figure IIIb). Beyond about Day 70, the fetus becomes increasingly cachectic and reddened in appearance due to haemolysis of fetal red blood cells. Eventually, the accumulated maternal leucocytes migrate through the endometrial epithelium and appear to attack the donkey trophoblast just prior to relaxation of the cervix and expulsion of the dead and autolysing conceptus at Day 80-95.[6]

The intense leucocyte reaction associated with the degeneration and abortion of the donkey-in-horse pregnancy is reminiscent of the leucocyte response that is restricted to the area around the invasive endometrial cups in normal intraspecies horse and donkey pregnancy. It provides a strong indication that immunological factors play an important role in the abortion process.

Figure IV

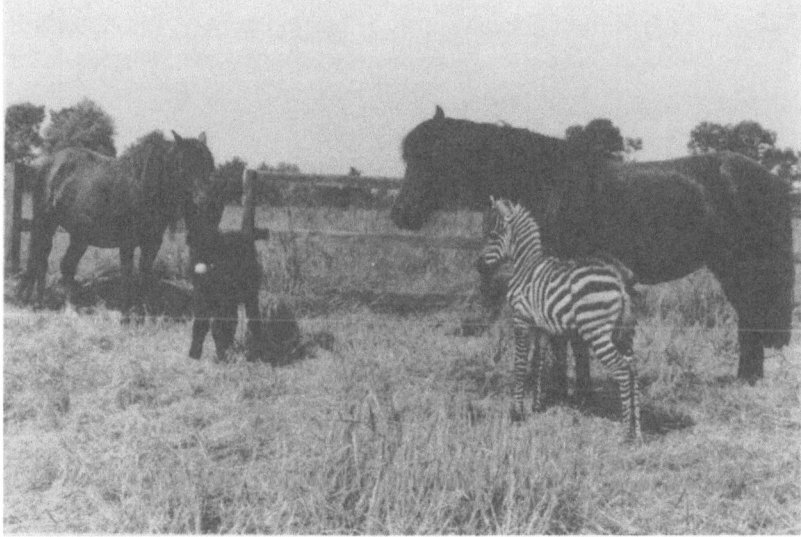

a) A Grant's zebra foal (2n=46) and a donkey foal (2n=62) with their domestic horse surrogate mothers (2n=64). No treatment was given to the mare carrying the zebra foal but the mare carrying the donkey was immunised 4 times with parental donkey lymphocytes between Days 21 and 54 of gestation.

Figure V

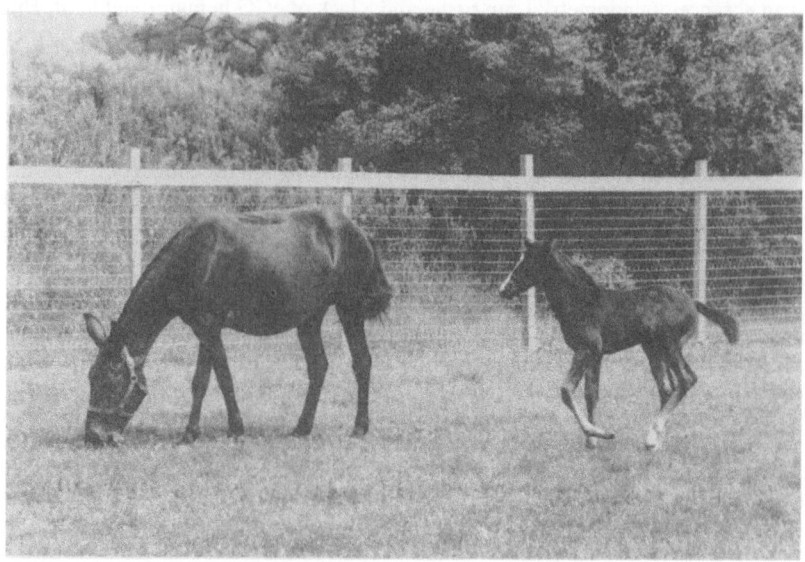

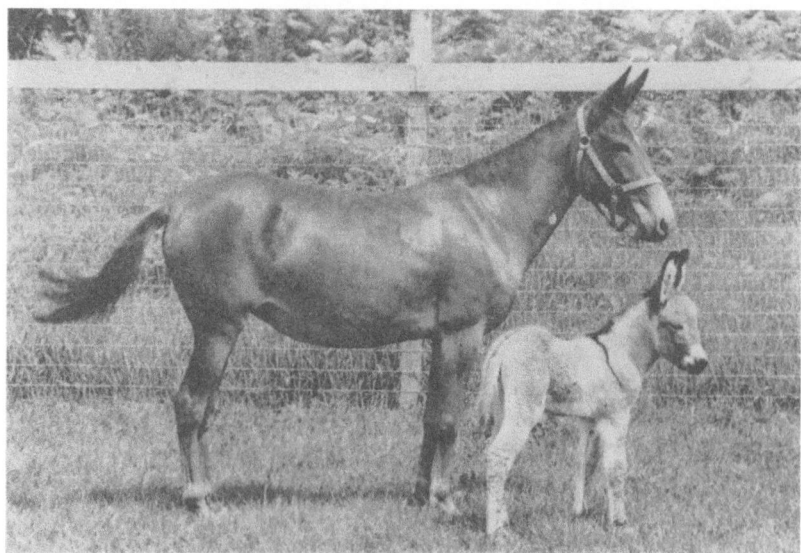

a) A horse and b) a donkey foal with their sterile, F1 hybrid mule surrogate mothers. Embryo transfer was performed on Day 7 after ovulation.

Hormonal replacement therapy

Endometrial cups are the sole source of eCG in equine pregnancy[12] and the complete lack of this glycoprotein hormone, together with lower than normal levels of progesterone, in the peripheral blood of mares carrying donkey conceptuses, suggested that hormone deficiency may play a part in the pregnancy loss. However, administration of either or both synthetic progestagen (allyl trenbolone) and large doses of exogenous eCG to a total of 11 mares carrying donkey pregnancies did not increase fetal survival rate.[6]

Genetic studies

The physiological and genetic basis of the failure of endometrial cup formation in the donkey-in-horse pregnancy was investigated by further between-species embryo transfer. Normal horse and donkey embryos were recovered non-surgically and transferred surgically to recipient mules which had been induced to ovulate synchronously with the donor animals by hormonal treatment. Pregnancies were established in 5 mules in this manner (4 horse and 1 donkey conceptuses) and of particular significance was the measurement of low levels of eCG between Days 40 and 85 of gestation in the serum of the mule carrying the donkey conceptus.[30] This demonstrated that endometrial cups had formed in this donkey-in-mule pregnancy as they also did in the 4 horse-in-mule pregnancies. Thus, in contrast to the horse, the uterus of the mule is an appropriate environment for invasion of both the donkey and horse chorionic girdle and the formation of endometrial cups. Live horse and donkey offspring were produced by the surrogate mule mothers (Figure V).

Immunotherapy

The failure of exogenous hormone therapy to prevent abortion in the donkey-in-horse pregnancy model prompted attempts at two immunological forms of treatment. In the first experiment large volumes of serum (Ω1 litre) from mares carrying normal intraspecies horse pregnancies were transfused intravenously into 6 mares carrying donkey pregnancies every 4-6 days between Days 40 and 80 of gestation. Three of the mares treated in this manner delivered live foals while the other three aborted in the characteristic manner between Days 80 and 100.[31] Two control mares carrying donkey conceptuses that were transfused with equivalent amounts of non-pregnant mare's serum both aborted.

Early reports of a beneficial effect from the immunisation of women suffering from recurrent spontaneous abortion with allogeneic leucocytes[32] prompted an attempt at similar treatment of 9 mares carrying donkey conceptuses. In this experiment 6 mares were immunised with lymphocytes from the genetic sire and dam of the transferred donkey embryo, and 3 with lymphocytes from unrelated male and female donkeys. In all cases, 4 injections, each of 200×10^6 washed lymphocytes, were given at approximately weekly intervals between Days 20 and 55 of gestation. Four of the 6 animals given parental lymphocytes and 2 of the 3 given unrelated lymphocytes remained pregnant to beyond Day 150, thereby increasing fetal survival rate to 67% (Figure IVb).[31]

Some of these successfully treated donkey-in-horse pregnancies were terminated experimentally between Days 145 and 160 of gestation. In all cases normal villus formation and placentation had occurred and there were no signs of abnormal maternal leucocyte accumulations at the allantochorion-endometrium border. Thus, the apparent success of the serum transfer and lymphocyte immunisation experiments was consistent with an immunological component to the abortion process. However, neither treatment worked in all cases.

Immunological memory

A striking observation in the donkey-in-horse pregnancy experiments was a phenomenon that closely resembles immunological memory. Second consecutive donkey pregnancies were established in mares which had either carried their first donkey foal to term, or had aborted it characteristically between Days 80 and 100. Mares which had aborted one donkey fetus aborted their second donkey conceptus earlier in gestation in 12 of 13 cases. On the other hand, all of 13 mares which had successfully carried their first donkey pregnancy to term, also carried their second pregnancies to term or to beyond Day 145. Many of the first successful pregnancies had been in mares treated by pregnancy serum infusion or by lymphocyte immunisation, but no treatments were given during the second pregnancies.[31]

Figure VI

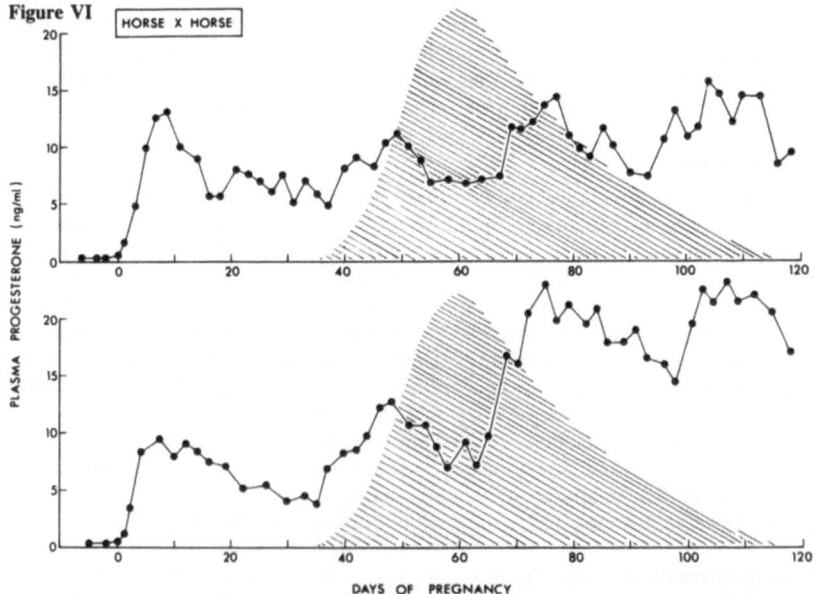

Peripheral plasma progesterone profiles measured in two mares carrying normal intraspecies horse pregnancies. Note the secondary rise in levels coinciding with the period of eCG secretion (diagrammatically hatched area) due to the development of secondary *corpora lutea* in the maternal ovaries.

This finding can be interpreted as a manifestation of the recall of, respectively, a destructive or protective immunity in the surrogate horse mothers. However, an alternative explanation is that some mares are genetically incapable of supporting a donkey pregnancy while others can do so even in the absence of eCG and in the face of peripheral plasma progesterone concentrations which are much lower than the values normally seen in intraspecies horse and donkey pregnancies (Figure VI/VII). The resolution of this question awaits further investigation.

Figure VII

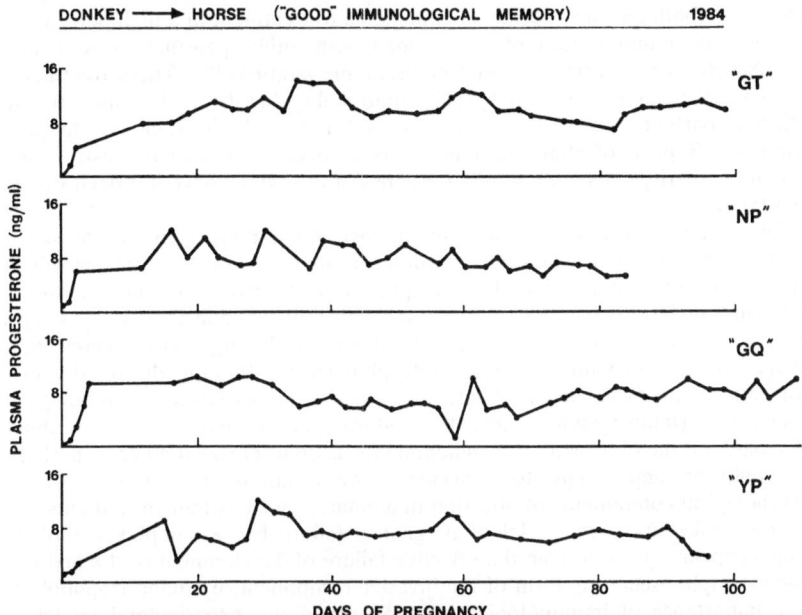

Peripheral plasma progesterone profiles in 4 mares carrying their second successful donkey conceptuses. Note the absence of a secondary rise in progesterone levels between Days 40 and 100 of gestation, which is a characteristic feature of normal intraspecies equine pregnancy. eCG was not detectable in the blood of these animals due to failure of endometrial cup development.

DISCUSSION AND CONCLUSIONS

The question arises as to how, if at all, the transferred xenogeneic donkey-in-horse model of early pregnancy failure relates to spontaneous or other experimental models of abortion in the human and in laboratory or domestic animal species.

Three rodent models have been explored as possible analogues of the recurrent spontaneous abortion syndrome in women.[33,34] In one of these, the *Mus musculus - Mus caroli* between-species pregnancy established by embryo transfer, it has been virtually impossible to achieve a term pregnancy by abrogation of immune effector mechanisms.[33] In the other intraspecies mouse models, beneficial effects of various immunisation schemes have been described.[34] However, no physiological or immunological defects have been demonstrated in these models, other than the possible deficit of uterine suppressor lymphocytes, and the increased overall rate of spontaneous fetal death and resorption affects only some of the individual conceptuses within the litter. Furthermore, strong environmental effects on litter size have been demonstrated in several strains of mice, including the CBA × DBA-2 cross.[35]

The clinical expression of recurrent spontaneous abortion in women is apparently both partner-specific and amenable to treatment in a high percentage of cases by immunisation of the women with either paternal or unrelated lymphocytes, or with trophoblast membrane preparations.[36,38] These treatments are controversial because no specific abnormality has been described in the affected partners, other than the observed repeated abortions in the first trimester. Reports of abnormal immune responsiveness in *in vitro* tests,[37] and genetic similarity between partners for genes of the MHC, have not been widely substantiated.[39]

The primary evidence for an immunological component to the recurrent spontaneous abortion syndrome in women is that a form of treatment which appears to have beneficial effect is purported to work via immunological mechanisms. However, other studies appear to achieve equivalent success rates with a variety of non-immunological treatment, including cervical cerclage,[40] exogenous human Chorionic Gonadotrophin (hCG) therapy during the first trimester[41] and even increased rates of clinical examination and psychological counselling (tender loving care, TLC) throughout gestation.[42] Given these findings, and the observed environmental effects on litter size in mice,[35] perhaps it would be appropriate to concentrate more attention in the future to psychological components of abortion in animal, as well as human, patients.

Our donkey-in-horse model of pregnancy failure has a complex pathology which appears to result from the selective failure of development of the mature, gonadotrophin-secreting form of the invasive component of equine trophoblast. The importance of immunological components in this experimental model of abortion is still an open question. But perhaps of greater significance to our understanding of the mechanisms involved in the maintenance of mammalian pregnancy is the demonstration that foals can survive *in utero* in the complete absence of chorionic gonadotrophin and in an environment which contains far less progesterone than normal (Figure VI). Both hormones are reputed to suppress cell-mediated immune responses and their deficiency serves to emphasise the underlying need for cellular cooperation between fetus and mother which results in a morphologically sound and functional placenta, if the former is to survive as an allograft in the latter.

ACKNOWLEDGEMENTS
This work was supported by grants from the U.S. Department Agriculture, the National Institutes of Health, the Dorothy Russell Havemeyer Foundation Inc., the Zweig Memorial Fund for Equine Research in New York State, the Horserace Betting Levy Board and the Thoroughbred Breeders' Association of Great Britain.

REFERENCES

1. Ewart JC. *A critical period in the development of the horse.* London: Adam & Charles Black, 1897.
2. Allen WR, Moor RM. The origin of equine endometrial cups. I. Production of PMSG by foetal trophoblast cells. *J Reprod Fertil* 1972; **29:** 313-316.
3. Antczak DF, Miller J, Remick LH. Lymphocyte alloantigens of the horse. II. Antibodies to ELA antigens produced during equine pregnancy. *J Reprod Immunol* 1984; **6:** 283-287.
4. Allen WR. Immunological aspects of the equine endometrial cup reaction. In: *Immunology of Trophoblast.* (Eds.) RG Edwards, CWS Howe, MH Johnson. Cambridge: Cambridge University Press, 1975; pp.217-253.
5. Gray AP. *Mammalian Hybrids.* Farnham Royal: Commonwealth Agricultural Bureaux, 1954; pp.45-59.
6. Allen WR. Immunological aspects of the endometrial cup reaction and the effects of xenogeneic pregnancy in horses and donkeys. *J Reprod Fertil* 1982; **Suppl 31:** 57-94.
7. Ewart JC. Studies on the development of the horse. I. The development during the third week. *Trans R Soc Edinb* 1915; **51:** 287-329.
8. Amoroso EC. Placentation. In: *Marshalls Physiology of Reproduction* Vol. II, (Ed.) AS Parkes. London: Longmans Green & Co, 1952; pp.127-311.
9. van Niekerk CH, Allen WR. Early embryonic development in the horse. *J Reprod Fertil* 1975; **Suppl. 23:** 495-498.
10. Allen WR, Hamilton DW, Moor RM. The origin of equine endometrial cups. II. Invasion of the endometrium by trophoblast. *Annat Rec* 1973; **117:** 475-501.
11. Cole HH, Hart GH. The potency of blood serum of mares in progressive stages of pregnancy in effecting the sexual maturity of the immature rat. *Am J Physiol* 1930; **93:** 57-68.
12. Cole HH, Goss H. The source of equine gonadotropin. In: *Essays in Honor of Herbert M Evans.* Berkeley: University of California Press, 1943; pp.107-119.
13. Amoroso EC. Endocrinology of pregnancy. *Br Med Bull* 1955; **11:** 117-125.
14. Clegg MT, Boda JM, Cole HH. The endometrial cups and allantochorionic pouches in the mare with emphasis on the source of equine gonadotropin. *Endocrinology* 1954; **54:** 448-463.
15. Samuel CA, Allen WR, Steven DH. Ultrastructural development of the equine placenta. *J Reprod Fert* 1975; **Suppl 23:** 575-578.
16. Urwin VE, Allen WR. Pituitary and chorionic gonadotrophic control of ovarian function during early pregnancy in equids. *J Reprod Fertil* 1982; **Suppl 32:** 371-382.
17. Bright S, Antczak DF, Ricketts SW. Studies on equine leucocyte antigens. In: *Infectious Equine Diseases.* (Eds.) JT Bryans, H Gerber. Princeton: Veterinary Publications, 1978; IV: pp.229-236.
18. De Weck AL, Lazary S, Buller S, Gerber H, Meister U. Determination of leukocyte histocompatibility antigens in horses by serological techniques. In: *Equine Infectious Diseases.* (Eds.) JT Bryans, H Gerber. Princeton: Veterinary Publications, 1978; IV: pp.221-227.
19. Allen WR. Maternal recognition of pregnancy and immunological implications of trophoblast-endometrium interactions in equids. In: *Maternal Recognition of Pregnancy.* (Ciba Fdn Series No. 64). Amsterdam: Excerpta Medica, 1979; pp.323-352.
20. Antczak DF. Lymphocyte alloantigens of the horse. III. ELY-2. 1: A lymphocyte alloantigen not coded by the MHC. *Animal Blood Groups and Biochem Genet* 1984; **15:** 103-115.
21. Allen WR, Kydd JH, Miller J, Antczak DF. Immunological studies on foeto-maternal relationships in equine pregnancy. In: *Immunological Aspects of Reproduction in Mammals.* (Ed.) DB Crighton. London: Butterworths, 1984; pp.183-193.

22. Crump A, Donaldson WL, Miller J, Kydd J, Allen WR, Antczak DF. Expression of Major Histocompatibility Complex (MHC) antigens on equine trophoblast. *J Reprod Fert* 1987; **Suppl 35**: 379-388.
23. Kydd JH, Allen WR. Suppressor activity in the equine endometrial cup reaction. In: *Proc IIIrd Int Congr Reprod Immunol (Toronto)*. (Eds.) DA Clark, BA Croy. Amsterdam: Elsevier, 1986; p.296 (Abstract).
24. Clark DA, Slapsys RM, Croy BA, Rossant J. Suppressor cell avtivity in uterine decidua correlates with success or failure of murine pregnancies. *J Immunol* 1983; **131**: 540-542.
25. Antczak DF, Poleman JC, Stenzler LM, Volsen SG, Allen WR. Monoclonal antibodies to equine trophoblast. *Trophoblast Res* 1987; **2**: 199-214.
26. Anderson DJ, Johnson PM, Alexander NJ, Jones WR, Griffin PD. Monoclonal antibodies to human trophoblast and sperm antigens: Report of two WHO-sponsored workshops, June 30th 1986, Toronto, Canada. *J Reprod Immunol* 1987; **10**: 231-257.
27. Antczak DF, Oriol JG, Donaldson WL, Poleman C, Stenzler L, Volsen SG, Allen WR. Differentiation molecules of the equine trophoblast. *J Reprod Fertil* 1987; **Suppl 35**: 371-378.
28. Antczak DF, Allen WR. Invasive trophoblast in the genus Equus. *Ann Immunol* 1984; **135D**: 325-331.
29. Summers PM, Shephard AM, Hodges JK, Kydd JH, Boyle MS, Allen WR. Successful transfer of the embryos of Przewalski's horses (*Equus przewalskii*) and Grant's zebra (*E. burchelli*) to domestic mares (*E. caballus*). *J Reprod Fertil* 1987; **80**: 13-20.
30. Davies CJ, Antczak DF, Allen WR. Reproduction in mules: Embryo transfer using sterile recipients. *Equine Vet J* 1985; **Suppl 3**: 63-67.
31. Allen WR, Kydd JH, Antczak DF. Maternal immunological response to the trophoblast in xenogeneic equine pregnancy. In: *Immunoregulation and Fetal Survival*. (Eds.) TJ Gill, T Wegmann. New York: Oxford University Press, 1987; pp.263-285.
32. Taylor C, Faulk WP. Prevention of recurrent abortion with leukocyte transfusions. *Lancet* 1981; **2**: 68-69.
33. Chaouat G. Genetic aspects of the CBA/DBA2 and B10X/X/B10A models of murine pregnancy failure and its prevention by lymphocyte immunisation. In: *Early pregnancy loss—mechanisms and treatment*. London: Royal College of Obstetricians and Gynaecologists, 1988; pp.89-102.
34. Crepeau MA, Yamashiro S, Croy BA. Anatomical and immunological aspects of fetal death in the *Mus musculus/Mus caroli* model of pregnancy failure. In: *Early pregnancy loss—mechanisms and treatment*. London: Royal College of Obstetricians and Gynaecologists, 1988; pp.69-83.
35. Hamilton MS, Hamilton BL. Environmental influences on immunologically associated spontaneous abortion in CBA/J mice. *J Reprod Immunol* 1987; **11**: 237-241.
36. Mowbray JF. Success and failures of immunisation for recurrent spontaneous abortion. In: *Early pregnancy loss—mechanisms and treatment*. London: Royal College of Obstetricians and Gynaecologists, 1988; pp.325-331.
37. Beer AE. Pregnancy outcome in couples with recurrent abortions following immunological evaluation and therapy. In: *Early pregnancy loss—mechanisms and treatment*. London: Royal College of Obstetricians and Gynaecologists, 1988; pp.337-349.
38. Johnson PM. Trophoblast membrane infusion (TMI) in the treatment of recurrent spontaneous In: *Early pregnancy loss—mechanisms and treatment*. London: Royal College of Obstetricians and Gynaecologists, 1988; pp.389-396.
39. Beer AE, Shekar SS, Quebbeman JF, Zhu X. Paternal and non-paternal leucocyte immunisation in women with recurrent spontaneous abortions: Immune responses and subsequent pregnancy outcome. In: *Reproductive Immunology: Materno-fetal relationship*. (Ed.) G Chaouat. Paris: Colloques Inserm, 1987; **154**: 161-178.
40. Edmonds DK. Use of cervical cerclage in patients with recurrent first trimester abortion. In: *Early pregnancy loss—mechanisms and treatment* London: Royal College of Obstetricians and Gynaecologists, 1988; pp.411-415.

41. Harrison RF. Early recurrent pregnancy failure: Treatment with human chorionic gonadotropin. In: *Early pregnancy loss—mechanisms and treatment*. London: Royal College of Obstetricians and Gynaecologists, 1988; pp.421-428.
42. Stray-Pederson B, Stray-Pederson S. Recurrent abortion: The role of psychotherapy. In: *Early pregnancy loss—mechanism and treatment*. London: Royal College of Obstetricians and Gynaecologists, 1988; pp.433-440.

Discussion

Chairman: Dr. W.R. Allen

Professor BEER: Did Dr. Antczak test any of the donkey trophoblast with his defined horse monoclonal antibodies to see if there was any cross-reacting antigenic expression?

Dr. ANTCZAK: Most of our antibodies were, in fact, raised against some endometrial cup tissue we recovered from an F1 hybrid hinny pregnancy and they therefore show reactivity for both horse and donkey molecules. Some molecules may differ between the two species and there may be allotypes of them that we cannot distinguish. We probably made antibodies against monomorphic portions of those molecules and we do not seem to have any polymorphic antibodies.

Dr. CHAOUAT: Because serum from pregnant mares is alloreactive and appears to increase the success rate in the donkey-in-horse model, have you used any horse alloantisera to look histologically at sections of donkey x donkey trophoblast?

Dr. ANTCZAK: We have looked but it is not possible to use alloantisera in immunohistochemical staining unless the specific antiserum has a titre in excess of 1:500.

Dr. CHAOUAT: But can't you extract and purify the specific antibody from the serum?

Dr. ANTCZAK: We have not done that experiment but probably should do so.

Dr. CHAOUAT: Because the serum treatment appears to react across the species barrier it becomes difficult to believe that it functions with classical Class 1 MHC reactivity. Perhaps the serum contains something else that has been conserved between the species which triggers a vital response. It would be very interesting to know where such a factor might react and to what extent.

Dr. ANTCZAK: The serum we used was from a normal horse x horse pregnancy. We didn't actually test the serum for antibody to MHC but it is very likely that it did contain high levels of alloantibody.

Dr. CHAOUAT: But one would like to know whether the protective effect of the infused serum comes from immunoglobulins, or whether some other factor is involved.

Dr. ANTCZAK: That is a good question, but it is just so difficult and costly to do these type of experiments.

Professor GILL: It seems to me that Dr. Antczak has a model, like that which Dr. Croy described earlier, in which there is some mechanism that is probably not immunological which destroys the embryo, and that there is then a response to the degenerating tissue. Will a mule accept a donkey embryo?

Dr. ANTCZAK: Yes it will.

Professor GILL: But I thought mules were sterile?

Dr. ANTCZAK: Mules are sterile in that they fail to produce viable oocytes. But they do possess an otherwise normal reproductive tract and some will ovulate spontaneously. We just transfer an embryo to these cycling animals and away they go in pregnancy.

Dr. ALLEN: Some mules are born with a few ova still remaining in primordial follicles in their ovaries. Although these ova are unable to be fertilised due to a block in meiosis, the animals will nevertheless pass through puberty and will exhibit relatively regular oestrous cycles thereafter. As we have shown, provided they receive the correct "maternal recognition of pregnancy" signal from an embryo transferred to their uterus, they will happily carry the pregnancy to term. However, there are other mules (about half the population) which are born with totally inactive (streak) gonads and which never cycle throughout their lives. Nevertheless, if one gives these animals exogenous progesterone they too can carry transferred embryos.

Dr. RHODES: Were the serum levels of eCG measured in the various pregnancies that were rescued by immunisation therapy? You showed a slide which indicated that progesterone concentrations were depressed but there was no information about eCG levels.

Dr. ALLEN: There was no eCG produced in any of the donkey-in-horse pregnancies.

Dr. RHODES: Yet they maintained the pregnancy?

Dr. ALLEN: We have had just one animal in 70 or 80 donkey-in-horse pregnancies we have created in which we measured a little "blip" of eCG secretion, for about 4 or 5 days. When we removed this conceptus surgically at Day 70 we found one small, necrotic endometrial cup. Thus, it appears that a small piece of chorionic girdle was successful in penetrating the maternal endometrium in this one animal. But in all the others there is a complete failure of girdle invasion and a resulting total absence of endometrial cups and eCG production. The fact that some mares can nevertheless carry their transferred donkey foals to term casts grave doubt on any useful function of eCG from the hormonal point of view.

Professor JENKINS: What about recurrent abortion in Thoroughbred mares? Is this being treated and what is the success rate?

Dr. ALLEN: I am hesitant to confess that we have, in fact, immunised 6 such mares during the past two years with lymphocytes from the mating stallion; and 5 of these animals have produced a foal or remain pregnant at the present time. In each case we checked that the mare did not have cytotoxic antibody against the particular stallion before commencing the immunisation schedule.

We would like to be encouraged by these preliminary results but we remain hesitant because of the wide range of pathological conditions, unrelated to immunology, that can exist in the uteri of such animals. Unlike women, the mare does not menstruate. Once she has had 6 or 7 foals in quick succession, coupled with occasional bouts of acute endometritis induced by bad vulval conformation and/or the bacterial challenge of mating, her endometrium can show a variety of chronic degenerative changes. In view of the diffuse, non-invasive nature of the equine placenta, a minimal or basic area of normal, functional endometrium is necessary to maintain a pregnancy to term. It is very difficult clinically to differentiate this sort of pathology from any potential immunological effect of lymphocyte immunisation.

Dr. PAGE FAULK: Your two forms of immunotherapy in the donkey-in-horse pregnancies involved passive transfer of pregnancy serum and active immunisation with paternal or third party white cells. Was there any variation in the results between these various modes of therapy?

Dr. ANTCZAK: We do not have the numbers to say.

Dr. BELL: In the donkey-in-horse model we saw a slide where there was no interdigitation between the trophoblast and the endometrium. Was there no glandular secretion from the endometrium in those regions as well?

Dr. ALLEN: On the contrary, there are excessive amounts of exocrine material between the trophoblast and endometrium in the failing donkey-in-horse pregnancy. The endometrial glands seem to become hyperactive but one also gains the impression, when looking at the interface with the electron microscope, that the donkey trophoblast is also releasing exocrine material which adds to the total.

Dr. BELL: In those animals treated with progesterone that did not remain pregnant, did their glandular histology revert back to the normal appearance of pregnancy?

Dr. ALLEN: We did not look at this specifically, but I would doubt it.

Dr. BELL: And is there no evidence in the donkey-in-horse model that the failure is one of recognition, say by the endometrium, of a particular type of trophoblast?

Dr. ALLEN: I would like to think that the underlying reason for the failure of the donkey-in-horse pregnancy is the failure of an important maternal immunological recognition message that results from the failure of endometrial cup development at the temporally important stage of gestation—Day 36. We have no real idea of the nature of the immunological stimulus provided by the endometrial cups but it does seem to be important in initiating all the subsequent structural changes associated with implantation and placentation.

Dr. BELL: If this is the case, could it be implied that pregnancy failure is a failure of the endometrium to recognise the donkey trophoblast, and the trophoblast to interact with the endometrium?

Dr. ALLEN: I think the former. Histologically, the endometrium appears quite unresponsive to the donkey trophoblast during the early stages and it seems unwilling to develop the necessary crypts or sulci to accommodate the villi of donkey trophoblast during implantation. Yet the horse endometrium will accommodate the trophoblast of the other bizarre, between-species pregnancies, such as the zebra-in-horse, which are genetically, and presumably antigenically, even more disparate than the donkey-in-horse situation. The one striking difference is the development of at least some endometrial cup activity in these other, successful xenogeneic gestations. The endometrial cups get destroyed very quickly but at least the surrogate mother received an antigenic signal during their development.

Professor CLARK: Does cyclosporin prevent graft rejection in the horse? If so, what about giving cyclosporin to mares carrying donkey fetuses? Secondly, if the leucocytes that infiltrate around the endometrial cups can be recovered, do they do anything which is remotely immunological? That is, do they have any properties of antigen-reactive cells?

Dr. ANTCZAK: We have not attempted cyclosporin. We would like to but the cost would be prohibitive. On your second point, about the endometrial cup leucocytes, this is currently under investigation. They are a very difficult population to get out clean since there is a mass of endometrial glands, endometrial cup cells and other tissues. Dr. Allen's graduate student, Julia Kydd, and a student in my laboratory in Ithaca, are experimenting with these cells and they do not seem to do much. They immunosuppress but, as an immunologist, I know that 10% of anything in tissue culture will suppress. The question is still very open at this stage.

We have started to build monoclonal antibodies against lymphocyte subsets in the horse. We do know that about half the cells around the endometrial cups are T-cells but we can't be any more specific than that; we don't have any markers for T4 or T8 in the horse.

Dr. PAGE FAULK: What is the proportion of T-cells in the peripheral blood of the horse if it is 50% around cups?

Dr. ANTCZAK: It is around 70:30. My figure of 50% T-cells around the endometrial cups is a very crude estimate. It is hard to do accurate morphometrics on the cups and there are a lot of plasma cells, and some eosinophils, in the population as well.

Dr. ALLEN: I should first like to thank the speakers. I think we all enjoyed their papers very much.

Beginning with Dr. Croy's contribution, it strikes me that she and ourselves are in the same, or a very similar, boat as regards the fundamental cause of the pregnancy failure in the two animal models. Both involve between-species differences in which there is considerable genetic, and presumably therefore, antigenic diversity between the mother and fetus. Yet in both models, the *Mus caroli* fetus in the *Mus musculis* uterus and the donkey fetus in the horse uterus, we are left wondering if the pregnancy failure is, indeed, immunologically based. On balance, Dr. Croy seems to conclude not, and she favours a significant developmental defect in placental structure and/or function. Dr. Antczak veers towards a similar conclusion in the horse model where we do know a very definite placental defect occurs—the donkey chorionic girdle fails to invade the surrogate maternal endometrium at Day 36. Yet for all that we must conclude that endometrial cups do not have any hormonal function in equine pregnancy which is vital. We now have over 20 donkeys born from mares which saw no eCG whatsoever throughout intrauterine life and which also survived in the face of very low levels of progesterone, the other main hormone involved in pregnancy maintenance which is reputed to exhibit immunosuppressive properties.

One big difference between the murine and equine models is survival rate in untreated animals; 100% loss in the mouse unless the extraspecific embryo is developing within an intraspecific trophoblast, compared to a 75-80% loss rate in the equids. It is frustrating for Dr. Antczak and me to have to admit that we have no idea at all at this stage why those 25% of mares should carry their xenogeneic donkey fetuses to term in the absence of any form of treatment—no hormones, no immunisation, nothing. And we try hard to give equal amounts of "tender loving care", or the lack of it, to all our patients.

But in favour of immunology, Dr. Antczak has described how we do have strong evidence for immunological memory in the donkey-in-horse model; memory for both rejective-type and protective-type maternal responses. And one further divergence between the mouse and equine models also points strongly towards immunology as playing at least some part in the process. When Dr. Croy immunises her recipient mothers with lymphocytes from the fetal strain the change one might expect to happen does; pregnancy failure is hastened. Yet when we immunise mares in the same manner, we would like to think that, like the situation in women who suffer repeated early pregnancy loss, the treatment enhances fetal survival.

Finally, when we turn to look at the other two animal models we have heard about in this session, Dr. Chaouat with his inbred strains of mice and Dr. Renard with the pigs, it seems clear that immunological factors associated with the MHC are involved. Thus, arguments exist for and against immunology in the animal models and we can now wait to learn about the possible involvement of immunology in the human model of pregnancy failure during the next two days.

SECTION 3

STUDIES OF THE NORMAL AND FAILING PLACENTA IN EARLY PREGNANCY

Placental pathology in spontaneous miscarriage

D. I. Rushton

INTRODUCTION

Spontaneous abortion is the major route by which natural selection operates in man with estimated pre-natal losses of fertilised ova based on human and animal data of at least fifty per cent.[1,2] The majority of these losses occur within the first few weeks of pregnancy and are the result of inherent defects within the conceptus, the most familiar being karyotypic abnormalities.[3] The latter may be considered as the extreme end of the spectrum of natural variation which in more subtle forms plays an essential role in evolution. As such it is logical to anticipate that, concurrent with these natural experiments, a process will have evolved that permits the early elimination of these abnormal conceptuses and return of the maternal organism to a fertile state.

The pathology of the aborted conceptuses may therefore be considered from two perspectives:- (i) that associated with the underlying inherent abnormality in the conceptus; (ii) that associated with the process and mechanisms of elimination of that conceptus from the uterus and the return of the latter to the pre-pregnant state. Unfortunately it is frequently assumed that knowledge of the former provides an explanation of the latter. Thus much data is available on the classification of the conceptus based upon the presence or absence of an embryo, or the presence or absence of developmental abnormalities in the embryo or fetus. Yet the demonstration of an abnormal karyotype or an anatomical abnormality does not necessarily equate with early pregnancy failure; indeed, if it did, the need for prenatal diagnostic services would be greatly reduced, if not eliminated.

Equally, it is well known that pregnancies may continue for several months in the absence of an embryo or in the presence of a dead embryo or fetus, thus indicating that neither embryo nor fetus are necessary (at least in the short term) for the establishment and/or continuation of pregnancy. It must follow that the placenta plays a key role in the maintenance of pregnancy and it is likely that it also has a major influence over the processes involved in the expulsion of the aborted conceptus. Since in the not too distant past the placenta was the obstetrician's favourite scapegoat to explain problems in the perinatal period, it is perhaps surprising that recently it has been virtually totally neglected in the consideration of early pregnancy wastage, though there is a considerable mass of accumulated pathological data.[4,5,6] Indeed, in a recent monograph on spontaneous abortion perusal of the index revealed only five entries relating to the placenta, two of which related to retained placenta and manual removal, the remaining three comprising less than 1% of the text.[7] Accepting the key role of the placenta and that it forms the interface with the maternal organism, it might be anticipated that it would be a valuable source of data both about the mechanisms and the causes of spontaneous abortion. The purpose of this presentation is to demonstrate that this is indeed the case, and that the simplistic view that spontaneous abortions consist of basically two populations, those with abnormal embryos or fetuses and those with normal embryos and fetuses, is both unscientific and erroneous.

The problems associated with the definition of spontaneous abortion and of studying a defined population have been alluded to earlier in these Proceedings. Such problems are greatly amplified by the time the pathologist becomes involved with aborted products of conception, principally as a result of the high degree of selection of material reaching the laboratory. This is determined by several factors including hospital admission policy, the population served and their awareness of early pregnancy wastage, the gestation at which abortion occurs and the interests of the clinicians and the pathologist.

MATERIALS AND METHODS

The data presented represents a preliminary report of the accumulated experience of an eleven year on-going study of a specified—though epidemiologically unrepresentative—population of women, the criteria for entry into the study being that the mothers were either past patients of Birmingham Maternity Hospital or that the abortion occurred to a patient booked for confinement in the hospital. Cases referred for pathological opinion from other units were excluded. The bias towards midtrimester abortions is self-evident in that few women losing their pregnancies before 6-8 weeks gestation required admission and only very occasionally were products of conception received from mothers aborting at home.

The specimens were all classified on the basis of the macroscopic and/or microscopic appearances of the placenta as described elsewhere[8] into three groups: group I—blighted ova, group II—macerated embryos and fetuses and group III—fresh embryos and fetuses. Though the embryos and fetuses were examined and have in some instances provided additional important information, the findings are outside the remit of this report. The proportion of cases falling into each group has remained remarkably constant[9] though in recent years there has been a decline in the macerated group, the reasons for which are uncertain.

Subclassification within the individual groups provides further insight into the nature and mechanisms of spontaneous abortions and emphasises that the arbitrary division of pregnancy into trimesters or into potentially viable and non-viable categories bears no relation to the biological processes involved in the success or failure of individual pregnancies.

RESULTS

During the eleven year period 1426 specimens fell into the defined population though it must be emphasised that an additional 10-15% of samples were inadequate to allow pathological classification. These were classified as follows (Table 1).

Table 1   Classification
1426 specimens

		No.	%
Group I	Blighted ova	672	47.1
Group II	Macerated	339	23.8
Group III	Fresh	415	29.1

Group I

672 cases (47.1%) were blighted ova. The majority showed a mixed histological pattern with fibrotic hypo- or avascular villi together with villi showing microscopic hydatidiform change. In 214 cases the majority of villi showed microscopic hydatidiform change (a term preferred by the author to hydropic change which is reserved for villous oedema in the presence of an intravillous circulation), the villi being avascular and sometimes visibly cystic to the naked eye, but with a characteristically attenuated trophoblast.

In 68 cases the villi were considered to show partial molar change, there being partial vascularisation together with cystic spaces within the stroma, these frequently having a flattened endothelial-like lining. Other villi in the same specimens showed either normal vascularisation or a fibrotic hypovascular stroma. In all cases identification of a chorionic plate was mandatory. A further 13 cases were classified as true moles on the basis of the uniformity of hydatidiform change, absence of vascular development, failure to demonstrate a chorionic plate and varying degrees of trophoblastic hyperplasia.

While these cases are of considerable biological interest they are not amenable to prevention or treatment (other than termination), the majority almost certainly being associated with karyotypic abnormalities.[10] They will not be considered further.

Group II

339 cases (23.8%) were macerated. These could be subclassified as follows (Table 2) and certain of these require further discussion.

Table 2   Macerated Fetuses
339 specimens

	No.	%
Maternal floor infarction	75	22.1
Malformations	38	11.2
Uteroplacental ischaemia	34	10.0
Chorioamnionitis	29	8.5
Hydrops	29	8.5
Retroplacental haemorrhage	19	5.6
Multiple pregnancies	10	3.0
Cord complications/abnormalities	10	3.0
Amniotic bands	5	1.5
Miscellaneous	6	1.8
No specific theory	84	24.8

(a) *MATERNAL FLOOR INFARCTION* (MFI)

This lesion, first described by Benirschke and Driscoll[11] was demonstrated in approximately one quarter of placentae in Group II. In the author's opinion the lesion is specific and follows cessation of the circulation through the villous vessels,[9] the extent of the lesion being related to the duration of retention of the conceptus after embryonic or fetal death. Its importance lies in the fact that it has almost certainly been mistakenly diagnosed for the much rarer disorder of massive perivillous fibrin deposition (MPF).[12] The characteristic features of MFI are that the perivillous deposition of fibrin begins in the basal plate and gradually extends towards the chorionic plate obliterating the intervillous space as it envelops the villi. Small groups of syncytial trophoblastic cells survive on free villi and sometimes apparently on the surface of the fibrin. Proliferation of the cytotrophoblast (cellules X) is not a feature. In contrast MPF affects the entire thickness of the placenta, initially in a patchy distribution, and is associated with very extensive cytotrophoblastic proliferation. Whereas in MFI the villi are invariably fibrotic with vascular obliteration throughout the placenta, those in MPF may retain vascular patency and in the non-affected areas the villi may be normally vascularised.

(b) *UTEROPLACENTAL ISCHAEMIA AND RETROPLACENTAL HAEMORRHAGE*

These cases show either a minimum of 5% villous infarction or an excavating, often old and laminated, haemorrhage on the maternal surface of the placenta, but exclude cases where fresh clot is simply adherent to the placental surface. In both these subgroups there may also be lesions in the placental bed, though it is impossible to determine the incidence of such changes because of incomplete pathological assessment, since in many cases appropriate tissue samples are not available. The lesions in the placental bed include fibrinoid necrosis and acute atherosis of the spiral arteries, findings of considerable interest as in later pregnancy they have been related to pre-eclampsia (PE)[13] and to intrauterine growth retardation (IUGR).[14] Since it is now known that the pathological changes in the placental bed in both PE and IUGR begin in early pregnancy it is interesting to speculate whether some of the aborted cases with vascular lesions represent latent cases of PE which are expelled before the disease becomes clinically manifest in the mother.[10,15] Overall, 16% of macerated fetuses were associated with infarction or retroplacental haemorrhage.

(c) *CHORIOAMNIONITIS*

Though much more frequent among Group III cases, inflammation of the membranes was present in 8.5% of macerated placentae. It is not yet clear whether chorioamnionitis and infection play a major role in these intrauterine deaths. In contrast, villitis of probable viral origin was seen in only 1% of cases.

(d) *MISCELLANEOUS*

Cord complications (3%) and multiple pregnancies (3%) are related in part in that monoamniotic twins with cord entanglements are not rare. Fetal abnormalities associated with amniotic bands are very much more common than in later pregnancy occurring in 1.5% of macerated fetuses.

Placental hydrops (8.5%) was generally associated with fetal hydrops and though the causes are diverse,[16,17,18] the presence of villous oedema with a well developed vascular network is common. There are, however, difficulties in diagnosis since immature villi may appear hydropic, while hydropic villi become progressively less so the longer the dead conceptus is retained *in utero*.

Group III

415 cases (29.1%) were fresh fetuses. These were further subclassified (Table 3) and the following subgroups merit further comment.

Table 3

Fresh Fetuses
415 specimens

	No.	%
Chorioamnionitis	125	30.1
Retroplacental haemorrhage	52	12.6
Uteroplacental ischaemia	24	5.8
Malformations	22	5.3
Multiple pregnancies	14	3.4
Hydrops	6	1.4
Miscellaneous	18	4.3
No specific pathology	154	37.1

(a) *CHORIOAMNIONITIS*

Almost one-third of fresh fetuses are aborted with placentae showing chorioamnionitis. In most cases no specific infection was identified since routine microbiological investigations were not performed, though there were examples of group B streptococcal, listerial, candidal and herpes simplex infections. In view of the very large number of potentially pathogenic organisms in the female genital tract, a wide spectrum of organisms may be the cause of ascending infections of the amniotic cavity. Some recent reports have emphasised specific organisms, e.g. Streptococcus milleri,[18,20] but in the vast majority of infected cases it is likely the commoner commensals of the lower genital tract will be involved. It is, however, of interest that among this group of mothers three have had recurrent midtrimester abortions with anatomically normal fetuses and severe chorioamnionitis with or without evidence of fetal infection. It seems likely that a significant number of cases of cervical incompetence result in the loss of conceptuses with amniotic cavity infection and in view of the controversy over the efficacy of treatment of cervical incompetence by cerclage it is perhaps worth asking whether incompetence of the cervix is mechanical or microbiological. I know of no study of cervical incompetence in which routine examination of the placenta has been performed in those cases where treatment failed.

(b) *UTEROPLACENTAL ISCHAEMIA AND RETROPLACENTAL HAEMORRHAGE*

Almost one-fifth of fresh fetuses and placentae could be subclassified into this category. The extent of placental infarction is frequently more extensive than in the macerated group and on microscopy the surviving villi show accelerated maturation and ischaemic damage. As in the macerated cases placental bed lesions are also present in a proportion.

(c) *MISCELLANEOUS*

Apart from abnormalities of placentation such as placenta praevia, placenta accreta, placenta membranacea and velamentous insertion of the cord which are more frequent, lesions, again notably amnionotic bands, are found similar to those in the macerated group.

DISCUSSION

The subclassification of the placental lesions demonstrated in this series of spontaneous abortions reveals considerable diversity both between groups and within groups emphasising the heterogenous nature of the aborted population, a feature which in the author's experience is frequently overlooked in clinical studies of spontaneous abortion and is generally not available in epidemiological studies.

Indeed, a major weakness of virtually all such studies is the lack of pathological data on the aborted conceptus. This is most strikingly obvious in mothers under investigation for recurrent or habitual abortion. It is more than remarkable that in a period of the human life span lasting between 20 and 28 weeks, depending on legal definitions of fetal viability, when the loss of fertilised ova of varying gestational ages may well equal or surpass the number of deaths from 28 weeks gestation to the maximum age reached by adults, that all such losses are frequently considered as a single population. Such an approach is comparable to the use of the crude death rate in a specific age group, together with minimal clinical data and no pathological data, to determine the incidence of carcinoma of the bronchus and the effectiveness of various regimens used in its treatment.

The data presented provide some insight into the complexity of early pregnancy wastage and also indicates some specific areas where there is a potential for therapeutic success, but much remains unexplained. In the majority of spontaneous abortions there is either no embryo or the embryo or fetus has been dead *in utero* for some time prior to expulsion. In the absence of an embryo, the villous circulation fails to develop, while after embryonic or fetal death the villous circulation ceases. Previously published data[9] suggest that the maintenance of a villous circulation is a prerequisite for trophoblastic survival and that trophoblastic failure subsequent to villous circulatory failure might be a mechanism by which these conceptuses are lost. In either case the failure is dependent upon the conceptus and not the maternal organism. It does not invoke the complexities of maternal recognition of an abnormality be it metabolic, chromosomal or anatomical. If the abortuses which are lost in very early pregnancy are included then it is likely that at least 80% of early pregnancy wastage could be mediated through trophoblastic failure, either as a primary event in the earliest losses where is would lead to failure of implantation, or secondary to circulatory failure in later abortions. This simplistic view does, of course, leave many unanswered questions, perhaps the most puzzling being why so many fetuses which are anatomically normal or have non-lethal malformations die *in utero*. The current data indicate that a significant proportion of these deaths might be the result of uteroplacental ischaemia while a few may be due to infection. Genetic disorders affecting vital processes of maturation may account for a proportion as may inherited biochemical disorders. Among those normal fetuses which are apparently alive until immediately prior to, or during abortion, the roles of infection and uteroplacental ischaemia clearly require further investigation and recent evidence on the value of eliminating Group B streptococci from the urine of women in the prevention of preterm labour may be pertinent in this respect.[21]

Later in this study group we are to hear about the value or otherwise of immunological regimens in the treatment of recurrent abortion. From the histopathological viewpoint these raise many difficulties, not the least of which is the fact that it has not yet been possible to identify a lesion or group of lesions which might be mediated through immunological interaction between the mother and conceptus in aborted material. It is not unreasonable to suppose, in view of the complexities of the immunological interrelationships between the conceptus and the maternal organism, that some pregnancies will be lost as a result of failure of these immunological processes. Since in our experience, not more than 1-2% of women who have one abortion will go on to become recurrent aborters and since few spontaneous abortions are examined pathologically, knowledge of the nature of the previous losses is inevitably either non-existent or very scanty by the time an index patient is identified. If the treatment succeeds then presumably the cause of the earlier losses will no longer be apparent, while if it fails it may be argued that perhaps the previous losses were not due to a cause amenable to the therapy being used. Thus, if we have no data on the nature of the earlier losses of recurrent aborters it is difficult, if not impossible, to determine the mechanism by which immunological, or for that matter any other therapy, improves the outcome in these unfortunate women.

This lack of data poses several important questions some of which I hope may be answered later in the meeting. These include:
(i) Is the treatment preventing immunological rejection by a specific biological mechanism assuming that rejection is the cause of abortion in these patients? Alternatively, is the treatment effective because the patients are receiving intensive medical care? It is well known, for example, that the number of cot deaths may be reduced by increasing the number of health workers caring for mothers with small infants, without introduction of any specific treatment.
(ii) If the treatment is effective how and where does it act?
(iii) Where should the histopathologist be looking for evidence of an immunological disorder: in the decidua, the placenta or the fetus?
(iv) What should he or she be looking for? The characteristic lesions associated with immunological rejection have not been demonstrated in aborted material.

Finally, may I suggest that there is a possible contender for this enigmatic pathological lesion. As one of its many functions trophoblast acts as an endothelial cell, lining the maternal component of the placental circulation. The surface layer, the syncytium, is continuously replaced from the cytotrophoblast and in normal pregnancies a balance is maintained. Under certain conditions notably hypoxia,[22,23] cytotrophoblastic proliferation may exceed that required to replace syncytium and the latter accumulates on the villous surface forming knots.[24] If syncytial loss were to exceed the ability of the cytotrophoblast to replace it, either because the turnover of syncytium was greatly increased or the cytotrophoblast was damaged, then the endothelial cell function would be compromised, and fibrin and platelets would be deposited on the villous surface. Once the trophoblast was covered by fibrin cytotrophoblastic proliferation could continue at least while the fetus remained alive, possibly stimulated by hypoxia due to the intervening layer of fibrin, and if the initial damage was to the cyto-trophoblast because the fibrin provided a barrier against further immunological onslaught. One lesion does fulfil these criteria—massive perivillous fibrin deposition. Is it the missing link? It is perhaps worthy of note that in the few women we have seen in which the placenta has shown MPF we have observed a tendency for it to recur in subsequent pregnancies. We have given some of these women low dose aspirin therapy in their next pregnancy with some success though at an anecdotal rather than a statistical level.

CONCLUSIONS

Pathological examination of the placenta from spontaneously aborted conceptuses provides insight into the complexity of the aborted population and our ignorance of the factors which may be involved in early pregnancy loss. It also suggests possible areas where treatment might be specific rather than empirical such as in uteroplacental ischaemia and infection.

In view of these findings, there is a need to consider all clinical and epidemiological studies of abortion with some scepticism since hard data on the nature of the aborted conceptus are almost invariably lacking, and where present it is not representative of the general population of women of reproductive age.

From the histopathological viewpoint there is as yet no firm evidence that clinically apparent spontaneous abortions result from a failure of the processes of immunological adaption that occur between the mother and her conceptus in normal pregnancy, though this clearly does not exclude the possibility of such a mechanism.

Since there are no biological barriers between midtrimester abortion and premature labour, treatments effective in preventing either may well be effective in both groups. Indeed, both prematurity and maternal hypertensive disease, the largest contributors to perinatal morbidity and mortality, undoubtedly stem in many instances from events occurring in these critical early weeks of pregnancy. The spontaneous abortion may yet reveal much of value to future obstetricians and neonatologists.

REFERENCES
1. Hafez ESE. Reproductive failure in domestic animals. In: *Comparative aspects of reproductive failure.* Ed. K Benirschke. Berlin: Springer-Verlag, 1967; pp.44-96.
2. Witschi E. Teratogenic effects from overripeness of the egg. In: *Congenital Malformations: Proceedings of the third international conference.* Eds. FC Fraser and VA McKusick. Amsterdam: New York Excerpta Medica, 1970; pp.157-169.

3. Simpson JL, Bombard A. Chromosomal abnormalities in spontaneous abortion: Frequency, pathology and genetic counselling. In: *Spontaneous and recurrent abortion.* Eds. MJ Bennett, DK Edmonds. Oxford: Blackwell Scientific Publications, 1987; pp.51-76.
4. Honoré LH, Dill FJ, Poland BJ. Placental morphology in spontaneous human abortuses with normal and abnormal karyotypes. *Teratology* 1976; **14:** 151-166.
5. Ornoy A, Salamon-Arnon J, Ben-Zur Z, Kohn G. Placental findings in spontaneous abortions and stillbirths. *Teratology* 1981; **24:** 243-252.
6. Rushton DI. Pathology of abortion. In: *Haines and Taylor's Obstetrical and gynaecological pathology.* Ed: H Fox. Edinburgh: Churchill Livingstone, 1987. pp.1117-1148.
7. Bennett MJ, Edmonds DK. *Spontaneous and recurrent abortion.* Oxford: Blackwell Scientific Publications, 1987.
8. Rushton DI. Simplified classification of spontaneous abortions. *J Med Genet* 1978; **15:** 1-9.
9. Rushton DI. The classification and mechanisms of spontaneous abortion. *Perspect Pediatr Pathol* 1984; **8:** 269-287.
10. Rushton DI. The nature and causes of spontaneous abortions with normal karyotypes. In: *Issues and reviews in teratology.* Volume 3. Ed. K Kalter. New York: Plenum Press, 1985; pp.21-63.
11. Benirschke K, Driscoll SG. *The pathology of the human placenta.* New York: Springer-Verlag, 1967; p.232.
12. Fox H. *Pathology of the Placenta.* London: WB Saunders, 1978; pp.95-101.
13. Robertson WB, Brosens I, Dixon G. Uteroplacental vascular pathology. *Europ J Obstet Gynec Reprod Biol* 1975; **5:** 47-65.
14. Sheppard BL, Bonnar J. The ultrastructure of the arterial supply of the human placenta in pregnancy complicated by fetal growth retardation. *Br J Obstet Gynaecol* 1976; **83:** 948-959.
15. Khong TY, Liddell HS, Robertson WB. Defective haemochorial placentation as a cause of miscarriage. A preliminary study. *Br J Obstet Gynaecol* 1987; **94:** 649-655.
16. Keeling JW. Fetal hydrops. In: *Fetal and neonatal pathology.* Ed. JW Keeling. London: Springer-Verlag, 1987; pp.211-228.
17. Machin GA. Diseases causing fetal and neonatal ascites. *Pediatr Pathol* 1985; **4:** 195-212.
18. Nakamura Y, Komatsu Y, Yano H, Kitazono S, Hosokawa Y, Fukuda S, Kawano S, Nagasue N, Matsunaga T, Aiko Y, Hashimoto T, Morimatsu M. Non immunologic hydrops fetalis. A clinico-pathological study of 50 autopsy cases. *Pediatr Pathol* 1987; **7:** 19-30.
19. MacGowan AP, Terry PB. Streptococcus milleri and second trimester abortion. *J Clin Pathol* 1987; **40:** 292-293.
20. Cox RA, Chen K, Coykendall AL, Wesbecher P, Herson VC. Fatal infection in neonates of 26 weeks gestation due to Streptococcus milleri. Report of two cases. *J Clin Pathol* 1987; **40:** 190-193.
21. Thomsen AC, Mørup L, Hanson KB. Antibiotics elimination of Group B streptococci in urine in prevention of preterm labour. *Lancet* 1987; **1:** 591-593.
22. Fox H. Effect of hypoxia on trophoblast in organ culture: a morphologic and autoradiographic study. *Am J Obstet Gynecol* 1970; **107:** 1058-1064.
23. Maclennan AH, Sharp F, Shaw-Dunn S. The ultrastructure of human trophoblast in spontaneous and induced hypoxia using a system of organ culture: a comparison with ultrastructural changes in pre-eclampsia and placental insufficiency. *J Obstet Gynaecol Br Commonw* 1972; **79:** 113-121.
24. Rushton DI. Placenta as a reflection of maternal disease. In: *Pathology of the placenta.* Ed. EVDK Perrin. New York: Churchill Livingstone, 1984; pp.57-88.

Discussion

Chairman: Professor W. B. Robertson

Dr B. STRAY-PEDERSON: I am a little worried about your conclusion from morphological appearances and the cause of the abortion, especially about your diagnosis of chorioamnionitis. We have investigated patients whom the pathologists had designated as having chorioamnionitis to an extensive degree by detailed microbiological screening and from the clinical course. We could see no indication that they have had any infections except in only a very few cases. Could it be that the migration of leucocytes is something which happens secondarily and not primarily?

Dr RUSHTON: Secondary to what?

Dr B. STRAY-PEDERSON: Secondary to the death of the fetus, for instance, to the associated necrosis. There are no correlations between the microbiological findings and the morphology.

Dr RUSHTON: In our study of later pregnancies, there is a relationship between the microbiology and chorioamnionitis if the baby is less than 2.5 kilogrammes and we have studied 200 consecutive cases. The other point which I didn't mention relating to chorioamnionitis, is that there is also increasing clinical evidence that chorioamnionitis can occur in intact sacs and organisms can be isolated from amniotic cavities which are needled when the sac is known to be intact. Another thing which I hadn't time to mention was that we have also done extensive studies on these fetuses and they have been quite clearly stimulated, at least most of them. About one-third of them had a congenital pneumonia, and I don't see how congenital pneumonia can occur without something getting into the lung to stimulate an inflammatory response. Furthermore, this is not simply due to inhalation of cells into the alveoli; it is an interstitial reaction within the lung which would not occur were it simply the aspiration of cells into the alveoli.

Dr CARP: You stated that there is probably not a lot of difference between fetal death in the first trimester or in the second trimester. Do you think that there is an essential difference between fetal death in the first or second trimester and with the blighted ova? If you think that there is not, do you have any idea when the embryo ceases to develop? I am asking this question because in our patients three-quarters of habitual aborters, of primary aborters at least, are primary

159

aborters of blighted ova. These are the ones that, paradoxically, seem to do best with immunisation.

Dr RUSHTON: The only thing I can say about that is, in respect of placental pathology in those that have a population of villi with what I call microscopic hydropic change, I believe that the embryo has probably died before and not later than five weeks of pregnancy, when the villus circulation becomes established. After that one cannot determine when fetal death occurs simply by examination, even if you have got the embryo and its measurements. You don't know if it was growth retarded before it died so you can't actually determine its age. I think this is something that the ultrasound people are going to have to tell us.

Professor ROBINSON: Could we ask Dr Michel who has been doing work on early ultrasound to comment on that?

Dr MICHEL: Yes, I think with anembryonic pregnancies and ultrasound, most of the time you don't see a fetal form at all, and you rely only on the menstrual history and the fact that the gestational sac does not increase in size from week to week. Then you can decide if it is a missed abortion or a blighted ovum. Even when you manage to take these sacs out, only rarely can you see a fetal form inside when the histologist identifies it. So, as far as blighted ova are concerned, I think that most of them do not have a fetal form, at least detectable with ultrasound examination.

Dr CARP: Did it ever happen?

Dr MICHEL: It did; I have had cases where you can just see an echo inside the sac but unfortunately we didn't get histological confirmation that there was fetal tissue, but you can see something inside the sac.

Dr RUSHTON: I would question whether it is an embryo, as it might have no amnion either, so that if there is no amnion it is unlikely that there was an embryo.

Professor BEARD: These are ultrasound studies from about six weeks, aren't they?

Dr MICHEL: Yes, as soon as the β-hCG is positive.

Early human trophoblast

Y. W. Loke

INTRODUCTION

Trophoblast represents that layer of the placenta which is in direct contact with maternal tissues and is, therefore, expected to play an important role in all aspects of fetal-maternal interaction. Although trophoblast comes to line the whole uterine cavity during gestation, it is at the placental implantation site where these cells are most numerous and where they penetrate deepest into decidua and myometrium. The present review will focus on some phenotypic and functional characteristics of these placental trophoblast populations during early pregnancy.

TROPHOBLAST POPULATIONS

The recent availability of monoclonal antibodies directed against trophoblast-associated molecules has greatly facilitated the identification of these cells so that their pattern of distribution in the placental bed can be readily appreciated.[1,2] The different locations where trophoblast contacts maternal tissues is represented diagrammatically in Figure I.

1) Enveloping each chorionic villus are two layers of trophoblast, an inner cytotrophoblast or Langhan's layer and an outer syncytiotrophoblast. The latter can also be seen to line the surface of the intervillous blood sinusoids and to dip into the openings of some uterine veins. The villous syncytiotrophoblast, therefore, is bathed in maternal venous blood and forms an important component of the haemochorial interface. Because of their location, these trophoblast cells are collectively known as villous trophoblast.

2) Some chorionic villi do not lie free in the blood sinusoids but serve to anchor the placenta onto the decidua basalis. From the tips of these anchoring villi, cytotrophoblast cells proliferate through the overlying syncytial layer to become cytotrophoblast columns. This trophoblast, together with all that to be described subsequently, are grouped as extravillous trophoblast.

3) From these columns, groups of irregularly-shaped cells spread downwards to form the cytotrophoblast shell which comes to intercede between the chorionic villi and the underlying decidua.

4) Cytotrophoblast cells, either singly or in small groups, continue to migrate into the decidua and even to reach the myometrium. These are the interstitial cytotrophoblast.

Figure I

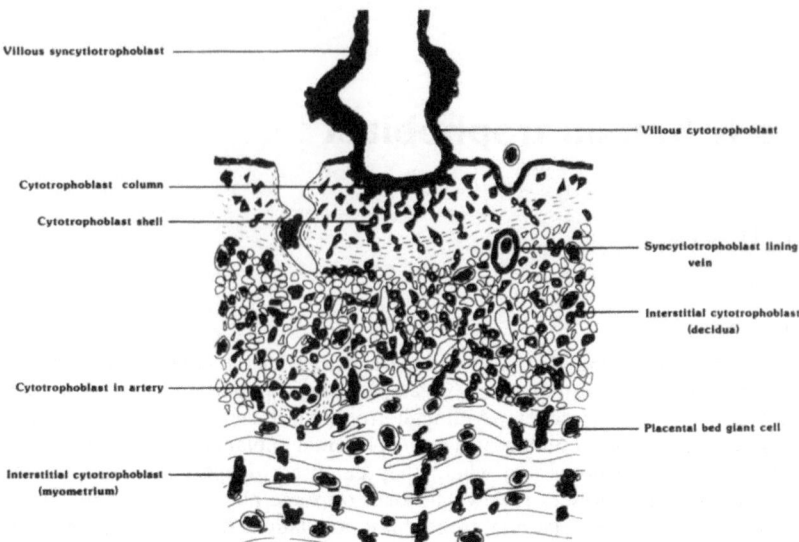

TROPHOBLAST POPULATIONS OF THE CHORIONIC VILLUS AND IN PLACENTAL BED

Villous syncytiotrophoblast

Villous cytotrophoblast

Cytotrophoblast column

Cytotrophoblast shell

Syncytiotrophoblast lining vein

Interstitial cytotrophoblast (decidua)

Cytotrophoblast in artery

Placental bed giant cell

Interstitial cytotrophoblast (myometrium)

Diagram showing pattern of distribution of trophoblast cells in placental implantation site.

5) Many of these interstitial cytotrophoblast cells remain as mononuclear cells, but some are transformed into multinuclear placental bed giant cells.

6) The walls of the uterine spiral arteries are frequently infiltrated by cytotrophoblast (mural trophoblast) which eventually replace all or part of the endothelial lining of the vessel (endovascular trophoblast). Clumps of these cells may even lie free within the lumen of the arteries (intravascular trophoblast). In these situations, cytotrophoblast comes into contact with maternal arterial blood. Cytotrophoblast cells clearly have remarkable penetrative ability. Not only can they invade decidua and myometrium, but they are also able to cross arterial walls, a property which is shared by malignant neoplasms.

In the same way as they have greatly facilitated the identification of trophoblast in tissue sections, as discussed in the preceding section, appropriate monoclonal antibodies have also been invaluable in distinguishing trophoblast from contaminating cells disaggregated from placental tissues[3] and also in a mixed cell culture.[4] This has permitted a proper assessment of the yield of trophoblast with different isolation and culture procedures. It is now accepted that standard techniques do not result in a pure trophoblast population and this point should be borne in mind in evaluating data when such cells are used for experiments. Recently, we have developed a culture method which consistently yields trophoblast cells of 80-90% homogeneity.[5] This has given us an opportunity to study these cells *in vitro*.

TROPHOBLAST SECRETORY ACTIVITY

It is well documented that most, if not all, of the main placental hormones and enzymes are secreted by villous syncytiotrophoblast. Some products, like human placental lactogen (hPL), are detected in these cells throughout pregnancy while others are restricted to certain stages of gestation. For example, human chorionic gonadotrophin (hCG) is produced predominantly during early pregnancy while placental alkaline phosphatase (PLAP) is synthesised later. Extravillous trophoblast, however, appears to be relatively unproductive with only a small population of cells exhibiting secretory activity. This is especially noticeable in endovascular trophoblast which has invaded the walls of uterine spiral arteries.[2] The demonstration of transcriptional activity in the form of mRNA for hCG and hPL in syncytiotrophoblast[6] indicates that these hormones represent endogenous synthesis and are not merely absorbed from maternal blood. Placental bed giant cells have not been observed to synthesise any hormones so they are not, in spite of being multinuclear, directly analogous to villous syncytiotrophoblast. The concentration of placental secretory activity mainly to the haemochorial interface is interesting and raises the question whether maternal serum factors may modulate trophoblast gene activity.

It is possible that extravillous trophoblast may be involved in the synthesis of different kinds of products. For example, the enzyme leucine aminopeptidase (LAP) has been detected in all extravillous trophoblast including placental bed giant cells.[2] LAP is thought to counter the hypertensive effects of renin-argiotension release, so its presence in the vicinity of the uterine spiral arteries could serve to regulate maternal blood pressure. Indeed, we have observed that trophoblast from patients with pre-eclampsia stained for this enzyme with less intensity than normal trophoblast. Prostaglandins have also been demonstrated in extravillous trophoblast,[7] and these cells are thought to secrete products responsible for the recruitment of uterine suppressor cells (see chapter by D.A. Clark). Thus, the extravillous trophoblast population may be the source of a different array of biologically and immunologically active molecules which function locally in the placental bed.

TROPHOBLAST ANTIGENICITY

A major effort in contemporary reproductive immunology is directed at the question of how the allogeneic placenta survives maternal immune attack during gestation. The antigenic status of trophoblast, which constitutes the ultimate fetal-maternal interface, has therefore received a great deal of attention. It is now generally accepted that villous trophoblast does not express HLA-A,B,C, HLA-DR, B_2 microglobulin or H-Y antigens.[8] Figure II shows cross-sections of first trimester chorionic villi stained with monoclonal antibody W6/32 which is directed against HLA Class I framework determinants. It can be seen that the two trophoblast layers are unstained while the cells of the villous mesenchyme are strongly reactive. Kirby and his colleagues[9] formulated the hypothesis, from observations on mouse trophoblast, that surface antigens are masked by a layer of immunologically inert sialo-mucin coating. However, a similar layer has never been convincingly demonstrated on human trophoblast, and data from antigen

Figure II

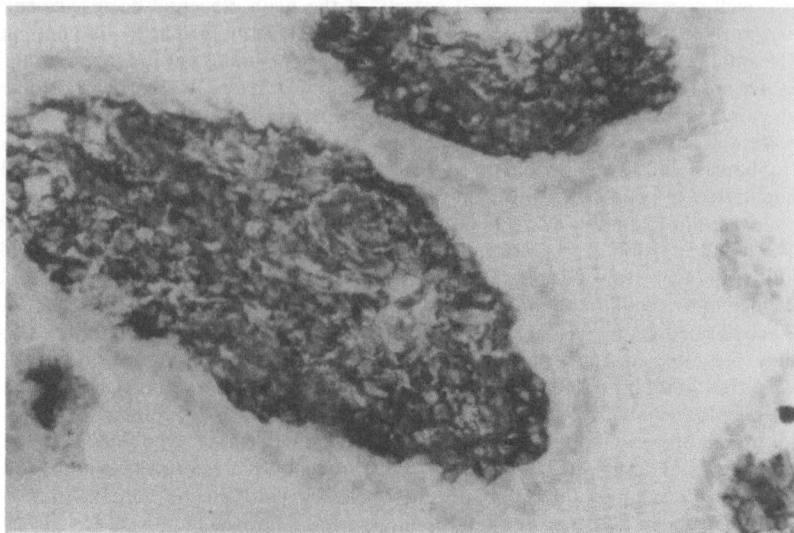

Frozen section of first trimester chorionic villi stained with monoclonal antibody W6/32 and localised by biotin-avidin-peroxidase. Villous mesenchymal cells are strongly reactive while overlying trophoblast layers are not stained.

'unmasking' experiments have been equivocal. Nevertheless, it should be noted that human syncytiotrophoblast does not have a highly sialylated cell surface,[10] and the carboxyl groups of the sialic acid residues may, in turn, be responsible for the high surface negative charge observed on the microvillous surface of these cells.[11,12] Since syncytiotrophoblast is in direct contact with maternal blood, these membrane features may provide an anti-thrombotic lining to prevent clotting of the slow-moving blood in the intervillous venous sinusoids like endothelium in blood vessels. The molecular hybridisation studies of Kawata and his colleagues[13] have shown that human trophoblast has very little HLA-A,B,C mRNA but did have appreciable quantities of B_2M mRNA compared to lymphocytes. This led to the conclusion that there is a selective transcriptional depression of HLA Class I molecules but not of B_2M so that the mechanism responsible for the absence of HLA antigens on trophoblast appears to be failure of synthesis rather than lack of insertion like the DAUDI lymphoblastoid cell line.

In contrast to villous trophoblast, extravillous trophoblast has been observed to express HLA Class I-like antigens, but not Class II.[14] Even the endovascular trophoblast which has invaded uterine arteries also expresses these antigens.[1] Thus, the haemochorial interface of the human placenta is immunologically less straightforward than originally envisaged, with maternal blood coming into contact with Class I positive extravillous cytotrophoblast on the arterial side, and with Class I negative villous syncytiotrophoblast on the venous side.

Currently, there is much discussion on the nature of the Class I antigen expressed by extravillous cytotrophoblast. This antigen is readily demonstrable by a monoclonal antibody W6/32 which is directed against framework epitopes of the Class I molecule, but these trophoblast cells fail to bind antisera to polymorphic determinants.[15] Another monoclonal antibody 61D2 directed at Class I common determinants, but perhaps at epitopes situated nearer the allotypic region of the heavy chain molecule, also does not stain extravillous trophoblast.[16] Our own unpublished data that human cytotrophoblast is lysed by W6/32 but not by human multispecific HLA antisera (Birkby *et al*, unpublished) are in accord with these immunohistological findings. These observations suggest that the HLA antigen expressed on extravillous trophoblast may be lacking the polymorphic regions. Supportive evidence for this conclusion was recently provided by Ellis and her colleagues[17] who demonstrated trophoblast antigen to have a molecular weight of 40,000 which is smaller than that of a conventional Class I molecule. Whether or not this could represent a non-classical HLA antigen analogous to the murine Qa or TLa or the rat Pa systems and the role it may play in human pregnancy, remain to be determined.

A further antigen which needs to be considered is the trophoblast-lymphocyte cross-reactive antigen (TLX) described by Faulk and his colleagues on syncytio-trophoblast.[18,19] The authors believe this is representative of a novel trophoblast alloantigenic system which is related to, but not the same as, HLA. It was further postulated that maternal recognition of incompatible TLX antigens on trophoblast could lead to the production of protective factors (e.g. blocking antibodies) beneficial to pregnancy. In this way, reproduction encourages antigenic heterogeneity and thus perpetuates genetic diversity in the population. It is this concept that has led to present regimes of treating habitually aborting women by immunising them with husband's lymphocytes[20] or, more recently, with purified syncytiotrophoblast plasma membranes in order to stimulate the patients to react, presumably, against this putative TLX antigen. It would be convenient if supportive evidence in the form of anti-trophoblast antibodies could be demonstrated in all pregnancy sera but, unfortunately, these have proved somewhat elusive.[21,22] There has been only one recent positive report.[23] We ourselves have observed a rising titre of anti-trophoblast antibodies throughout gestation which is mainly IgM (Grabowska *et al*, unpublished). Immunoglobulin class and subclass restriction is well documented in murine pregnancy (see chapter by W.D. Billington). It would be of interest to see if human anti-trophoblast antibodies follow the same pattern.

Besides TLX, the interesting feature about anti-trophoblast antisera generated in animal species, both polyclonal and monoclonal, is their cross-reactivities with certain tissues but not with others. One such reaction is found against certain cell lines[24,25] and also with a variety of human cancers.[26,27] In addition, anti-trophoblast antisera are seen to recognise antigens on cells transformed by retroviruses[28] together with the corollary observation that antisera generated against retroviral polypeptide sequences will immunoblot a variety of proteins extracted from human trophoblast.[29,30,31] What role these retroviral-encoded products play in pregnancy is unclear. At present, there is a great deal of interest in oncogenes and their biological functions. In this context, it may be mentioned that transcriptional activity of several oncogenes like c-myc, c-sis, c-fos and c-fms have been found to be exceptionally high in human trophoblast cells.[32,33,34] This raises the intriguing possibility that proteins encoded by oncogenes may be responsible for the pseudo-malignant growth properties and invasive behaviour of trophoblast as they are thought to do in cancer cells. The similarities between trophoblast and cancer are really quite impressive (Table 1). We are increasingly inclined to believe that the interaction between trophoblast and mother is more akin to the tumour-host than to the graft-recipient relationship.

Table 1

Similarities between trophoblast and neoplastic cells

1) *Behaviour*
   a) Both cell types have invasive properties.
   b) Trophoblast cells are disseminated in maternal blood like cancer metastases.

2) *Cell surface*
   a) Both cell types have high membrane sialic acid.
   b) Villous trophoblast cells do not express MHC antigens.
      Many neoplastic cells are also deficient in MHC antigens.
   c) Trophoblast and neoplastic cells share similar surface antigens.
   d) Are retro-virus antigens expressed on trophoblast cells?

3) *Products*
   Many neoplasms produce trophoblast proteins like:-
   a) Human chorionic gonadotrophin (hCG)
   b) Placental alkaline phosphatase (PLAP)
   c) Trophoblast-specific B_1-glycoprotein.

CONCLUSION

It will be appreciated from the preceding review that placental trophoblast encroaches onto maternal territory over an extensive area, coming directly into contact with maternal blood and a variety of uterine tissues. These trophoblast cells can be broadly divided into villous and extravillous populations, each with its own distinctive characteristics. They are highly interesting cells and their study may well have relevance beyond the confines of reproductive biology.

ACKNOWLEDGEMENTS

We are grateful for financial support from the American Friends of Cambridge University, Cancer Research Campaign, Medical Research Council, Wellcome Trust and World Health Organization. We would like to thank our obstetric colleagues and staff at Addenbrooke's Hospital for collecting placental material.

REFERENCES
1. Butterworth BH, Khong TY, Robertson WB, Loke YW. Human cytotrophoblast populations studied by monoclonal antibodies using single and double biotin-avidin-peroxidase immunocytochemistry. *J Histochem Cytochem* 1985; **33**: 977-983.
2. Loke YW, Butterworth BH. Heterogeneity of human trophoblast populations. In: *Immunoregulation and Fetal Survival* Eds. TJ Gill and TG Wegman. Oxford: Oxford University Press, 1987; pp.197-209.

3. Butterworth BH, Loke YW. Immunocytochemical identification of cytotrophoblast from other mononuclear cell populations isolated from first-trimester human chorionic villi. *J Cell Science* 1985; **76:** 189-197.

4. Loke YW, Butterworth BH, Margetts JJ, Burland K. Identification of cytotrophoblast colonies in cultures of human placental cells using monoclonal antibodies. *Placenta* 1986; **7:** 221-231.

5. Loke YW, Burland K. Human trophoblast cells cultured in modified medium and supported by extracellular matrix. *Placenta*; In press.

6. Hoshina M, Boothby M, Boime I. Cytological localization of chorionic gonadotrophin and placental lactogen mRNAs during development of the human placenta. *J Cell Biol* 1982; **93:** 190-198.

7. Duneas J, Nguyen SH, Wegmann R, Panigel M. Localisation de la prostaglandine déhydrogenasé dans le placenta et les tissus déciduaux humains. *Cell Mol Biol* 1984; **30:** 485-488.

8. Galbraith RM, Kantor RRS, Gerrara GB, Ades EW, Galbraith GMP. Differential anatomical expression of transplantation antigens within the normal human placental chorionic villus. *Am J Reprod Immunol* 1981; **1:** 331-335.

9. Kirby DRS, Billington WD, Bradbury S, Goldstein DJ. Antigen barrier of the mouse placenta. *Nature* 1964; **204:** 548-549.

10. Whyte A. Biochemistry of the human syncytiotrophoblast plasma membrane. In: *Biology of Trophoblast.* Eds. YW Loke and AWhyte. Amsterdam: Elsevier Science Publishers; 1983, pp.513-553.

11. Kawagoe K, Kawana T, Sakamoto S. Ultra-structural demonstration of the negative surface charge on human trophoblast. *Acta Histochem Cytochem* 1980; **13:** 254-269.

12. King BF. The distribution and mobility of anionic sites on the surface of human placental syncytial trophoblast. *Anatom Record* 1981; **199:** 15-22.

13. Kawata M, Parnes JR, Herzenberg LA. Transcriptional control of HLA-A,B,C antigen in human placental cytotrophoblast isolated using trophoblast- and HLA-specific monoclonal antibodies and the fluorescence-activated cell sorter. *J Exp Med* 1984; **160:** 633-651.

14. Sunderland CA, Redman CWG, Stirrat GM. HLA-A,B,C antigens are expressed on non-villous trophoblast of the early human placenta. *J Immunol* 1981; **127:** 2614-2615.

15. Redman CWG, McMichael AJ, Stirrat GM, Sutherland CA, Ting A. Class I major histocompatibility complex antigens on human extra-villous trophoblast. *Immunology* 1984; **52:** 457-468.

16. Wells M, Hsi B-L, Faulk WP. Class I antigens of the major histocompatibility complex on cytotrophoblast of the human placental basal plate. *Am J Reprod Immunol* 1984; **6:** 167-174.

17. Ellis SA, Sargent IL, Redman CWG, McMichael AJ. Evidence for a noval HLA antigen found on human extravillous trophoblast and a choriocarcinoma cell line. *Immunol* 1986; **59:** 595-601.

18. McIntyre JA, Faulk WP. Allotypic trophoblast—lymphocyte cross-reactive (TLX) cell surface antigens. *Human Immunology* 1982; **4:** 27-35.

19. McIntyre JA, Faulk WP. HLA and the generation of diversity in human pregnancy. Immunology of human placental proteins. *Placenta Supplement 4*; **1:** 1-11.

20. Mowbray JF, Gibbings C, Liddell H, Reginald PW, Underwood J, Beard RW. Controlled trial of treatment of recurrent spontaneous abortion by immunisation with paternal cells. *Lancet* 1985; **1:** 941-943.

21. Johnson PM, Cheng HM, Stevens VC, Matangkasombut P. Antibody reactivity against trophoblast and trophoblast products. *J Reprod Immunol* 1985; **8:** 347-352.

22. Nickson DA, Sutcliffe RG. A search for antibodies in term maternal sera to solubilized syncytiotrophoblast surface components. A passive haemagglutinin assay yields negative evidence. *J Reprod Immunol* 1986; **9:** 302-312.

168   Study Group: Early Pregnancy Loss

23. Davies M, Browne CM. Anti-trophoblast antibody responses during normal human pregnancy. *J Reprod Immunol* 1985; **7**: 285-297.
24. McIntyre JA, Faulk WP. Cross-reactions between cell surface membrane antigens of human trophoblast and cancer cells. *Placenta* 1980; **1**: 197-207.
25. Whyte A, Ragge N, Loke YW, Thiry L. Human syncytiotrophoblast membrane proteins defined using heterologous antiserum. *Clin Exp Immunol* 1985; **59**: 227-234.
26. Loke YW, Whyte A, Davies SP. Differential expression of trophoblast-specific membrane antigens by normal and abnormal human placentae and by neoplasms of trophoblastic and non-trophoblastic origin. *Int J Cancer* 1980; **25**: 459-461.
27. Johnson PM, Cheng HM, Molloy CM, Stern CMM, Slade MB. Human trophoblast-specific surface antigens identified using monoclonal antibodies. *Am J Reprod Immunol* 1981; **1**: 246-254.
28. Thiry L, Sprecher-Goldberger S, Hard RC, Bossens M, Buekens P. Heterologous antiserum to human syncytiotrophoblast membrane is cytotoxic to retrovirus-producing cells and to some cancer cell lines. *Am J Reprod Immunol* 1981; **1**: 240-245.
29. Jerabek LB, Mellors RC, Elkon KB, Mellors JW. Detection and immunochemical characterization of a primate type C retrovirus-related p30 protein in normal human placentas. *Proc Nat Acad Sci* 1984; **81**: 6501-6505.
30. Suni J, Narvanen A, Wahlstrom T, Aho M, Pakhanen R, Vaheri A, Copeland T, Cohen M, Oroszian S. Human placental syncytiotrophoblast Mr 75,000 polypeptide defined by antibodies to a synthetic peptide based on a cloned human endogenous retroviral DNA sequence. *Proc Nat Acad Sci* 1984; **81**: 6197-6201.
31. Wahlstrom T, Nieminen P, Narvanen A, Suni J, Lehtovirta Saksela E, Vaheri A. Monoclonal antibody defining a human syncytiotrophoblast polypeptide immunologically related to mammalian retrovirus structural protein p30. *Placenta* 1984; **5**: 465-474.
32. Muller R, Tremblay JM, Adamson ED, Verma IM. Tissue and cell type specific expression of two human c-onc genes. *Nature* 1985; **304**: 454-456.
33. Pfeifer-Ohlsson S, Goustin AS, Rydnert J, Wahlstrom T, Bjersing L, Shehelin D, Ohlsson R. Spatial and temporal pattern of cellular myc oncogene expression in developing human placenta: implications for embryonic cell proliferation. *Cell* 1984; **38**: 585-596.
34. Goustin AS, Betscholtz C, Pfeifer-Ohlsson S, Persson H, Rydnert J, Bywater M, Holmgren G, Heldin C-H, Westermark B, Ohlsson R. Coexpression of the *sis* and *myc* proto-oncogenes in developing human placenta suggests autocrine control of trophoblast growth. *Cell* 1985; **41**: 301-312.

Discussion

Chairman: Professor W. B. Robertson

Professor KENNEDY: Is anything known about the fate of those trophoblastic cells which migrate as far as the myometrium? What happens when parturition occurs?

Dr LOKE: I don't know, but my impression is that many of them become placental bed giant cells indicating that they are trying their best to become multinuclear like syncytiotrophoblasts, but they can't quite make it. In other words, they cannot quite achieve terminal differentiation and that is why these placental bed giant cells are non-productive, unlike syncytiotrophoblast, in spite of their multinuclear nature.

Professor ROBERTSON: The interesting thing is that they disappear about a week post-partum and where they go nobody knows; it is like asking where the flies go in winter.

Professor GILL: There is no answer to that question, but I would like to ask one of Dr Loke. Do I understand properly that when you stain the trophoblastic villus, that there are no W6/32 positive cells in the syncytiotrophoblast or the cytotrophoblast, but as the trophoblast migrates into the decidua and then into the myometrium there is a gradual transition of the staining so that they do stain for W6/32?

Dr LOKE: Yes.

Professor STIRRAT: In relation to that impression, one has got to be very careful nowadays in making claims about MHC status based on monoclonal antibody staining; one has really got to be able to show that the molecules are there or that the genes are there. I know that you have tried to do that, but that is what is required of us and it is extremely difficult. I think that more and more stringency, quite rightly, is required before one calls a cell MHC Class I or Class II positive because it shows such with a monoclonal antibody. You have really got to do the biochemistry or the gene probing.

The Decidua in Early Pregnancy

J. N. Bulmer, A. Ritson

INTRODUCTION

The decidua is the transformed stromal part of gestational endometrium. Endometrial stromal cells, which have been primed by oestrogen, enlarge and store glycogen under the influence of progesterone. Decidualisation occurs only in those species with haemochorial placentation and hence is likely to play a key role,[1] but despite various investigational approaches, the function of decidua remains unclear. Recent studies have focused on the possible role of decidua in maternal immune acceptance of the feto-placental unit. Immunohistochemical studies have allowed *in situ* characterisation of decidual cell populations throughout pregnancy. However, functional studies continue to be limited by poor documentation of cells under investigation.

DECIDUAL LEUCOCYTES IN EARLY HUMAN PREGNANCY

Decidualised endometrial stromal cells may be recognised without difficulty by their large size and glycogen content but distinction of other cell types in decidua is less clear. A wide range of monoclonal antibodies (mAbs) has been used to characterise leucocytic populations in human decidua. However, although specimens from elective pregnancy terminations and pregnancy hysterectomies are generally readily available, specimens from pregnancies of less than 6 weeks' menstrual age are rarely available and hence information about implantation and this crucial early phase of placental development remains scanty.

Two major leucocytic populations have been identified in first trimester human decidua. Macrophages are scattered throughout, with aggregates around spiral arteries and adjacent to endometrial glands.[2] They are often closely associated with extravillous trophoblast in decidua basalis.[3] The main phenotypic characteristics of decidual macrophages in early pregnancy are summarised in Table 1.[2-8] Macrophages are present in large numbers in decidua throughout pregnancy and they are also the predominant maternal leucocytic population at the ectopic implantation site in tubal pregnancy.[9]

The second major leucocyte population in early pregnancy decidua comprises lymphocytes. These have an unusual antigenic phenotype (summarised in Table 2)[5,10-12] and their distribution mirrors that of the so-called endometrial stromal granulocytes (EGs).[12,13,14] These latter cells are characterised by the presence of

Table 1

Phenotypic characteristics of dedicual macrophages

Antigen/mAb/enzyme	CD number	
Leucocyte common antigen	45	+
Leu-M3	14	+
Dako-macrophage		+
OKM1	11b	−
Leu-M1	15	−
HLA-DR		+
HLA-DP		+
HLA-DQ		+
p150,95	11c	+
OKT4	4	+
NA1/34	1	−
non-specific esterase		+
acid phosphatase		+

phloxinophilic cytoplasmic granules and are a prominent feature of late secretory phase endometrium and first-trimester decidua. Recent studies of formalin-fixed paraffin-embedded decidua and of decidua cell suspensions have provided good evidence that EGs are leucocytic cells, most probably within the spectrum of large granular lymphocytes (LGL).[12] Both EGs and decidual LGL (CD2+, CD3−,

Table 2

Phenotypic characteristics of dedicual granulated lymphocytes (endometrial granulocytes)

Antigen/mAb	CD number	
Leucocyte common antigen*	45	+
NA1/34, anti-leu-6	1	−
Dako-T11, anti-leu-5	2	+
UCHT1, OKT3	3	−
OKT4, anti-leu-3	4	−
Dako-T1, anti-leu-1	5	−
Dako-T2	7	+
Dako-T8, OKT8	8	−
OKT9 (transferrin receptor)		−
OKT10	38	+
anti-leu-7		−
anti-leu-11	16	−
NKH1		++
Class II MHC		−
interleukin 2 receptor	25	−
MT1*		+
UCHL1*		+

*mAbs applicable to formalin-fixed paraffin-embedded sections

NKH1++) are present in large numbers in decidua during the first trimester but thereafter decline. At term, classical CD2+, CD3+ T lymphocytes may be detected, but the unusual CD2+, CD3−, NKH1++ population cannot be identified. It is not known whether the EGs lose their cytoplasmic granules as pregnancy advances or whether the population is destroyed. Analogously the CD2+, CD3−, NKH1++ lymphocytes may acquire the CD3 antigen and lose the NKH1 antigen in later pregnancy, thus preventing their distinction from classical T lymphocytes.

KINETICS OF DECIDUAL LEUCOCYTE POPULATIONS

As already stated, decidual macrophages may be detected throughout pregnancy, whilst LGL are prominent only in the first trimester. Immunohistochemical studies of non-pregnant endometrium have provided some data about recruitment and differentiation of human endometrial leucocytes.[15,16,17] The results of our studies of 44 samples of normal non-pregnant human endometrium are summarised in Table 3.

Table 3

Leucocytes in non-pregnant human endometrium

	Macrophages	T cells (CD2+ CD3+)	'T lineage' cells (CD2+ CD3−) NKH1++
STRATUM BASALIS	++	++	−
STRATUM FUNCTIONALIS			
proliferative	+++	+	−
early secretory	+++	++	−
mid-secretory	+++	++	++
late secretory	+++	+	+++
EARLY PREGNANCY	+++	+	++++

Macrophages were present throughout the menstrual cycle and in post-menopausal endometrium. There was no apparent variation with cycle stage in our studies, although a pre-menstrual increase in endometrial macrophages has been reported.[16] In contrast, lymphocyte populations varied according to cycle stage. Classical T cells (CD2+, CD3+) were rare in proliferative endometrium but gradually increased in numbers in the early and mid-secretory phases. However, in late secretory phase endometrium, particularly in areas of predecidual change, classical T cells were scanty. An additional population of CD2+, CD3− lymphocytes was detected from the mid-secretory phase onwards, showing a substantial increase premenstrually. The distribution of these cells mirrors that of the EGs and these studies provide supportive evidence that they are granulated lymphocytes. It remains to be established whether there is influx of CD2+, CD3− lymphocytes from blood, or whether they differentiate *in situ*, either from primitive bone-marrow-derived precursors or from CD2+, CD3+ T cells which decline in numbers as the CD2+, CD3− cells increase. These remaining questions may be answered by *in vitro* decidualisation of endometrium obtained at various stages of the menstrual cycle.[18]

FUNCTIONAL ASPECTS OF DECIDUAL LEUCOCYTES

The function of the two major leucocyte populations in human decidua remains to be fully established. The presence of decidual macrophages throughout gestation suggests a fundamental role in normal pregnancy. The expression of Class II MHC antigens and their close association with extravillous trophoblast may indicate an immune function and first trimester human decidua has been shown to have antigen-presenting ability.[19] Suppressor function has also been attributed to macrophages in human[20] and murine[21] decidua mediated by secretion of prostaglandin E_2. However, the 'macrophages' in human decidua have not been fully characterised; populations under study are often impure and suppression has also been attributed to 'true' decidualised endometrial stromal cells.[20]

CD2+, CD3−, NKH1++ granulated lymphocytes are prominent in mid- and late-secretory phase endometrium and in first-trimester decidua. Thereafter, they decline in numbers and are scanty in the second half of pregnancy. This distribution suggests a role in implantation and early placental development. A soluble suppressor factor which blocks lymphocyte responses to interleukin 2 has been reported to be produced by a small granulated lymphocyte in murine decidua.[22] Both 'large' and 'small' suppressor cells have been detected in human decidua but the cells have not been characterised either morphologically or phenotypically.[23] In particular, 'large' cells could represent decidual macrophages, endometrial gland epithelium or decidual cells. The lack of phenotypic clarification of cells under investigation does not allow satisfactory correlation of results from different groups. Furthermore, different methods of tissue disaggregation and cell separation may yield varying cell populations. Our approach to functional studies of early human decidua has been to characterise cell populations by their surface antigenic phenotype so that functional data may be related to cell populations which have already been documented within decidual tissue sections.

1. Preparation of cell suspensions

Studies of the function of decidual cell types are largely dependent on preparation of cell suspensions from decidual tissue. Mechanical and enzymatic methods of preparation have been employed but the effect of the tissue dispersal method on the cellular composition of the resulting suspension has received little attention. Lala *et al*[20] used collagenase digestion for tissue disaggregation and reported that a large proportion of cells in human decidua expressed lympho-myeloid markers. A detailed study of the effect of dispersal technique on cell suspension composition[24] has shown that enzyme digestion preferentially selects for infiltrating bone marrow derived cells and does not reflect the proportion of cells in the intact tissue, an observation also made for murine decidua.[25] Mechanical disaggregation yields different results; suspensions obtained by sieving or teasing of decidual tissue are rich in decidualised stromal cells and contain only 25% bone-marrow-derived cells.[24] Thus, mechanically disaggregated suspensions contain cell proportions which are more representative of those in the intact tissue.

The dispersal method should thus be selected according to the type of cell required for study. It should also be noted, however, that the disaggregation method may alter cell function. Clark *et al*[26] have reported loss of suppressor function in lymphocytes isolated from early murine decidua using collagenase digestion as opposed to mechanical dispersal. However, the duration of enzyme treatment was not documented and the full significance of these results remains to be established.

2. Separation of decidual LGL

For meaningful functional studies of decidual cell populations, it is necessary to further fractionate cell suspensions to isolate individual cell types. We have developed a density gradient centrifugation method for the isolation of granulated lymphoid cells from human decidua.[27] The decidual tissue is minced and serially digested for 30 minutes with type II collagenase. The resulting cell suspension is cultured on plastic for one hour to remove adherent cells and then layered over a three step discontinuous Nycodenz gradient comprising 10 ml each of 5%, 10% and 20% Nycodenz (Nygaard, Denmark). The gradient is centrifuged at 1500g for 30 minutes. A broad band of cells is consistently obtained in the low density area of the gradient. Histochemical and immunocytochemical studies have shown that this band is enriched for granulated lymphocytes with up to 82% purity, as detected by Giemsa and toluidine blue staining and by the mAbs Dako T11 and NKH1.

3. In vitro functional assays

Decidual cell suspensions enriched for granulated lymphoid cells have been subjected to a variety of functional assays in an attempt to determine a physiological role in early pregnancy.

a) *Proliferation in response to mitogens*

Decidual cell suspension enriched for granulated lymphocytes (decidual LGL) were cultured with between 0 and 50 µg/ml PHA or ConA. Control peripheral blood lymphocytes (PBL) produced a good proliferative responses, as assessed by uptake of tritiated thymidine. Decidual LGL, however, showed no proliferative response to either mitogen. Decidual LGL and control PBL were then cultured with varying concentrations of recombinant interleukin-2 (IL2) both in the presence and absence of mitogen. Control PBL showed a good response to both mitogen and interleukin 2 but decidual LGL showed minimal response only at 200 HMU/ml IL-2 and above (less than 10% of the PBL response at 50 HMU/ml.

b) *Cytotoxicity assays*

Decidual LGL were also analysed for natural killer (NK) activity against the NK susceptible target cell K562. Unfractionated decidual cell suspensions, decidual LGL and peripheral blood lymphocytes were tested in a standard 18 hour ^{51}Cr release assay. Effector to target cell ratios ranged from 1:1 to 50:1. Decidual LGL showed cytotoxic activity at all effector:target ratios tested, the percentage of specific killing ranging from 12 to 35%. These semi-purified decidual LGL cells showed higher levels of killing than unfractionated decidual cell suspensions, thus implying that NK activity was confined to the EG population. However, unfractionated PBL showed higher levels of killing than either decidual cell populations, the specific killing ranging from 29% to 52%. Decidual granulated lymphocytes therefore possess NK activity but are relatively poor effectors in a K562 chromium release assay.

c) *Suppressor activity*

The suppressor activity of decidual lymphocytes has also been investigated. Unfractionated decidual cell suspensions, semi-purified decidual LGL and PBL were cultured for 24 hours at 2×10^6 cells/ml. The supernatants were collected and their effect on PBL response to mitogen assessed by culturing unrelated PBL at 1×10^6/ml with either 10 µg/ml PHA or 50 µg/ml Con A. Decidual LGL, unfractionated decidual cell, or PBL supernatant was then added to all except control cultures. The proliferative response of the PBL was assessed by tritiated thymidine uptake. A level of 'non specific' suppression was shown by the PBL supernatants. In all cases in which paired unfractionated decidual cell supernatants were tested in parallel with semi-purified decidual LGL, the unfractionated cell supernatant showed higher levels of suppression than the purified cell supernatant. The level of suppression due to the unfractionated decidual cells was significantly higher than 'non-specific' suppression due to PBL supernatants. However, semi-purified decidual LGL often failed to show significant suppression above the level shown by control PBL. Thus, it appears that suppressor activity is present within early human decidua but this suppression cannot be attributed solely or even principally to decidual granulated lymphocytes.

COMMENTS ON THE FUNCTION OF DECIDUAL GRANULATED LYMPHOCYTES

The distribution of granulated lymphoid cells within the uterine lining implies that they may play an important role in early pregnancy. Studies of abnormal pregnancies, particularly of recurrent spontaneous abortions are hampered by poor tissue preservation, although useful information could be obtained from immunocytochemical studies of suitably preserved tissues. Morphologically, decidual granulated lymphocytes resemble large granulated lymphocytes (LGL) and they also carry cell surface antigens, such as CD2, CD7 and OKT10, which are associated with NK cells.[10,15,28] They label very intensely with the NK cell marker NKH1[5] but decidual LGL fail to express the 'classical' NK cell markers Leu 11 (CD16), Leu 7 or OKM1 (CD11b).[5,10] Decidual LGL do not proliferate in response to PHA or Con A. This is another feature of NK cells, but in contrast with classical NK cells, decidual LGL do not respond to high dose IL-2. The intense labelling with NKH1 is an interesting feature of decidual LGL. Lanier *et al*[29] recently reported a small sub-population of peripheral blood LGL which was also intensely NKH1-positive but CD16 negative. These cells were poor effectors in a K562 chromium release assay, as we have found for decidual LGL. Alterations in the phenotype, proportions and function of certain NK cell subsets in the peripheral blood of pregnant women have been reported.[30] NK cell activity has also been reported in decidua from early murine pregnancy.[31] It is possible that decidual LGL represent a type of NK cell, possibly a developing cell population.

Suppressor activity has long been ascribed to human decidual tissue.[32] In our studies, culture supernatants from unfractionated decidual cells have been more suppressive than those from semi-purified decidual LGL. Culture supernatants from explants of the same specimens of first trimester human decidua used to prepare cell suspensions have been shown to exhibit profound suppression of PBL mitogen responses (Ritson & Bulmer, unpublished observations). This pattern of suppressive activity, present in undispersed fragments of decidua, to a lesser extent in decidual cell suspensions and often absent in semi-purified decidual LGL, could be explained if suppression were due to decidualised endometrial stromal cells which are largely absent from the purified decidual LGL and present in relatively small numbers in the enzymatically-dispersed unfractionated decidual cell suspensions. It is also conceivable that the preservation of cellular relationships is necessary for suppression to occur, hence explaining the higher levels shown by explant supernatants. The diminished suppressor activity exhibited by unfractionated decidual cell suspensions and purified lymphocytes could also be due to the effects of tissue dispersal by collagenase digestion.[26] However, the serial digest technique should minimise cell damage due to enzyme[24] and Clark *et al*[26] failed to document the duration of exposure to collagenase or other enzymes. Nevertheless, the problem of the effect of dispersal techniques on cell function requires careful consideration and merits further investigation.

Several groups have investigated suppressor activity of cell populations in human decidua. Daya *et al*[23] and Clark *et al*[33] reported 'large' and 'small' suppressor cells in both human and murine decidua. These cells have not been fully characterised, although they are claimed to be lymphocytes. Suppressor activity has also been attributed to other cells in human and murine decidua. Lala *et al*[20] reported suppressor activity in populations of decidual macrophages, an observation also made by Tawfik *et al*.[21]These groups also detected suppressor activity in large decidual stromal cells. In both cases the activity was found to be partially removed by indomethacin and therefore was attributed to prostaglandin E_2. In addition, the cells were found to mediate suppressive mechanisms other than prostaglandin, which were not affected by indomethacin. The possibility that endometrial gland epithelial cells may be responsible for immunosuppressive effects also merits consideration. Supernatants produced by short term culture of epithelial cells separated from non-pregnant human endometrium have been reported to inhibit mixed lymphocyte reactivity.[34] The functional activity of epithelial cells in decidualised endometrium in early pregnancy has not been investigated, although endometrial epithelial cells may constitute a contaminating cell in studies of other cell types.

CONCLUSIONS

It appears from our studies and those of other groups that decidual tissue in early human pregnancy is capable of mediating suppressor function. However, the cell type responsible for this suppression remains to be established with certainty; this will be achieved only by careful phenotypic and morphological characterisation of cells under study. The problems of the variable cell populations yielded by different dispersal techniques and the effect of enzymatic digestion on cell function also require a systematic approach.

Despite the enormous progress which has been made in recent years, there remains a gap in our knowledge of endometrial cell populations and their function in the earliest stages of pregnancy. We have little idea of the fundamental differences which must exist between endometrium in the last week of a normal cycle and endometrium when conception and implantation have occurred. Despite progress in the treatment of recurrent spontaneous miscarriage,[35,36] there is a deficiency of information regarding local intrauterine and placental changes accompanying such pregnancy loss. A similar dearth of data is available for the endometrial changes accompanying very early pregnancy loss within a week or two of implantation. Furthermore, our knowledge of normal endometrial leucocyte populations could be applied to investigation of endometrium in primary unexplained infertility in which a deficiency of E-rosette receptor bearing lymphocytes has been reported.[37] Understanding of the local immune mechanisms which may mediate successful pregnancy has been expanded. Similar techniques should now be applied to pregnancy abnormalities.

ACKNOWLEDGEMENTS

This work was supported by grants from Yorkshire Regional Health Authority and Birthright.

REFERENCES
1. Robertson WB. *The Endometrium*. London: Butterworths Press, 1981; pp.7-44.
2. Bulmer JN, Johnson PM. Macrophage populations in the human placenta and amniochorion. *Clin Exp Immunol* 1984; **57**: 393-403.
3. Bulmer JN, Smith J, Morrison L, Wells, M. Maternal and fetal cellular relationships in the human placental basal plate. *Placenta* 1987; In press.
4. Bulmer JN, Morrison L, Smith JC. Expression of class II MHC gene products by macrophages in human uteroplacental tissue. *Immunol* 1987; In press.
5. Ritson A, Bulmer JN. Endometrial granulocytes in human decidua react with a natural killer cell marker, NKH1. *Immunol* 1987; In press.
6. Sutton L, Mason DY, Redman CWG. HLA-DR positive cells in the human placenta. *Immunology* 1983; **49**: 103-112.
7. Kabawat SE, Mostoufi-Zadeh M, Driscoll SG, Bhan AK. Implantation site in normal pregnancy. A study with monoclonal antibodies. *Am J Pathol* 1985; **118**: 76-84.
8. Nehemiah JL, Schnitzer JA, Schulman H, Novikoff AB. Human chorionic trophoblasts, decidual cells and macrophages: a histochemical and electron microscopic study. *Am J Obstet Gynecol* 1981; **140**: 261-268.
9. Earl U, Lunny DP, Bulmer JN. Leucocyte populations in ectopic tubal pregnancy. *J Clin Pathol* 1987; **40**: 901-905.
10. Bulmer JN, Sunderland CA. Immunohistological characterization of lymphoid populations in the early human placental bed. *Immunology* 1984; **52**: 349-357.
11. Bulmer JN, Johnson PM. The T-lymphocyte population in first-trimester human decidua does not express the interleukin-2 receptor. *Immunology* 1986; **58**: 685-687.

12. Bulmer JN, Hollings D, Ritson A. Immunocytochemical evidence that endometrial stromal granulocytes are granulated lymphocytes. *J Path* 1987; In press.
13. Bulmer JN, Hagin SV, Browne CM, Billington WD. Localization of immunoglobulin-containing cells in human endometrium in the first trimester of pregnancy and throughout the menstrual cycle. *Eur J Obstet Gynecol Reprod Biol* 1986; **23:** 31-44.
14. Dallenbach-Hellweg G. *Histopathology of the endometrium.* Berlin: Springer-Verlag, 1981; pp.22-88.
15. Bulmer JN, Johnson PM, Bulmer D. Leucocyte populations in human decidua and endometrium. In: *Immunoregulation and fetal survival.* Eds. TG Gill III, TG Wegman. New York: Oxford University Press, 1987; pp.111-134.
16. Kamut BR, Isaacson PG. The immunocytochemical distribution of leucocytic subpopulations in human endometrium. *Am J Pathol* 1987; **127:** 66-73.
17. Morris H, Edwards J, Tiltman A, Emms M. Endometrial lymphoid tissue: an immunohistological study. *J Clin Pathol* 1985; **38:** 644-652.
18. Daly DC, Maslar IA, Riddick DH. Prolactin production during *in vitro* decidualization of proliferative endometrium. *Am J Obstet Gynecol* 1983; **145:** 672-678.
19. Oksenberg JR, Mor Yosef S, Persitz E, Schenker Y, Mozes E, Brautbar C. Antigen-presenting cells in human decidual tissue. *Am J Reprod Immunol Microbiol* 1986; **11:** 82-88.
20. Lala PK, Parchar RS, Kearns M, Johnson S, Scodras JM. Immunologic aspects of the decidual response. In: *Reproductive Immunology 1986.* Eds. DA Clark, BA Croy. Amsterdam: Elsevier Science Publishers, 1986; pp.190-198.
21. Tawfik OW, Hunt JS, Wood GW. Implication of prostaglandin E_2 in soluble factor-mediated immune suppression by murine decidual cells. *Am J Reprod Immunol Microbiol* 1986; **12:** 111-117.
22. Clark DA, Slapsys R, Croy BA, Krcek J, Rossant J. Local active suppression by suppressor cells in the decidua: a review. *Am J Reprod Immunol* 1984; **5:** 78-83.
23. Daya S, Clark DA, Devlin C, Jarrell J, Chaput A. Suppressor cells in human decidua. *Am J Obstet Gynecol* 1985; **151:** 267-270.
24. Ritson A, Bulmer JN. Extraction of leucocytes from human decidua: a comparison of dispersal techniques. *J Immunol Methods* 1987; In press.
25. Gambel P, Rossant J, Hunziker RD, Wegmann TG. Origin of decidual cells in murine pregnancy and pseudopregnancy. *Transplantation* 1985; **39:** 443-445.
26. Clark DA, Brierly J, Slapsys R, Daya S, Damji N, Chaput A, Rosenthal K. Trophoblast dependent and trophoblast independent suppressor cells of maternal origin in murine and human decidua. In: *Reproductive Immunology 1986.* Eds. DA Clark, BA Croy. Amsterdam: Elsevier Science Publishers, 1986; pp.219-226.
27. Ritson A, Bulmer JN. The isolation and characterisation of granulated lymphocytes from first trimester human decidua. Submitted.
28. Reynolds CW, Ortaldo JR. Natural killer activity: the definition of a function rather than a cell type. *Immunol Today* 1987; **8:** 172-174.
29. Lanier LL, Le AM, Civin CI, Loken MR, Phillips JH. The relationship of CD16 (Leu 11) and Leu 19 (NKH-1) antigen expression on human peripheral blood NK cells and cytotoxic T lymphocytes. *J Immunol* 1986; **136:** 4480-4486.
30. Gregory CD, Lee H, Scott IV, Golding PR. Phenotypic heterogeneity and recycling capacity of natural killer cells in normal human pregnancy. *J Reprod Immunol* 1987; **11:** 135-145.
31. Croy BA, Gambel P, Rossant J, Wegmann TG. Characterization of murine decidual natural killer [2](NK) cells and their relevance to the success of pregnancy. *Cell Immunol* 1985; **93:** 315-326.
32. Golander G, Zakuth V, Shechter Y, Spirer Z. Suppression of lymphocyte reactivity *in vitro* by a soluble factor secreted by explants of human decidua. *Eur J Immunol* 1981; **11:** 849-851.

33. Clark DA, Chaput A. Local intrauterine suppressor cells and suppressor factors in survival of the fetal allograft. In: *Reproductive Immunology: Materno-Fetal Relationship*. Ed. G Chaouat. Paris: INSERM, 1987; pp.77-88.
34. Johnson PM, Risk JM, Bulmer JN, Niewola Z, Kimber I. Antigen expression at maternofetal interfaces. In: *Immunoregulation and Fetal Survival*. Eds. TJ Gill III, TG Wegmann. New York: Oxford University Press, 1987; pp.181-196.
35. Mowbray JF, Underwood JL. Immunisation with paternal cells for recurrent spontaneous abortion. In: *Reproductive Immunology: Materno-Fetal Relationship*. Ed: G Chaouat. Paris: INSERM. 1987; pp.179-186.
36. Beer AE, Shekar SS, Quebbeman JF, Zhu X. Paternal and non-paternal leucocyte immunisation in women with recurrent spontaneous abortions: immune responses and subsequent pregnancy outcome. In: *Reproductive Immunology: Materno-Fetal Relationship*. Ed. G Chaouat. Paris: INSERM, 1987; pp.161-178.
37. Soffer Y, Caspi E, Weinstein Y. Endometrial cell mediated immunity and contraception: new perspectives. In: *Immunological factors in human contraception*. Field Educational Italia Acta Medica, 1983; pp.161-167.

Discussion

Chairman: Professor W. B. Robertson

Dr BELL: This granulated cell type, that is defined by Cesar Marcus, is it found in any other part of the body, particularly in mammary glands, where you get involution and re-epithelialisation? As fas as I remember, these cells, in terms of their appearance, seem to be associated with a period of involution, particularly growth and involution, and re-epithelialisation in the endometrium. Is it a question, perhaps of looking for suppressive action of these cells that may actually be associated with the fate of the glandular epithelium, and in that respect they may be found in other tissues?

Dr BULMER: They haven't been reported in other tissues, and I haven't had a chance to look for them in other tissues, but I do think you are probably right that they don't have very much to do with suppression or killing, and that anything we can detect like that may not actually be what their role is *in vivo*.

Dr BELL: In your slide you show the cells evenly distributed but is there in your experience an association with the involuted glandular structures?

Dr BULMER: They tend to aggregate around vessels and this aggregation has been taken to mean that they are either coming out from vessels, or they are cells responding to something coming out from the vessels. However, they are found also in the aggregates of lymphocytes which are seen around glands, so they could well have something to do with glandular activity.

Professor SZULMAN: Dr Bulmer, I wonder whether you take into account the fact that decidual tissue is very prone to necrosis, and that in every normal pregnancy there will be areas of necrosis, which are more common than non-pathologists realise, and a good deal of what one sees in the way of lymphocytic and macrophagic reaction may simply be in response to the necrosis. Not only do you find necrosis at the time of implantation, but also throughout pregnancy and some of the necrotic areas are quite big holes.

Dr BULMER: I have thought of that. The granulated cell population is well known to be present in the second half of the cycle and in early pregnancy and is not specifically related to areas of necrosis. In fact, in areas of necrosis the cells are conspicuous by their absence. It may well be, and this is the problem of studying any spontaneous abortion by any of these techniques, that you just don't know whether or not you see is just an infiltrating cytotoxic population. All I can say is that these are normal pregnancies but we can't guarantee that there is no necrosis but when you look at the tissues you see no evidence that these granulated cells are in any way related to areas of necrosis. I have examined also several intact implantations.

Professor SZULMAN: May the cells be on the way to the area of implantation?

Dr BULMER: Well in that case why do you see them in the late secretary phase of the cycle where they are well described and why would you then not see them after the first trimester when they decline but you still see necrosis?

Professor SZULMAN: I am not speaking of complete and total necrosis, but I wondered if this were not part of the complicated latticework.

Early pregnancy failure: biochemical and biophysical assessment

J. G. Grudzinskas, I. Stabile and S. Campbell

INTRODUCTION

Vaginal bleeding and abdominal pain occur commonly in the first trimester, clinically presenting as threatened miscarriage (TMC) or suspected ectopic pregnancy. Threatened miscarriage is estimated to occur in up to 25 percent of all pregnancies, an incidence which has remained unaltered for decades.[1,2] Vaginal examination to assess the state of the cervix may permit an immediate diagnosis of evolving miscarriage if the cervix is dilated, but if the cervix is closed, the duration and extent of bleeding is notoriously unreliable in predicting the outcome of these pregnancies.[3] Evaluation of hormones and proteins produced by the placenta such as human chorionic gonadotrophin (hCG) and human placental lactogen (hPL), by the *corpus luteum* such as oestradiol (E2) and progesterone (P), and by the fetus such as alphafetoprotein (AFP) have not contributed greatly to improving diagnostic precision because of the overlap in values of these substances in normal and abnormal pregnancies. The introduction of, firstly, static B-scanning, and later real-time ultrasonography have made it possible to determine reliably the presence of a live fetus after six weeks' gestation and hence alter the clinical management of women with TMC.[5] If fetal life is confirmed ultrasonically in the first trimester, 95 to 98 percent of these women will progress to normal outcome of pregnancy.[6] The risk of spontaneous miscarriage increases with maternal age and decreases with advancing gestational age.[7,8] We have evaluated the usefulness of high-resolution abdominal ultrasound examination[9] in addition to the measurement of hormones and proteins of placental origin[10] in a cohort of women with vaginal bleeding and abdominal pain in early pregnancy.

CLINICAL ASPECTS

In 158 of the 624 women studied we failed to find any clinical, biochemical or ultrasonic evidence of pregnancy, the most common diagnoses being follicular/luteal cysts (n=32), and pelvic inflammatory disease (n=26). Abnormalities were not detected in the remaining 100 women whose symptoms settled spontaneously. Pregnancy was confirmed at ultrasound examination in 466 patients; Table 1 summarises the clinical outcome of these patients. In 60 women a diagnosis of

Table 1
Clinical outcome in study group (N=466)

	Number (percent)
Intrauterine pregnancy:	406
Normal progress beyond 20 weeks	227 (48.7)
Elective termination of pregnancy	26 (5.6)
Subsequent spontaneous abortion	6 (1.3)
Anembryonic pregnancy	67 (14.4)
Complete abortion	4 (0.9)
Incomplete abortion	41 (8.8)
Missed abortion	34 (7.3)
Hydatidiform mole	1 (0.2)
Extrauterine pregnancy:	60
Tubal	58 (12.4)
Ovarian	1 (0.2)
Cornual	1 (0.2)

ectopic pregnancy was made. A live fetus of normal size for gestational age was identified in 259 of the 406 women with threatened miscarriage, of whom 10% requested termination of their pregnancy. In 227 of the remaining 233 women the pregnancies continued uneventfully beyond 26 weeks gestation.

ULTRASONIC OBSERVATIONS
The ultrasonic findings at first presentation in this group of 406 women are summarised in Table 2. It is noteworthy that ultrasound was accurate in the prediction of the diagnosis at first presentation and the subsequent course of pregnancy in all but 4 of the 6 women who aborted a live fetus, and 2 of 4 with a low-lying placenta. In the women with anembryonic pregnancies the absence of a fetal pole was noted at first presentation. However, in 10 women a repeat examination, considered necessary because a gestational sac volume of less than 2.5 ml was noted, confirmed the diagnosis a week later. This condition was confirmed by the absence of fetal or embryonic parts at subsequent histological examination.

Table 2
Ultrasound observations at first U/S examination in 406 women with intrauterine pregnancy and vaginal bleeding

	Number	(Normal outcome %)
Live fetus appropriate size	189	(97.4)
Second empty sac	16	(100.0)
Intrauterine haematoma	22	(100.0)
Low lying placenta	4	(50.0)
Elective TOP	26	(0)
Anembryonic (gestational sac ≥ 2.5 ml)	67	(0)
Crumpled fetus with no FH	34	(0)
Oligohydramnios	2	(0)
Hydatidiform mole	1	(0)
Thick irregular echoes in the uterine cavity	41	(0)
Endometrial echoes not seen	4	(0)

Figure I

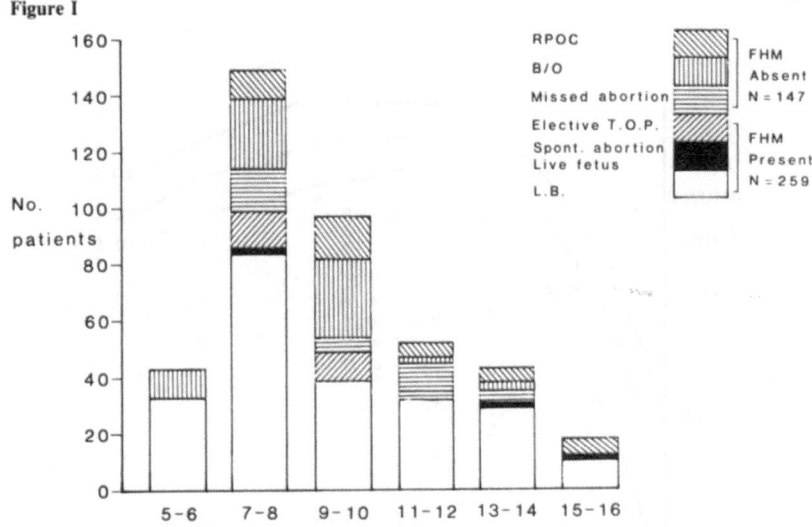

Gestational age in weeks

Pregnancy outcome and the detection of fetal life in 406 women with intrauterine pregnancy complaining of painless vaginal bleeding in relation to the gestational age. (RPOC, retained products of conception; B/O blighted ovum; TOP, termination of pregnancy; LB, live birth; FHM, fetal heart movement).

Figure I demonstrates the state of the pregnancy in 406 women with threatened miscarriage at the time of the first ultrasound examination in relation to pregnancy outcome. Once a live pregnancy had been demonstrated, other abnormalities were looked for that could possibly account for the bleeding. These abnormalities fell into two groups. In 16 women a second empty gestational sac (double sac), which was always smaller than the first, could be seen. In 22 women an intrauterine haematoma could be seen. The volumes of the haematoma, which were determined weekly varied from 0.7 to 16 ml, and were not followed by miscarriage. Oligohydramnios was evident in two women before 13 weeks' gestation. Both of these patients aborted in the second trimester, at 23 and 25 weeks respectively.

HORMONE AND PROTEIN MEASUREMENTS

Serum hCG levels in the women with anembryonic pregnancy are shown in Figure II. Fifty-eight of the 61 women in whom hCG measurements were assessed before 13 weeks, had a depressed hCG level (<10th centile) at the time of their ultrasound scan. Similarly 9 of the 15 patients scanned at or before 7 weeks had depressed SP1 levels. However, up to 15 weeks' gestation, 27 patients with anembryonic pregnancy had normal SP1 levels, depressed or absent SP1 levels being seen in the remaining 50 women. Serum PAPP-A levels were depressed in 49 of the 67 women.

Figure II

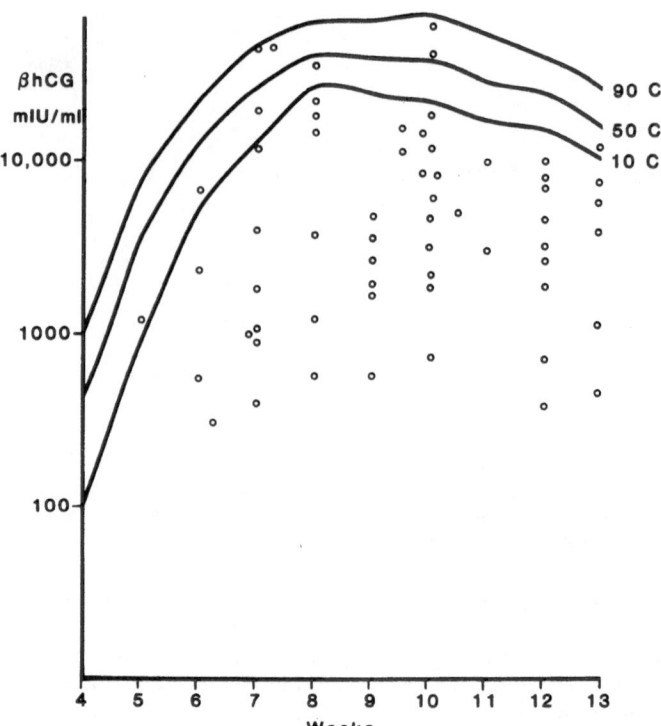

hCG measurements in 61 of the 67 patients with anembryonic pregnancy studied at 5 to 13
weeks' gestation (o), superimposed on the normal range (10th, 50th and 90th centiles
determined from 488 samples in 227 patients with TMC and normal outcome of pregnancy).
A further 6 patients at more than 14 weeks' gestation are not shown here.

Since ultrasound can reliably diagnose all cases of anembryonic pregnancy after
7 weeks' gestation (or when the gestational sac is 2.5 ml), hCG and SP1
measurements obtained before this time were analysed in the assessment of the
prognostic value of this test. Considering only the samples taken at or before 7
weeks' gestation (Table 3), the sensitivity and predictive value positive of a

Table 3

Circulating hCG, and SP1 in the prediction of
anembryonic pregnancy prior to 7 weeks (N=15)

	Sensitivity (%)	PV Pos (%)	PV Neg (%)
Depressed but detectable hCG	66.6	66.6	97.8
Depressed or absent SP1	60.0	56.3	97.3

depressed but detectable hCG level was 66%, while a normal result excluded this condition in 97.8% of cases. The sensitivity of a depressed or absent SP1 level was 60% and the predictive value of an abnormal result for an anembryonic pregnancy was 56%. The predictive value negative was 97.3%.

Figure III

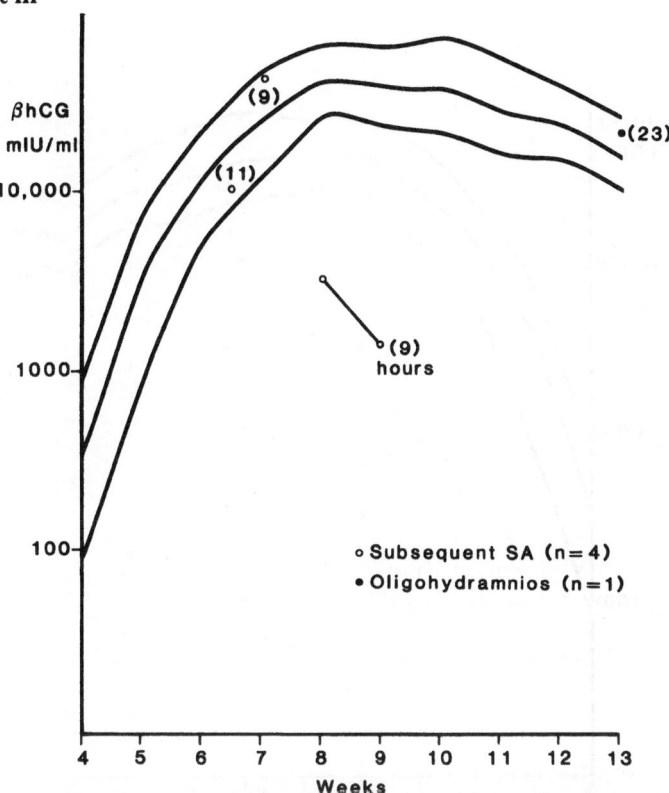

hCG measurements in 4 of the 6 women who aborted during the first trimester superimposed on the normal range (10th, 50th and 90th centiles determined from 488 samples in 227 patients with TMC and normal outcome of pregnancy). The remaining 2 women were sampled after 16 weeks (results not shown). In one patient aborting a few hours later falling hCG levels are noted.

Four of the 6 women who subsequently aborted had hCG estimations performed during the first trimester of pregnancy (Figure III). The other two women were scanned and sampled after 16 weeks. Only one patient had depressed hCG levels (also depressed PAPP-A, but normal SP1). All 6 patients who subsequently aborted had normal SP1 levels including the two women with oligohydramnios noted at ultrasound examination. PAPP-A levels were normal in all but one patient (who also had low hCG levels), who aborted a few hours after the scan had demonstrated a live fetus. Falling levels were noted in one patient, who aborted two hours after the blood sample was taken. The time interval from the final blood sample and scan prior to abortion ranged from 2 to 10 weeks in the remaining four patients. In each case normal PAPP-A levels were seen.

Figure IV

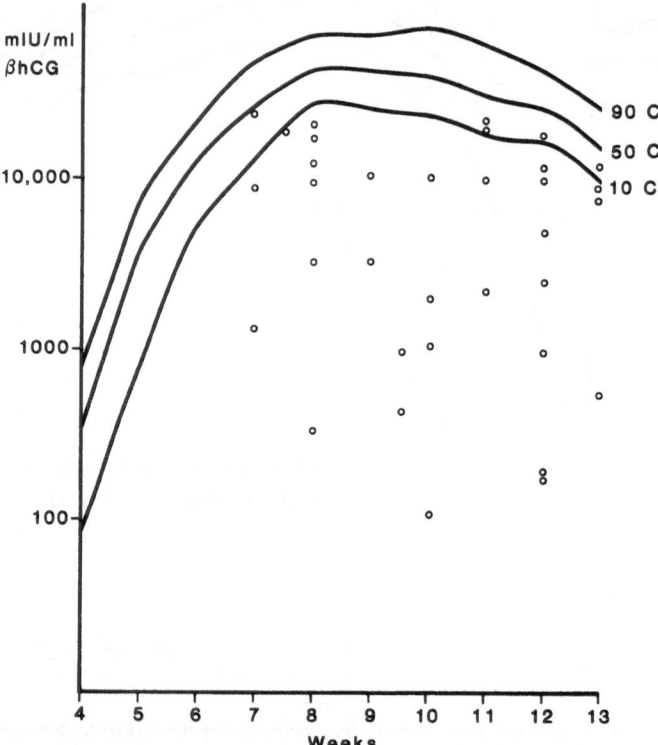

hCG measurements in 34 patients with a missed abortion studied at 7 to 13 weeks gestation superimposed on the normal range (10th, 50th and 90th centiles determined from 488 samples in 227 patients with TMC and normal outcome of pregnancy).

Serum hCG levels in 34 women with missed abortion are shown in Figure IV. All but five patients had depressed levels of hCG (<10th centile), but the levels were always above 100 IU/l at the time of presentation. Similar observations were made with respect to PAPP-A levels, whereas only 56% of the patients had depressed SP1 values.

Figure V

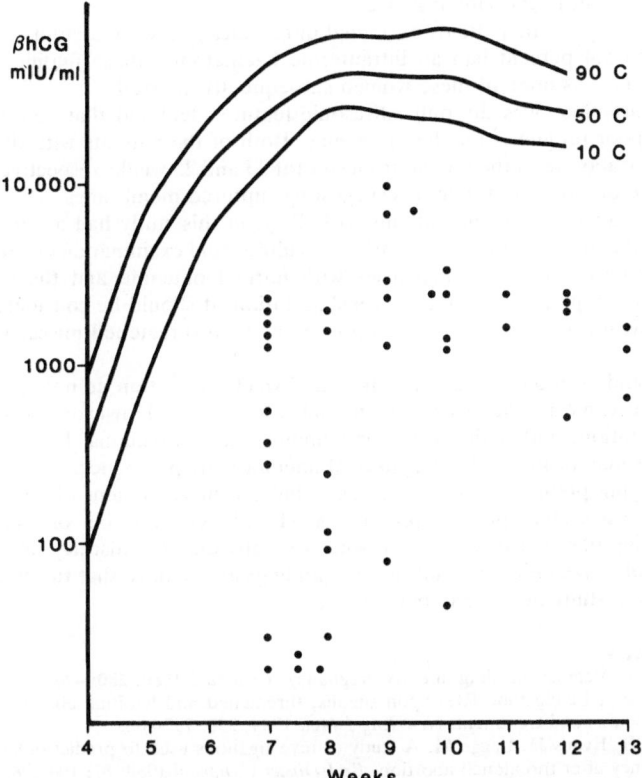

hCG measurements in 41 women with an incomplete abortion superimposed on the normal range (10th, 50th and 90th centiles determined from 488 samples in 227 patients with TMC and normal outcome of pregnancy). The 4 patients with a complete abortion are not shown here.

Circulating levels of hCG in women with complete (N=4) and incomplete miscarriage (N=41) are shown in Figure V. All patients had depressed but detectable levels of hCG (<10th centile). Similar findings were observed with respect to PAPP-A, whereas 7 of the patients had normal circulating SP1 levels.

DISCUSSION

Our prospective study provides guidelines for the role of ultrasonography and hormonal measurements in the differential diagnosis and management of women with vaginal bleeding and pain in early pregnancy. Pregnancy will continue in about half the women who present with bleeding in the first trimester, 7 to 10 weeks' gestation being the commonest time for such women to present. It is noteworthy that spontaneous abortion, once a live fetus has been identified, is an uncommon event in this circumstance.

In 3.9 percent of the patients examined ultrasonically a second empty sac was present and 5.4 percent had an intrauterine haematoma, these findings being benign features as none of these women subsequently aborted.

Oligohydramnios was the only ultrasonic feature identified that consistently predicted poor prognosis for the pregnancy. Both of the patients with this rare abnormality aborted in the second trimester (at 23 and 25 weeks respectively), in the absence of any clinical features suggesting ruptured membranes.

Overall, 36 percent of the patients with TMC in this study had a non-viable pregnancy diagnosed at first presentation. As ultrasound examination can reliably distinguish between most pregnancies with normal outcome and the complications of early pregnancy after 7 weeks' gestation, it should be considered the primary investigation for any women presenting with threatened miscarriage at this time.

Protein and hormone measurements after 7 weeks' gestation do not appear to provide the clinician with useful additional information. However, prior to 7 weeks' gestation, and if the ultrasound findings are ambiguous, hCG or SP1 estimations may facilitate the diagnosis of anembryonic pregnancy.

Encouraging preliminary results suggest that the measurement of circulating pregnancy associated plasma protein A (PAPP-A) may be of value in distinguishing between those women who will subsequently miscarry and those who will not.[4] We failed to confirm these findings and believe that this is due to differences in study design and patient selection.

REFERENCES
1. Editorial: Vaginal bleeding in early pregnancy. *Br Med J* 1980; **280:** 470.
2. Hertig AT, Livingstone RG. Spontaneous, threatened and habitual abortion: their pathogenesis and treatment. *New Eng J Med* 1944; **230:** 797-806.
3. Duff GB, Evans JJ, Legge M. A study of investigations used to predict outcome of pregnancy after threatened abortion. *Br J Obstet Gynaecol* 1980; **87:** 194-198.
4. Westergaard JG, Teisner B, Sinosich MJ, Madsen LT, Grudzinskas JG. Does ultrasound examination render biochemical tests obsolete in the prediction of early pregnancy failure? *Br J Obstet Gynaecol* 1985; **92:** 77-83.
5. Mantoni M. Ultrasound signs in threatened abortion and their prognostic significance. *Obstet Gynecol* 1985; **65:** 471-475.
6. Christiaens CG, Stoutenbeek P. Spontaneous abortion in proven intact pregnancies. *Lancet* 1984; **2:** 571-572.
7. Wilson RD, Kendrick V, Wittmann BK, McGillivray B. Spontaneous abortion and pregnancy outcome after normal first-trimester ultrasound examination. *Obstet Gynecol* 1986; **67:** 352-355.
8. Gilmore DH, McNay MB. Spontaneous fetal loss rate in early pregnancy. *Lancet* 1984; **2:** 107.
9. Stabile I, Campbell S, Grudzinskas JG. Ultrasonic assessment of complications during first trimester of pregnancy. *Lancet* 1987; **2:** 1237-1240.
10. Stabile I, Campbell S, Grudzinskas JG. Ultrasound and circulating placental protein measurements in complications of early pregnancy. *Br J Obstet Gynaecol*; In press.

Discussion

Chairman: Professor W. B. Robertson

Dr ALLEN: Are you suggesting, or do your data not indicate, that it is necessary to have a viable fetus for the production of a polypeptide hormone by the placenta, hCG as an example, or, indeed, any of the other hormones you were talking about? To put it another way, is the placenta, where there is a blighted embryo, as extensive as one would expect were there an embryo there before abortion occurs?

Professor GRUDZINSKAS: Our evidence seems to imply that if the fetus or embryo plays any role in the synthesis of hormones, or of proteins of unknown functions, it would do so only in the earliest weeks of pregnancy. The levels are apparently in the normal range for such pregnancies until about seven or eight weeks. Thereafter, when the pregnancy is anembryonic the levels start to fade out to below the tenth centile. Protein synthesis or hCG synthesis, for example, in the earliest weeks, in the first third or quarter of pregnancy, might be entirely independent of the presence of the embryo or fetus. Alternately, the embryo or fetus is there, albeit developing abnormally, and its trophic effect on the trophoblast diminishes as it undergoes resorption. But, the embryo or fetus is not necessary for hCG synthesis by the placenta, as evidenced by trophoblastic disease where there are very high levels of hCG.

Dr ALLEN: That is what was bothering me.

Professor SZULMAN: Would the speaker care to speculate briefly on what actually precipitates the exfoliation of the conceptus?

Professor GRUDZINSKAS: I am persuaded by the classical literature which would suggest that the primary cause of failure of pregnancy is some sort of gross deficiency of the embryo or fetus. I am still to be persuaded that it should be anything other than some sort of karyotypic abnormality.

Professor SZULMAN: What I actually mean is why is it that the fetus dies at six weeks and exfoliation takes place at twelve, thirteen, fourteen of fifteen weeks?

Professor GRUDZINSKAS: I am sorry. As far as anembryonic pregnancy or blighted ova are concerned, I think that we have hinted already that the placenta can be a law unto itself. It can function, at least in a limited capacity, independently and a mole is a good example of this. As far as missed abortion is concerned, from a clinical impression only, in the majority of women in whom the embryo or fetus has perished expulsion of the dead embryo or fetus occurs soon after that.

Professor SZULMAN: Well, it is surprising that in my experience how late expulsion does occur; four, five, six or seven weeks is quite common and, as I will try to show tomorrow, in partial mole it can be anything from ten to fifteen weeks which to me is astonishing.

Dr RUSHTON: That is exactly the point I was making, that in the long-retained ones they develop maternal floor infarction which is a progressive condition which actually obliterates the intervillous space.

Professor SZULMAN: In some.

Dr RUSHTON: Yes, in some. It is a matter of the conceptus surviving long enough to do this and I look upon it as a natural mechanism which makes the placenta rigid and also reduces the blood supply to the intervillous space. So, when the conceptus is expelled the mother is protected, if you look upon spontaneous abortion as a natural process as I tend to do, in getting rid of an abnormal pregnancy. There has been one study to show that there is a risk of developing afibrinogenaemia from a pregnancy that is retained for too long. On the other hand, if the placenta is retained longer the amount of bleeding on delivery is less than when either a recently-dead or fresh conceptus is delivered.

Haemostasis and fibrinolysis in human normal placentae: possible role in early pregnancy failure

W. Page Faulk

INTRODUCTION

For many years it has been known that blood clotting is a cardinal feature of placental histology.[1] No reasonable explanation ever has been put forward for the abundant presence of fibrin in and around chorionic villi.[2] Similarly, no mechanism has been advanced to explain what either initiates or controls placental haemostasis[3] and no data have been produced to indicate that specific fibrinolytic enzyme systems are involved. Nonetheless, it generally is accepted that haemostasis[4] and fibrinolysis[5] are necessary reactions to establish and maintain normal placentation.[6]

The purpose of this investigation was to utilise specific antibodies by means of immunohistological techniques to determine if key components of the haemostatic and fibrinolytic systems were identifiable in normal human placentae. In addition, antibodies to the recently described Protein C anticoagulant pathway were used to study a possible control mechanism of haemostasis within placental tissues. The results provide convincing data that all three systems of haemostasis, fibrinolysis and Protein C pathways are involved in human normal placentation. This puts forward the testable hypothesis that imbalances in these interacting systems could contribute to abnormal placentation. This hypothesis is presently being tested.

MATERIALS AND METHODS

Characteristics of the antibodies used in this investigation are listed in Table 1. Western blot analysis, various immunoassays and functional tests were used to assess the specificity of all antibodies. The study was performed on twenty normal spontaneously delivered placentae. Studies on tissues obtained by caesarean section, and from premature and pathological deliveries will be reported in a separate publication. The intention of this present report is to detail the location and distribution of certain haemostatic and fibrinolytic factors in normal term placentae delivered spontaneously. The immunohistological reaction procedures have been described in detail elsewhere.[7] Briefly, biopsies were taken midway

193

through the central codyledon and snap frozen in liquid nitrogen. Sections were prepared with the use of a cryostat and air dried. No fixation was used.

Table 1

Antibodies used in this investigation

Anti-	Commercial Source	Species	Specificity test
C3c	Cytotech	Mouse	Immunochemical
VII	Behring	Rabbit[1]	Western blot
IX	Hybritech	Mouse	Functional test
X	Nordic	Rabbit	Western blot
Thrombin[2]	American Dx	Mouse	ELISA
Fibrinogen	Chemicon	Mouse	ELISA
Fragment D	Behring	Rabbit	Immunoelectrophoresis
Protein C	American Dx	Mouse	Immunochemical
Plasminogen	Dakopatts	Rabbit	ELISA
α_2-plasmin inhibitor	American Dx	Mouse	ELISA
Rabbit IgG	Protos	F(ab')$_2$ Goat FITC conjugate	ELISA
Mouse IgG	Protos	F(ab')$_2$ Goat RITC conjugate	ELISA

[1]Rabbit antibodies were used for double antibody experiments; for example, when C3c was studied with Factor VII or when fibrinogen was studied with Fragment D. Otherwise, the corresponding monoclonal was used.

[2]Two epitopes were studied: EST-1 (a neoantigen made available by antithrombin III binding) and EST-4 (an antigen blocked by antithrombin III binding).

The microscopy techniques used in this study have been previously described.[8] Use was made of epi-illumination and interference optics.[9] A Leitz microscope fitted with an HBO 100 mercury-arc lamp was used. The microscope contained a FITC filter complex (I-2) consisting of a 450-490 nm excitation filter, 510 nm dichroic mirror, and 515 nm barrier filter which allowed greater than 515 nm to pass. There was also a RITC filter complex (N2.1) consisting of a 515-560 excitation filter, 580 nm dichroic mirror, and 580 nm barrier filter which allowed 580 nm to pass. The microscope was connected to a Leitz camera in which ASA 200 daylight 35 mm Ektachrome film Kodak was used.

RESULTS

The C3c product of complement activation was identified on trophoblastic basement membranes (TBM), as reported previously.[10] Monoclonal antibody to Factor VII reacted around fetal stem vessels, but also was identified on TBM. When C3c and Factor VII were studied together, they were found to co-localise on the same segments of TBM (Table 2). Factor IX was not always identified.

Factor X was found on TBM. The occasional absence of Factor IX and presence of Factor VII suggests that Factor X was deposited here as a result of clotting activation via the extrinsic pathway. Factor X sometimes was co-localised with the EST-1 epitope of thrombin (Table 2). The EST-4 epitope was not reactive, indicating that TBM thrombin was bound by antithrombin III.[11]

Table 2

Antigenic Co-localisation on TBM[1]

Factor VII and C3c
Factor X and thrombin [2]
Fibrinogen and Fragment D
Plasminogen[3] and α_2-plasmin inhibitor

[1]Localisation other than trophoblastic basement membranes (TBM) are in the Results section.
[2]Epitope EST-1
[3]Binding by inhibitor means antigen was plasmin, not plasminogen.

Fibrinogen was identified in syncytiotrophoblastic microvilli and occasionally on TBM. Double antibody experiments with antibody to fibrinolytic Fragment D often identified this fragment on TBM (Table 2). The localisation of both the parent molecule and its specific enzymatic degradation product to the same regions suggest that a certain amount of proteolysis occurs on TBM. If this is true, it must be tightly regulated, because thrombin is present with its inhibitor, and, as will be seen below, plasmin is also present with its inhibitor.

If fibrin deposition on TBM is not controlled, nutrient transport would presumably be impaired. There are at least two control systems represented in chorionic villi. First, monoclonal antibodies to Protein C identified this anti-coagulant in some trophoblast as well as in fibrinoid areas and on segments of TBM. Second, plasminogen was identified in the same areas, but, double antibody experiments with alpha-2-plasmin inhibitor revealed the inhibitor to co-localise with plasminogen (Table 2), indicating the plasminogen had been activated to plasmin.[12] Plasmin(ogen) has also been reported within tropho-blast[7], fibrinoid areas[13] and intervillous fibrin.

DISCUSSION

Faulk and Johnson[7] and Johnson and Faulk[14] showed that products of activated C3 are found on TBM of mature and immature chorionic villi. This pattern of deposition subsequently was reported to be amplified in placentae from diabetic[15] and/or pre-eclamptic pregnancies.[16] Increased complement deposition in pathological pregnancies has been interpreted as representing a heightened and perhaps disturbed immunological relationship between mother and tropho-blast.[17] The results of double antibody experiments reported here show C3c and Factor VII in identical locations on some segments of TBM, suggesting the possibility that C3c might have been produced by the serine protease activity of activated Factor VII. If true, existing ideas about placental immunopathy require modification.

The presence of Factor VII suggests most placental fibrin is deposited in and around villi as a consequence of activation of the extrinsic clotting pathway. and around villi as a consequence of activation of the extrinsic clotting pathway. Tissue factor activated Factor VII apparently triggered the local assembly of the activated Factor X-Factor V-Ca^{++}-phosholipid-prothrombin convertase complex, as represented by the presence of Factor X on TBM. This interpretation is strengthened by our recent finding that Factor V is present in cytotrophoblast contiguous with TBM, but is absent from both syncytiotrophoblast and other subsets of cytotrophoblast.[18] The prothrombin convertase complex probably was functional, because monoclonal antibodies showed thrombin on TBM. The thrombin probably was functional, because the present antibody results showed fibrin generated from fibrinogen, which was also demonstrated on TBM.

This study provides evidence in placentae for two control systems which are known to effect both the rate of fibrin deposition and the remodelling of deposited fibrin. First is thrombomodulin-bound thrombin which activates Protein C that inactivates activated Factor VIII and Factor V.[19] The co-factor for this reaction is Protein S, which falls to almost undetectable concentrations in blood during normal pregnancies.[20] The trophoblast and basement membrane associated thrombin and Protein C found in this investigation indicate that the Protein C anticoagulant pathway is represented and functioning in placentae during normal pregnancy. Second is the fibrinolytic enzyme system which is initiated by plasminogen activators and modulated by alpha-2-plasmin inhibitor.[5] A type of plasminogen activator inhibitor is uniquely produced by trophoblast.[21] The trophoblast and basement membrane associated plasminogen/plasmin and alpha-2-plasmin inhibitor found in this investigation indicate that the fibrinolytic enzyme system is represented and functioning in placentae during normal pregnancy.

The results of this study put forward evidence for the first time that pivotal components of the haemostatic, fibrinolytic and Protein C pathways are intimately involved with trophoblast and trophoblastic basement membranes in human placentae. This raises questions about how and why they are involved in the materno-trophoblastic relationship. A testable explanation for their involvement relates to the need for allogeneic recognition in human pregnancy,[22] and the possible lack of allogeneic recognition in primary recurrent spontaneous abortions.[23] Products of allogeneic recognition reactions can cause several cell types to produce tissue factor,[24] which is a potent initiator of coagulation. Similarly, endothelial cells can be stimulated to produce tissue factor by immune complexes,[25] interleukin-1[26] or endotoxin.[27] Haemostasis is not the only haematological reaction to be triggered by immunological recognition, because antibody[28] or thrombin[29] stimulation can cause endothelial cells to produce platelet-activating factor, and thrombin stimulated endothelium produces both plasminogen activators and plasminogen activator inhibitors.[30] Thus, the allogeneic recognition reaction of normal pregnancy could recruit haemostatic and fibrinolytic reactions that ensure a stable implantation, and inadequate allogeneic responses could fail to recruit such reactions and result in failed pregnancies.

ACKNOWLEDGEMENTS
These ideas have been discussed with my colleagues Professor Nils Bang and Dr. John McIntyre, also with postdoctoral fellows Dr. Patrizia Gargiulo and Dr. Carlos Labarrere. Miss Patricia Gulley gave technical assistance.

REFERENCES

1. Astedt B, Lecander I, Brodin T, Lundblad A, Low K. Purification of a specific placental plasminogen activator inhibitor by monocolonal antibody and its complex formation with plasminogen activator. *Thromb Haemost* 1985; **53:** 122-126.
2. Boyd JD, Hamilton WJ. *The Human Placenta*. London: Heffer, 1970.
3. Camussi G, Aglietta M, Malavasi F, Tetta C, Piacibello W, Sanavio F, Bussolino F. The release of platelet-activating factor from human endothelial cells in culture. *J Immunol* 1983; **131:** 2397-2403.
4. Cochrane CG. Initiating events in immune complex injury. In: *Progress in Immunology*. Ed. B Amos. New York: Academic Press, 1971. pp.143-153.
5. Colucci M, Balconi G, Lorenzet R, Pietra A, Locati D, Donati MB, Semararo N. Cultured human endothelial cells generate tissue factor in response to endotoxin. *J Clin Invest* **71:** 1893-1896.
6. Comp PC, Thurnau GR, Welsh J, Esmon CT. Functional and immunologic Protein S levels are decreased during pregnancy. *Blood* 1986; **68:** 881-885.
7. Dawes J, James K, Micklem LR, Pepper DS, Prowse CV. Monoclonal antibodies directed against human alpha-thrombin and the thrombin-antithrombin III complex. *Thromb Res* 1984; **36:** 397-409.
8. Esmon CT. The regulation of natural anticoagulant pathways. *Science* 1987; **235:** 1348-1351.
9. Faulk WP, Fox H. Reproductive Immunology. In: *Clinical Aspects of Immunology* 4th edition. Eds. P Lachmann, K Peters. Oxford: Blackwell Scientific Publications, 1981; pp.1104-1150.
10. Faulk WP, Hijmans W. Recent developments in immunofluorescence. *Prog Allergy* 1972; **16:** 9-39.
11. Faulk WP, Hsi BL. Immunopathology of human pregnancy. In: *Haines & Taylor's Obstetrical and Gynaecological Pathology*. Ed. H Fox. Edinburgh: Churchill Livingstone. 1987.
12. Faulk WP, Jarret R, Keane M, Johnson PM, Boackle RS. Immunological studies of human placentae: complement components in immature and mature chorionic villi. *Clin Exp Immunol* 1980; **40:** 229-305.
13. Faulk WP, Johnson PM. Immunological studies of human placentae: identification and distribution of proteins in mature chorionic villi. *Clin Exp Immunol* 1977; **27:** 365-375.
14. Faulk WP, McIntyre JA. Trophoblast survival. *Transpl* 1981; **32:** 1-5.
15. Faulk WP, McIntyre JA. Immunological studies of human trophoblast: markers, subsets and functions. *Immunol Rev*1983; **75:** 372-408.
16. Fox H. Perivillous fibrin deposition in the human placenta. *Am J Obstet Gynecol* 1967; **98:** 245-251.
17. Galbraith RM, Sinha DP, Galbraith GMP, Faulk WP. Immunohistological studies of placentae from insulin dependent diabetic women. In: *Carbohydrate Metabolism in Pregnancy and the Newborn*. Eds. HW Sutherland, JM Stowers. Edinburgh: Churchill Livingstone, 1984; pp.23-33.
18. Hsi BL, Faulk WP, Yeh CJG, McIntyre JA. Immunohistology of clotting factor V in human extra-embryonic membranes. *Placenta*; In press.
19. Johnson PM, Faulk WP. Immunological studies of human placentae: identification and distribution of proteins in mature chorionic villi. *Immunol* 1978; **34:** 1027-1035.
20. Matter L, Faulk WP. Fibrinogen degradation products and Factor VIII consumption in normal pregnancy and pre-eclampsia: role of the placenta. In: *Hypertension in Pregnancy*. Eds. J Bonnar, I McGillivray, EM Symonds, 1980; Lancaster: MTP Press. pp.357-369.
21. Kruithof EKD, Tran-Thang C, Gudinchet A, Hauert J, Nicolosco G, Genton C, Welti H, Bachmann F. Fibrinolysis in pregnancy: a study of plasminogen activator inhibitors. *Blood* 1987; **69:** 460-466.

198   *Study Group: Early Pregnancy Loss*

22. Moe N, Jorgensen L. Fibrin deposits on the syncytium of the normal human placenta: evidence for their thrombogenic origin. *Acta Path Microbiol Scand* 1968; **72:** 519-541.
23. Moe N. Deposits of fibrin and plasma proteins in the normal human placenta: an immunofluorescence study. *Acta Path Microbiol Scand* 1969; **76:** 74-88.
24. Prescott SM, Zimmerman GA, McIntyre TM. Human endothelial cells in culture produce platelet-activating factor (1-alkyl-2-acetyl-sn-glycerol-3-phosphoryl-choline) when stimulated with thrombin. *Proc Nat Acad Sci USA* 1984; **81:** 3534-3538.
25. Rothberger H, Zimmerman TS, Vaughan JH. Increased production and expression of tissue thromboplastin-like procoagulant activity in vitro by allogeneically stimulated human leucocytes. *J Clin Invest* 1978; **62:** 649-655.
26. Schorer AE, Kaplan ME, Rao GHR, Moldow CF. Interleukin-1 stimulates endothelial cell tissue factor production and expression by a prostaglandin-independent mechanism. *Thromb Haemost* 1986; **56:** 256-259.
27. Sinha DP, Wells M, Faulk WP. Immunological studies of human placentae: complement components in pre-eclamptic chorionic villi. *Clin Exp Immunol* 1984; **56:** 175-184.
28. Stirling Y, Woolf L, North WRS, Seghatchian MJ, Meade TW. Haemostasis in normal pregnancy. *Thromb Haemost* 1984; **52:** 176-180.
29. Van Hinsbergh VWM, Sprengers ED, Kooistra T. Effects of thrombin on the production of plasminogen activators and PA inhibitor-1 by human foreskin microvascular endothelial cells. *Thromb Haemost* 1987; **57:** 148-153.
30. Wun T-C, Capuano A. Initiation and regulation of fibrinolysis in human plasma at the plasminogen activator level. *Blood* 1987; **69:** 1354-1362.

Discussion

Chairman: Professor W. B. Robertson

Professor GRUDZINSKAS: May I make a comment? I would like to challenge Page Faulk because he has shown the first slide several times and mostly got away with it. I submit that the slide from which Page Faulk says there is evidence of activation of the complement system is a dud, unless the antibody against C3c is actually monoclonal.

Dr PAGE FAULK: I mentioned at the outset that all these antibodies I am talking about are monoclonal antibodies.

Professor GRUDZINSKAS: Thank you, then it is not a dud!

Professor ROBERTSON: It is quite obvious from only one day of this symposium so far that what we know about the complex subject of early pregnancy wastage is far outweighed by what we don't know. The speakers in this session have, by implication, emphasised the pressing need for more detailed studies of the pregnant uterus and its contents in the early stages of gestation. Dr. Rushton has illustrated the heterogenous nature of the pathology of miscarriages, Dr Loke the many unsolved characteristics of trophoblast, both villous and the migratory extravillous variety, while Dr Bulmer has revealed all too plainly how little we know about the functions of decidua and its cell population. Professor Grudzinskas, understandably unable to tell us much about the functions of pregnancy-associated hormones and proteins, has made a case for their assessment in certain circumstances as an aid in the diagnosis of abnormal early pregnancy. Dr Page Faulk, not surprisingly, has come up with yet another new idea that abnormalities in the haemostatic and fibrinolytic mechanisms at the interface between fetal and maternal tissues may account for the failure of some pregnancies. To me, as a morphologist, it is a pity we have heard little on the subject of abnormalities of placentation, particularly of the establishment of the uteroplacental circulation,[1] that may be an important factor in precipitating the demise of the conceptus.

REFERENCE
1. Khong TY, Liddell HS, Robertson WB. Defective haemochorial placentation as a cause of miscarriage: a preliminary study. *Br J Obstet Gynaecol* 1987; **94**: 649-655.

SECTION 4

FACTORS WHICH MAINTAIN PREGNANCY AT AND IMMEDIATELY AFTER IMPLANTATION

Chairman's introductory remarks

Chairman: Professor D. A. Clark

We are going to discuss the various aspects of early pregnancy failure. Data from both human and animal studies show that early loss of embryos in the pre- and peri-implantation phase exceeds the loss due to the abortion of an established and diagnosed pregnancy. The loss rate is higher whenever the pre-implantation embryo is cultured *in vitro* prior to implantation. Furthermore, damage suffered by the pre-implantation or early implanting embryo may have a delayed expression such as in spontaneous abortion. It is therefore highly relevant to the subject of human pregnancy failure to deal now with physiologic and pathologic mechanisms which can affect early pregnancy. The selection of topics for this session has taken into account our growing awareness of the need to integrate both immunologic and non-immunologic concepts for a full understanding of the basis for problems that occur clinically.

Chairman's introductory remarks

Chairman: (re-elect) C. A. Clark

Antigen expression by cells of the conceptus before, during and after implantation

W. D. Billington

INTRODUCTION

Knowledge of the antigenic status of the cells of the conceptus is being sought largely by workers in the fields of developmental biology and reproductive immunology. The former are seeking to determine whether cell surface molecules are useful markers of differentiation and involved in cellular recognition and interaction whilst the latter are attempting to elucidate their role in signalling the presence of a viable embryo and establishing a feto-maternal immunological dialogue that may be necessary for the maintenance of pregnancy. As long ago as 1951, Brambell and his colleagues[1] asserted that immune responses must play a part in the production and survival of the young in man and other mammals. More than thirty years later, the precise nature and extent of these responses are still far from clear, with the notable exception of the transfer of maternal immunoglobulins for the protection of the neonate against environmental pathogens.

The great majority of studies on the antigens of the conceptus have examined the cell surface expression of histocompatibility antigens. This has emanated from the long-held view, initiated by Medawar in 1953, that the conceptus must be regarded as an intra-uterine foreign graft, owing to the inheritance of paternal genes not shared by the mother.[2] The path of transplantation immunology has therefore been followed in order to seek an explanation for the apparently paradoxical success of the engrafted conceptus. Although there is now evidence that antigen systems other than the classical histocompatibility antigens can play a part in tissue recognition and rejection,[3] rather little is yet known of any such systems expressed on the conceptus. However, the identification of antigens by monoclonal antibodies (mAbs) generated from lymphoid cells obtained from syngeneically mated mice,[4] as well as from mice immunised with human trophoblast membranes,[5] indicates that maternal immune responses to embryonic non-histocompatibility antigens may occur and be of relevance in normal pregnancy.[6] At the present time it is possible to explore the reasons for the non-rejection of the conceptus to a large degree only within the context of the major histocompatibility complex (MHC) antigens. This short review therefore summarises the information to date on MHC antigen expression throughout embryonic development, from the fertilised oocyte to the fully differentiated cells of the fetus and, especially, the placenta. Most of the data on the early embryo have been obtained from studies on the mouse, whilst information on the later stages of development has accumulated from investigation of mouse, rat and human material.

MHC ANTIGENS ON THE MOUSE PRE-IMPLANTATION EMBRYO

Although the presence of minor histocompatibility (non-H-2) antigens had been documented by many workers it was for long believed that MHC antigens were not expressed on pre-implantation embryos. This was, however, demonstrated to be due to the use of poorly defined antisera and assays of insufficient sensitivity to detect low levels of expression and/or low surface density of these antigens.[7,8] The initial findings of MHC antigens on the trophectoderm of the blastocyst were made possible by the use of radiolabelled antiglobulin[7] and electron-microscope immunoperoxidase[8] assays. This has been confirmed by later similar studies[9] which have additionally shown the antigens to be expressed on the 8-cell, but not the 2-cell, embryo. There is a more recent claim that MHC antigen expression occurs on the unfertilised oocyte and the 1-cell and 2-cell embryo, detectable by an enzyme-linked immunosorbent assay (ELISA) utilising monoclonal antibodies.[10] Papain-stripping of antigens from blastocysts led to their reappearance after a short period in culture, indicating active synthesis rather than cytophilic absorption of the antigens. The authors assume that their findings of early expression relate to the high sensitivity of the ELISA assay. This interesting study should be repeated using careful specificity controls with F1 hybrid embryos to determine whether paternally encoded MHC antigens are expressed. It should also be determined whether the H-2 antigens detected are of the adult molecular form or have a different structure.

The presence of MHC antigens on the pre-implantation embryo may have little relevance to maternal immune recognition since there is no evidence for the existence of Class II MHC positive antigen presenting cells (APC) in the lumen of the uterus at this time. In this context it is also of interest that MHC antigens are lost from the trophectodermal cell surface of the blastocyst following oestrogenic activation for implantation.[7,8] By the time of first cellular contact of mother and embryo there are thus no MHC recognition molecules present.

POST-IMPLANTATION EMBRYONIC DEVELOPMENT

For technical reasons, it has not proved possible to study antigen expression on the intact embryo in the immediate post-implantation period. Use has been made of the ability of the blastocyst to attach to substrates *in vitro* and undergo two-dimensional outgrowth to produce trophectodermal and inner cell mass derived cell populations during a 3-5 day culture period.[11] Under these conditions, MHC antigens are detectable at low levels on the cells derived from the inner cell mass but not from the trophoblast,[12] although the latter do express non-H-2 antigens of both maternal and paternal origin.[12,13]

207 Antigen expression in the conceptus

The next stage of mouse embryonic development convenient for study is the 7-day conceptus, consisting of an embryonic sac, destined to give rise largely to the fetus, and an encapsulating trophoblastic component with a proliferating cap of cells, the ectoplacental cone (EPC) trophoblast, that invades the uterus and ultimately forms the main part of the placenta. Most studies have been carried out on the EPC and sac cultured *in vitro* for 3-5 days. These have shown that MHC antigens are absent from the outer trophoblastic giant cells of the EPC but are present on the smaller, diploid trophoblast cells of the EPC core, as well as on the embryonic sac cells.[14] Non-H-2 antigens are expressed on all cell populations. The most important feature is that the conceptus at this stage is surrounded by a trophoblastic barrier devoid of MHC antigens. Allowing for the further differentiation of cells in culture following explantation at 7 days, the time of first appearance of MHC antigen positive embryonic cells correlates well with the detection of low levels of Class I mRNA from day 9.[15] It would seem that there is no significant Class I gene transcription in the post-implantation embryo before organogenesis and that this remains very low (more than 50 times less than in adult spleen cells) until at least 13 days of gestation.[15] This would thus rule out the proposed role for MHC antigens in early morphogenesis.[16]

The ectoplacental cone subsequently undergoes rapid proliferation and differentiation *in vivo* to establish the anatomically complex haemochorial placenta with three major trophoblastic sub-populations. Almost all studies of antigen expression on placental trophoblast have been carried out on cell suspensions or adherent cultures *in vitro*. Without the use of definitive cell markers this has led to difficulties in the interpretation of the results obtained. It has not so far proved possible to map the expression of MHC antigens by immunohistology on cryostat sections of the mouse placenta, owing to the fact that the appropriate monoclonal antibodies have been of mouse origin and the placenta has considerable quantities of endogenous maternal immunoglobulin, resulting in excessive non-specific background staining. This could possibly be overcome by avidin-biotin labelling using direct biotinylation of the mAbs. Notwithstanding the difficulties, there is now compelling evidence for MHC antigen expression on the spongiotrophoblast cells of the placenta in direct cellular contact with the maternal decidual cells. In contrast, the labyrinthine trophoblast, the main area of feto-maternal physiological exchange, and the trophoblastic giant cells of the placenta, have little or no expression. These conclusions have been reached independently by groups employing both poly-specific and monoclonal reagents directed against paternal H-2 specificities in different binding assays on cells *in vitro*.[17,18,19] These paternal MHC antigens are exposed to the maternal environment *in situ* since injection of radiolabelled mAbs into the circulation of pregnant females leads to their binding to the placental trophoblast.[20,21] It is also conceivable that the level of MHC antigen expression is much greater on trophoblast cells *in vivo* than is apparent from the *in vitro* studies since it is now clear that interferons (IFNs) of several types can significantly enhance Class I antigen expression on trophoblast cell cultures[19,22] and interferons are found in normal mouse placentae.[23]

MHC ANTIGENS ON THE RAT CONCEPTUS

The availability of xenogeneic (mouse) mAbs directed against polymorphic determinants of rat Class I MHC molecules has recently enabled an immuno-histological analysis of the rat conceptus without the technical problems described above for the mouse placenta. Paternally encoded Class I (RT1A) antigens have been detected on the spongiotrophoblast, but not the labyrinthine trophoblast, of the mature rat placenta.[24] Sections of the early post-implantation conceptus showed no labelling with the anti-Class I mAb. The first detectable expression occurred on the presumptive spongiotrophoblast cell layer at day 9 of gestation. Soon after this time, large numbers of endovascular cells lining the blood vessels in the decidua and myometrium became strongly labelled, thus identifying them as fetal. Cellular continuity with the presumptive spongiotrophoblast layer was seen in the central area of the placenta, providing definitive proof that these endovascular cells are fetal trophoblast and not hypertrophied maternal endothelial cells, as debated in the earlier literature.[25] As in the mouse, the onset of Class I gene expression in the fetal organs does not begin until late in their development (Burrows and Billington, unpublished results).

SUSCEPTIBILITY OF THE RODENT CONCEPTUS TO MATERNAL IMMUNE REJECTION

The accumulated evidence in rat and mouse indicates that the early post-implantation conceptus is not vulnerable to maternal recognition and rejection. The outer trophoblastic cell populations encapsulating the embryonic tissues are lacking in Class I MHC antigens. In any case, there are no potentially susceptible embryonic cells at this stage, as mentioned above. However, in both species there emerges a population of Class I antigen-bearing trophoblast cells that comes to comprise a major component of the mature placenta. The question is whether these cells are potential targets for immune destruction. It has not so far proved possible to provide a definitive answer. This is because of the difficulty in obtaining purified populations of trophoblast for appropriate *in vitro* cytotoxicity assays. Ectoplacental cone trophoblast, which can be cultured uncontaminated by other cells, is insusceptible to cell-mediated lysis.[26] Mouse placental cell cultures show a considerable degree of lysis under similar conditions[27] but it not yet confirmed that the trophoblastic population (spongiotrophoblast) is affected. Cultured mouse trophoblastic cells have been shown to be lysed by anti-paternal antibody and complement[19] but endogenous mouse complement would almost certainly be ineffective and in any case anti-paternal alloantibody is detectable in only a small minority of pregnant mice.[28] It is also a persuasive fact that experimentally induced immunity, involving the presence of cytotoxic T cells and antibody, has no apparent adverse effects on the course of pregnancy.[29]

IMMUNOREGULATORY MECHANISMS FOR SURVIVAL OF THE CONCEPTUS

The simplest explanation for the survival of the conceptus as an intra-uterine allograft is that maternal immunocompetent cells do not gain access to the fetal circulation, at least in any significant numbers, and that those trophoblastic cell populations of the placenta that express paternal Class I MHC antigens are in some way resistent to immune-mediated lysis *in vivo*. Any eventual demonstration of susceptibility of purified trophoblastic cell populations *in vitro* might therefore have little biological relevance.

It is quite clear that allogeneic pregnancy does not induce a classical immunological rejection reaction in the mother, even after multiparity.[28,36] If paternal MHC antigens are in an exposed position on fetal cells (trophoblast) this implies some form of afferent modulation of the maternal immune response to these antigens. Two major forms of immunoregulatory control have been proposed. The first involves trophoblast-secreted factors that have been shown to deviate both cell-mediated and humoral immune responses, both *in vitro* and *in vivo*.[30] The second implicates a population of maternal decidua-associated suppressor cells.[31] The latter are of two types: non-T lymphocytes secreting a soluble factor capable of blocking the action of interleukin-2, and prostaglandin (PGE_2) producing cells, which are either decidual cells or macrophages. There is evidence indicating that some of these regulatory control systems are also able to inhibit the efferent pathway of the immune response. They would therefore be capable of protecting the conceptus in an experimentally immunised female, perhaps in conjunction with the pregnancy-associated serum molecules that have also been shown to exhibit efferent blocking activities.[28] It remains to be determined whether these, or any other forms of immunoregulation, are essential for the success of pregnancy or whether some innate properties of the trophoblast cell membrane *in vivo*, rendering this fetal barrier tissue resistant to immune destruction, alone are sufficient.

MHC ANTIGENIC STATUS OF THE HUMAN CONCEPTUS

Until recently, the only data available on MHC antigen expression on human tissues were from the study of material from 6 weeks of gestation onwards. The earliest evidence, employing fetal cells grown in culture and polyspecific human isoantisera in mixed agglutination assays, demonstrated that HLA antigens were present on diverse cell types, with the exception of trophoblastic syncytia, by the 6th week.[32] Extensive studies on trophoblast from 6 weeks to term have confirmed that the syncytiotrophoblast fails to express Class I MHC antigens but have shown that non-villous trophoblast can be stained in immunohistology by mAbs directed against a monomorphic (framework) determinant of the Class I molecule.[5] These trophoblastic populations do not, however, stain with mAbs directed against polymorphic determinants of the Class I molecule specific for the fetal allotype.[33] It is an important task to determine the precise nature of the molecular structure on the non-villous trophoblast. Should it be a novel non-HLA antigen that cannot be recognised by the maternal immune system the survival of the human conceptus may result simply from the unique antigenic nature of the trophoblastic barrier tissue. This would then imply that there is no requirement for any complex immunoregulatory control mechanisms in human pregnancy. Pregnancy failure could not then result from breakdown of these mechanisms.

There is a recent report that unfertilised and *in vitro* fertilised human oocytes, including some that produced abnormally developing cleavage-stage embryos, fail to express Class I MHC antigens.[34] In view of the technical difficulties seen in the mouse studies it will be necessary to confirm whether the indirect immuno-fluorescence assay used with the human oocytes is sufficiently sensitive to detect any low levels of expression of these antigens. Absence of MHC antigens also from human sperm[35] indicates that they can have no involvement in the process of fertilisation.

IMPLICATIONS OF LACK OF CELL SURFACE MHC ANTIGENS

If Class I MHC antigens are not expressed on the human pre-implantation embryo or, as in the mouse, are transiently expressed and lost from the trophectoderm by the time of blastocyst attachment, this would argue against the hypothesis that successful implantation requires this form of immunological recognition. There is universal agreement that Class II MHC antigens are absent from the pre-implantation embryo as well as from all populations of trophoblast in both mouse and man. Recognition of *any* molecular structure by the maternal immune system would therefore have to involve Class II positive antigen presenting cells (APC) from another source. There is no evidence for APCs in the uterine lumen, ruling out any form of immune recognition of the pre-implantation embryo. In the post-implantation period there would be APCs in the decidual tissue that could process any non-MHC antigens on the trophoblast for maternal immune recognition and induction of a response. However, the absence of classical Class I antigens on the human trophoblast would, assuming that the dogma of MHC restriction applied, prevent the co-recognition of any other trophoblast cell surface antigens by any pre-existing maternal cytotoxic T cells, although in fact these appear not to be present in normal pregnancy.[36] Immune attack on a potential target antigen might therefore have to be instigated by natural killer (NK), or similar, perhaps LAK, cells. Little is known of this form of cellular immunity *in vivo* in pregnancy, but it is worth noting that IFN-boosted NK cells can kill human trophoblast *in vitro*.[37]

CONCLUSIONS

Survival of the allogeneic conceptus depends upon a barrier of trophoblastic cells. In the early post-implantation period the outermost populations of trophoblast fail to express Class I or Class II MHC antigens. Class I gene transcription does not begin until organogensis is well advanced, at least in the mouse. None of the trophoblast populations at any stage of gestation appear susceptible to immune destruction *in vivo*. The extent to which this depends upon an absence of cell surface antigens capable of eliciting a maternal immune reaction and acting as targets for lytic mechanisms or, alternatively, upon a complex immunoregulatory system deviating responses at the afferent or efferent levels remains to be determined. Only then will it be possible to establish whether pregnancy failure can be due to perturbation of maternal immune control. The validity of current immunotherapeutic approaches to recurrent spontaneous miscarriage must be assessed within this context.

REFERENCES
1. Brambell FWR, Hemmings WA, Henderson M. *Antibodies and Embryos.* London: The Athlone Press, University of London, 1951.
2. Medawar PB. Some immunological and endocrinological problems raised by the evolution of viviparity in vertebrates. *Symp Soc Exp Biol* 1953; **7**: 320-338.
3. Lalezari P. Organ-specific and systemic alloantigens: interrelationships and biologic implications. *Transplant Proc* 1980; **12**: 12-21.
4. Hamilton MS, Vernon RB, Eddy EM. A monoclonal antibody, EC-1, derived from a syngeneically multiparous mouse alters *in vitro* fertilization and development. *J Reprod Immunol* 1985; **8**: 45-49.
5. Bulmer JN, Johnson PM. Antigen expression by trophoblast populations in the human placenta and their possible immunobiological relevance. *Placenta* 1985; **6**: 127-140.
6. Hamilton MS. Maternal immune responses to oncofetal antigens. *J Reprod Immunol* 1983; **5**: 249-264.
7. Hakansson S, Heyner S, Sundqvist KG, Bergstrom S. The presence of paternal H-2 antigens on hybrid mouse blastocysts during experimental delay of implantation and the disappearance of these antigens after onset of implantation. *Int J Fertil* 1975; **20**: 137-140.
8. Searle EF, Sellens MH, Elson J, Jenkinson EJ, Billington WD. Detection of alloantigens during preimplantation development and early trophoblast differentiation in the mouse by immunoperoxidase labeling. *J Exp Med* 1976; **143**: 348-359.
9. Warner CM, Spannaus DJ. Demonstration of H-2 antigens on preimplantation mouse embryos using conventional antisera and monoclonal antibody. *J Exp Zool* 1984; **230**: 37-52.
10. Goldbard SB, Gollnick SO, Warner CM. Synthesis of H-2 antigens by preimplantation mouse embryos. *Biol Reprod* 1985; **33**: 30-36.
11. Jenkinson EJ. The *in vitro* blastocyst outgrowth system as a model for the analysis of peri-implantation development. In: *Development in Mammals* Vol. 2. Ed: MH Johnson. Amsterdam: North-Holland Publishing Co., 1977; pp.151-172.
12. Sellens MH. Antigen expression on early mouse trophoblast. *Nature* 1977; **269**: 60-61.
13. Carter J. Expression of maternal and paternal antigens on trophoblast. *Nature* 1976; **262**: 292-293.
14. Sellens MH, Jenkinson EJ, Billington WD. MHC and non-MHC antigens on mouse ectoplacental cone and placental trophoblastic cells. *Transplantation* 1978; **25**: 173-179.
15. Ozato K, Wan Y-J, Orrison BM. Mouse major histocompatibility class I gene expression begins at midsomite stage and is inducible in earlier-stage embryos by interferon. *Proc Natl Acad Sci USA* 1985; **82**: 2427-2431.
16. Ohno S. The original function of MHC antigens as the general plasma membrane anchorage site of organogenesis-directing proteins. *Immunol Rev* 1977; **33**: 59-69.
17. Jenkinson EJ, Owen V. Ontogeny and distribution of major histocompatibility complex (MHC) antigens on mouse placental trophoblast. *J Reprod Immunol* 1980; **2**: 173-181.
18. Lala PK, Chatterjee-Hasrouni S, Kearns M, Montgomery B, Colavincenzo V. Immunobiology of the feto-maternal interface. *Immunol Rev* 1983; **75**: 87-116.
19. Zuckermann FA, Head JR. Expression of MHC antigens on murine trophoblast and their modulation by interferon. *J Immunol* 1986; **137**: 846-853.
20. Singh B, Raghupathy R, Anderson DJ, Wegmann TG. The placenta as an immunobiological barrier between mother and fetus. In: *Immunology of Reproduction.* Eds. TG Wegmann and TJ Gill. Oxford: Oxford University Press, 1983. pp.229-230.
21. Lala PK, Kearns M, Colavincenzo V. Cells of the feto-maternal interface: their role in the maintenance of viviparous pregnancy. *Am J Anat* 1984; **170**: 501-517.

22. Drake BL, King NJC, Maxwell LE, Rodger JC. Class I MHC antigen expression on early murine trophoblast and its induction by lymphokines in vitro. *J Reprod Immunol* 1987; **10:** 319-328.
23. Fowler AK, Reed CD, Giron DJ. Identification of an interferon in murine placentas. *Nature* 1980; **286:** 266-267.
24. Billington WD, Burrows FJ. The rat placenta expresses paternal class I major histocompatibility antigens. *J Reprod Immunol* 1986; **9:** 155-160.
25. Bridgman J. A morphological study of the development of the placenta of the rat. *J Morphol* 1948; **83:** 61-86; 195-224.
26. Jenkinson EJ, Billington WD. Differential susceptibility of mouse trophoblast and embryonic tissue to immune cell lysis. *Transplantation* 1974; **18:** 286-289.
27. Smith G. In vitro susceptibility of mouse placental trophoblast to cytotoxic effector cells. *J Reprod Immunol* 1983; **5:** 39-47.
28. Bell SC, Billington WD. Anti-fetal alloantibody in the pregnant female. *Immunol Rev* 1983; **75:** 5-30.
29. Mitchison NA. The effect on the offspring of maternal immunization in mice. *J Genet* 1953; **51:** 406-420.
30. Chaouat G. Placental immunoregulatory factors. *J Reprod Immunol* 1987; **10:** 179-188.
31. Clark DA, Damji N, Chaput A, Daya S, Rosenthal KL, Brierley J. Decidua-associated suppressor cells and suppressor factors regulating interleukin-2: their role in survival of the fetal allograft. In: *Progress in Immunology*, Vol. VI. Eds. B. Cinauer, RG Miller. New York: Academic Press, 1986. pp.1089-1099.
32. Seigler HF, Metzgar RS. Embryonic development of human transplantation antigens. *Transplantation* 1970; **9:** 478-486.
33. Redman CW, McMichael AJ, Stirrat GM, Sunderland CA, Ting A. Class I major histocompatibility complex antigens on human extra-villous trophoblast. *Immunology* 1984; **52:** 457-468.
34. Dohr GA, Motter W, Leitinger S, Desoye G, Urdl W, Winter R, Wilders-Truschnig MM, Uchanska-Ziegler B, Ziegler A. Lack of expression of histocompatibility leukocyte antigen class I and class II molecules on the human oocyte. *J Immunol* 1987; **138:** 3766-3770.
35. Anderson DJ, Bach DL, Yunis JE, De Wolf WC. Major histocompatibility antigens are not expressed on human epididymal sperm. *J Immunol* 1982; **129:** 452-454.
36. Sargent IL, Redman CWG. Maternal cell-mediated immunity to the fetus in human pregnancy. *J Reprod Immunol* 1985; **7:** 95-104.
37. Pross H, Mitchell H, Werkmeister J. The sensitivity of placental trophoblast cells to intraplacental and allogeneic cytotoxic lymphocytes. *Amer J Reprod Immunol Microbiol* 1985; **8:** 1-9.

Discussion

Chairman: Professor D. A. Clark

Professor BEER: Dr. Billington, the experiments showing MHC antigen expression on human embryos were all done on polyploid embryos that had multiple polar bodies. I think as a result of their being abnormal embryos it is really premature to say anything about the lack of MHC antigen expression on normal embryos. Have any studies been done on the normally fertilised egg?

Dr BILLINGTON: There is other data from two sources, ovarian biopsy material, and also from those oocytes aspirated for IVF. One assumes that many of these oocytes would be normal. The absence of MHC antigens on the oocytes is consistent with the pre-implantation embryo data, at least those which have been published. I understand that they have actually looked at non-polyploid embryos and found a lack of MHC expression.

Dr CHAOUAT: Some unpublished studies of IVF pre-embryos which were not transferred because there was an excess number, showed a lack of MHC by molecular biology test methods.

Dr BILLINGTON: One must add the caveat learned from studies of antigens on the inner cell mass, and that is, of course, the sensitivity of the assay may be important. If we simply use light microscope immunoperoxidase, or indirect immunofluorescence, even using highly specific monoclonal antibodies, we may not detect antigen. It is necessary to use the electron microscope to be really sure.

Professor KLEIN: I wonder on what you base your conclusion concerning expression of minor histocompatibility antigens. It is very difficult (impossible until now) to get antibodies against these antigens. If you have some antibodies, how do you know that they are against minor histocompatibility antigens? Concerning the expression or lack of expression of Class I MHC, why do you think it matters? If there is no Class II, then the Class I cannot simulate an immune response.

Dr BILLINGTON: To answer your second point, there are maternal macrophages in the uterine lining which are Class II bearing cells in intimate apposition with the fetal membranes. These cells may "help" induce an immune response to Class I.

Professor KLEIN: The Class I and Class II might have to be on the same cell.

Dr BILLINGTON: They might, but not necessarily. To answer your first question, certainly as far as the minor H antigens are concerned, their definition is not very well developed. The data that I have given to you are those generated very largely by Susan Heyner and in work by Liz Simpson using monospecific reagents against certain minor H specificities. I certainly agree these are not well defined at the present time.

Professor STIRRAT: You referred to the debate about whether Class I MHC in human trophoblast is a classical or non-classical Class I antigen, which has arisen from biochemical data. You did not produce any biochemical data in relation to the rodent to define what antigens were being recognised by the anti-MHC antibody.

Dr BILLINGTON: Yes. The only information we have on that is information on monoclonal antibody that was used, which has been fairly well characterised by John Faver, and which has specificity for one particular MHC type in the rat. Using the F1 placenta you can be sure at least that it is identifying the pattern of a Class I antigen epitope. Now whether that is a classical Class I antigen would depend on full biochemical analysis. There have been some sequencing studies carried out on the molecule immunoprecipitated by that monoclonal antibody. It appears to have all the characteristics of Class I so far.

Dr LOKE: In one of your earlier slides did you imply that the down regulation of MHC antigens on the pre-implantation blastocyst is mediated by maternal oestrogen?

Dr. BILLINGTON: If you test the blastocysts that have been activated for implantation by oestrogen, you observe the loss from the cell surface of a variety of antigen systems. The inference is that oestrogen is directly or indirectly affecting regulation and/or expression of those antigens.

Host immunoregulatory mechanisms and the success of the conceptus fertilised in vivo and in vitro

D. A. Clark

INTRODUCTION

In their classic article published in the *Lancet* in 1975, Roberts and Lowe asked, "Where have all the conceptions gone?"[1] They estimated from epidemiological data that 80% of conceptions were lost before term. As only 1/7-1/10 clinically diagnosed pregnancies abort, approximately 75% of conceptions must be lost before the woman is known to be pregnant. Confirmation of this figure comes from laboratory measurements of early pregnancy factor (EPF) that appear in the woman's blood within 24 hours of conception, and persist so long as the conceptus is viable.[2,3] Using the EPF assay, Rolfe estimated that approximately 75% of conceptions were lost in the first 14 days.[3] Based on the combined use of EPF and βhCG (which becomes positive after implantation), it can be estimated that of 100 fertilised embryos, 20-30 will not implant, 20 may make a transient attempt to implant (as reflected by a single low level, spike of βhCG-like material in blood or urine), and 5-10 may persist as true chemical pregnancies for a few days and silently abort; an additional 5-10 will abort after the diagnosis of pregnancy is made clinically (20 days post-conception and 14 days after implantation) by conventional βhCG testing and absent menses.[3-11] From the studies of Hertig and others,[12,13] one anticipates a 50% incidence of lethal genetic and anatomical abnormalities in the early conceptus, and these embryos will comprise a major part of the 75% total mortality. Such defectiveness is random and not likely to explain recurrent loss manifest as apparent infertility or recurrent abortion. It must be noted that the proportion of early embryos lost may vary considerably with the population being studied. In older patients and in infertile couples, the occult abortion rate may be higher[8] whereas in other groups, the total early loss may be as low as 25%.[11]

With the advent of *in vitro* fertilisation (IVF) to treat "unexplained" infertility, it has become apparent that fertilisation is indeed possible for a majority of affected couples, but the rate of failure to implant is increased at least 2-fold (i.e. 80-90% fail). Of those IVF embryos that establish a pregnancy, 30-50% abort, a figure that is also 2-3 greater than expected.[14-16] Assuming lethal genetic defects

215

will occur randomly at a frequency of 50%, replacing 4 IVF embryos ensures a 93.8% probability that there will be at least 1 "normal" conceptus in the recipient's uterus. It follows that both in normal fertile couples and in infertile patients (including those treated by IVF), non-genetic factors may be causing a proportion of pregnancy failures. It is our hypothesis that physiological and toxicological events may be responsible. To test this idea, our strategy has been to define the normal physiological parameters of early successful pregnancy and then to determine what is abnormal in the situation of early pregnancy failure.

It is not feasible to study the events of implantation and early pregnancy physiology at the tissue and cellular level using human material. Fortunately, a few informative animal models exist. In the laboratory mouse the genetics are defined, immunological assays well established, and techniques for reproductive biological studies have been developed. The frequency of chromosomal abnormalities in mouse gametes is much lower (10-15%) than in humans.[18] Transfer of *in vivo*-generated blastocysts from one mouse to a recipient has a 70-90% success rate if the recipient is hormonally conditioned.[17] The success rate tends to improve with experience. Approximately 10% resorption (abortion) is expected, usually occurring after the 5th post-implantation day. *In vitro* fertilised mouse eggs have been reported by Abe *et al* to have only 20% rate of implantation followed by a 40% resorption rate, similar to human IVF-ET results.[19] If mouse eggs were fertilised *in vivo*, but then were removed and cultured *in vitro*, the implantation rate was also low, (only 30%) with a 65% resorption rate.[20] However, when the *in vivo*-fertilised eggs were incubated in the uterus of another mouse and then removed and transferred to the recipient, the implantation rate remained low (suggesting trauma, toxicity, or perhaps dysynchrony between the stage of development of the conceptus and the recipient uterus, as will be discussed), but the resorption rate was only 9%.[20] Exposure to a physiological environment during the pre-implantation phase of development therefore produced implantations with a higher probability of survival.

The embryo may be viewed as a "seed" which must establish itself in a suitable "soil" in order to grow and develop (Figure I). Failure of this process may occur due to defects in the "seed". Gross defects such as anatomical and chromosomal anomalies have already been mentioned. More subtle genetic defects are also possible. There may also be defects in the "soil". The uterine lining must be suitably conditioned by gestational hormones. Too much oestradiol[21,22] or too little progesterone[22,23] may lead to failure. The interaction between the embryo and uterus must also be synchronised.[24] Mistiming will prevent successful implantation, and might also affect post-implantation survival as reflected by spontaneous abortion of those embryos that do manage to implant.

The co-ordinated interaction between embryo and uterine lining is particularly interesting as it is in this interaction that the explanation for early pregnancy failure may lie. The synchrony required to avoid failure at implantation may be conceptually regarded as having two components. A passive requirement for matching of surface receptors may be one.[25] The other is active interaction. These effects may in turn be either stimulatory or inhibitory, and may be immunological or non-immunological. While the schema illustrated by Figure I

Figure I

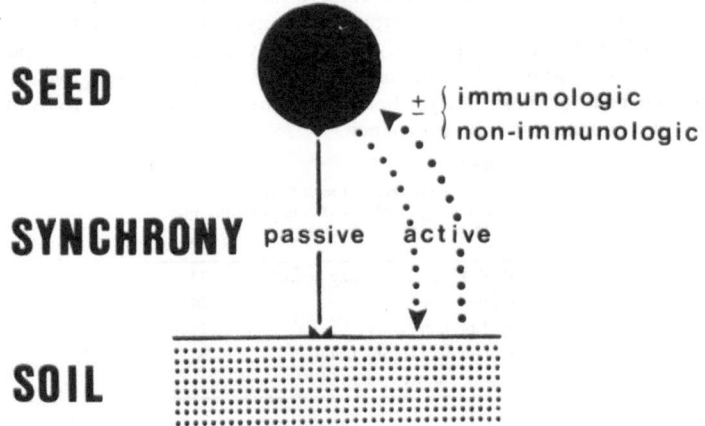

SEED

SYNCHRONY passive active

SOIL

$+ \begin{cases} \text{immunologic} \\ \text{non-immunologic} \end{cases}$

A simple schematic model of factors determining the outcome of early pregnancy. For explanation, see text.

provides a useful framework for analysis, anatomy of the embryo-uterine interaction changes sufficiently during development, that it is useful to consider the interactions shown in Figure I that may be relevant in each of three distinct phases of early pregnancy depicted in Figure II.

Figure II

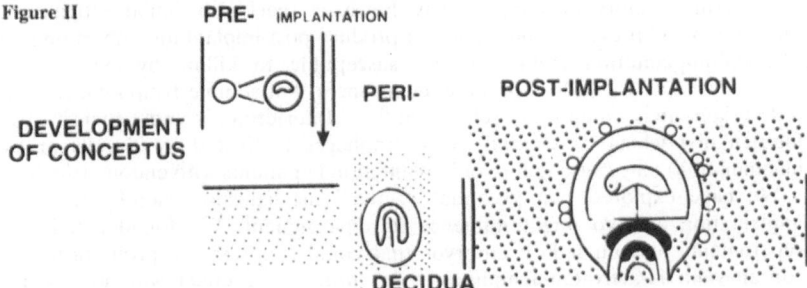

PRE- IMPLANTATION

PERI-

POST-IMPLANTATION

DEVELOPMENT OF CONCEPTUS

DECIDUA

Changes in the nature of the conceptus-maternal uterus interaction in early pregnancy. The model is based on the mouse where implantation occurs 4.5 days after conception and the transition from pre-implantation phase to post-implantation phase (with development of placenta and fetus proper) occurs at approximately 9.5 days. In humans, implantation occurs on day 6, and by day 14 (when the next menses would normally onset) placental development and fetal development can be seen.

PRE-IMPLANTATION INTERACTIONS

The pre-implantation embryo may release a variety of soluble factors that alter the maternal environment. Some of these are listed in Table 1 and further details may be found in the chapter by Kennedy (this volume). In the cow, molecules released by the pre-implantation embryo stimulate the uterus to release substances that in turn act to prevent luteolysis that would terminate the pregnancy.[26] O'Neill has suggested the PAF may activate platelets in the uterus to enhance implantation.[27] Ovum factor, SP1, histamine releasing factor(s), and suppressor factor(s) have not yet been shown to have significant roles in determining the outcome of early pregnancy.[28-31]

Table 1

Some soluble factors found in supernatants of human eggs within 48 hours of fertilisation

Factor	Reference
PAF (Platelet activating factor)	27
Ovum factor	28
SP 1 protein	29
Histamine-releasing factor	30
Suppressor activating (EPF?)	31

Maternally-derived factors may directly affect the embryo prior to implantation. For example, non-immunological tubal factors appear able to enhance the growth of rabbit blastocysts and their development both *in vitro* and *in vivo*.[32] The pre-implantation embryo may also express cell surface antigens (see David Billington, this volume). Although there has been some evidence that the female rodent can develop an immune response within 1-2 days of mating,[32-34] there is no convincing data to suggest such immunity benefits or harms the pre-implantation zygote. IgA antibodies in uterine secretions reactive with sperm or embryonic antigens may, however, react with similar antigens on the embryo and prevent implantation or produce post-implantation abortion.[35,36] The pre-implantation embryo is not susceptible to killing by cytotoxic T lymphocytes (CTL) under normal circumstances, but soluble lymphokines of T cell origin may inhibit development.[37,38] Interferon is not toxic[39] but interleukin-1 which is released by macrophages (activated by T cells or by inflammation) may cause failure of implantation in patients with endometriosis.[40]

We have explored two potential "active" mechanisms whereby the pre-implantation embryo might influence its environment. We found activity in supernatants of human IVF embryos that could suppress the proliferation of concanavalin A-activated lymphocytes *in vitro*.[41] The effect was not species specific and acted like a chalone, i.e. the growth of a variety of cells was inhibited.[42] Inhibitory activity has been associated with two molecular species of 1300 kd and 3700 kd molecular weight.[43] In two independent studies, it was found that overall only 1/63 women cleaving IVF embryos with non-suppressive supernatants became pregnant in contrast to 47/209 women receiving embryos with suppressive supernatants. However, interpretation of this association has been complicated by the fact that the IVF culture medium alone may be suppressive, particularly if incubated at 37C or supplemented with adult human serum, and that suppression may be found in the supernatant of embryos that fail to fertilise, fail to cleave, or are polyspermic. Furthermore, HPLC fractionation of non-suppressive supernatant from cultures containing cleaving embryos suggests that immunosuppressive molecules may be present but are masked by lymphocyte stimulating factors of broad molecular weight distribution.[43] These stimulatory type molecules that reverse suppression appear to distinguish embryos unlikely to establish a pregnancy from those that will. We suspect that release of these molecules may be indicative of "leaky" embryos. As we have recently been able to produce mouse embryos by IVF that have suppressive and non-suppressive supernatants, the molecular mechanisms and biological significance of suppression/stimulation can be investigated free of the problems associated with human experimentation.

The second aspect of pre-implantation embryo-uterine interaction we have studied concerns the "soil", i.e. immunosuppressive activity of the uterine lining cells. In the mouse, suppressive activity occurs at oestrus (the time of ovulation and mating) and persists until metoestrus.[44] The suppressor cell is large in size, lacks MAC-1 and Fc receptors, but bears the T cell marker Lyt 2.[44] A fluctuating suppression of CTL generation may be found in the lymph nodes draining the uterus synchronous with the oestrus cycle but shows a 24 hour lag compared to the uterine endometrium (DA Clark and J Brierley, unpublished). Large non-specific suppressor cells also occur in the luteal phase of the human menstrual cycle, but their surface phenotype has not yet been established.[45] In the mouse, mating whether fertile or sterile, triggers the hormonal changes of pregnancy. With these changes, suppressor cell activity in the uterine lining is increased.[44] Prior to implantation in the mouse, suppressor activity begins to decrease and at implantation and in the peri-implantation period (the first 4-5 days after implantation) suppressive activity is minimal.[46] The suppression found in the pre-implantation endometrium can be transiently reversed by injection into the uterine lumen of a variety of media and cell culture supernatants (DA Clark and J Brierley, unpublished). Traumatisation of the hormonally primed uterus leads to a decidual response similar to that triggered by implantation itself. However, the cells from artificial deciduomata are highly suppressive (with the suppressor cell being large in size) in contrast to the minimal degree of suppressive activity associated with peri-implantation uterine lining.[47] By ligating one uterine tube to prevent conception and then mating the mice, we have found that under natural circumstances a fertilised egg is required to reverse suppression. This reversal is confined to the uterine horn with implantations. (Figure III).

Figure III

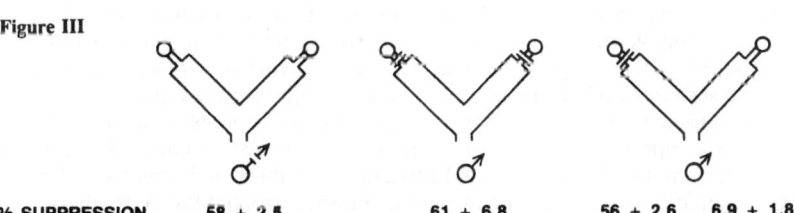

| % SUPPRESSION | 58 ± 2.5 | 61 ± 6.8 | 56 ± 2.6 | 6.9 ± 1.8* |

Effect of conceptual mating on intrauterine suppressor cell activity. Mating scheme shown in the left hand and middle panel induce pseudo pregnancy without an intrauterine conceptus. Only the right-sided uterine horn will contain implantations.

The rationale for reversal of suppression at the time of implantation is uncertain. Loss of intrauterine suppression may be related to the migration of suppressor cell activity to the uterine draining lymph nodes. Alternatively, it may be necessary to eliminate cells that could also suppress the growth of the implanting embryo. In this regard it is interesting that O'Neill has reported that uterine secretions in the mouse are inhibitory to blastocyst growth but this inhibition decreases at the time of implantation.[48]

IMPLANTATION AND PERI-IMPLANTATION PHASE

Many of the cellular and molecular aspects of implantation have been reviewed by Kennedy (this volume). The antigenic changes have been described by David Billington (this volume and see also Reference no. 37). Several aspects of the peri-implantation phase of pregnancy have been particularly interesting to us.

An influx of NK cells and asialo-GM1+ cells occurs 2 days after implantation and treatment of CBA/J females carrying CBA × DBA/2 fetus with anti-asialo-GM1 antibody on Day 6.5 of gestation has been reported to decrease the rate of abortion that occurs after Day 10.5 of gestation.[49] By Day 10.5 there is evidence of developmental retardation of the embryos and an infiltration by NK-type cells.[50,51] Further, indomethacin, a drug that activates macrophages to a cytotoxic state, produces abortion in the peri-implantation period and an infiltration with non-specific killer cells.[52,53] These data suggest that non-antigen specific host effector mechanisms may be particularly important mediators of embryo damage immediately following implantation and that the consequences of this toxicity may be manifest later in pregnancy. Further support for this idea is provided by very recent data showing that antibody to IL2-receptor that blocks allograft rejection is ineffective in preventing abortion (DA Clark, unpublished), and by the finding that *in vivo* T cell depletion with anti-L3T4 + anti-Lyt 2 does not prevent abortion (see Chaouat, Clark and Wegmann, this volume). Similar conclusions about the potentially important role of non-specific effector mechanisms in abortion have been derived from studies in the *Mus caroli-Mus musculus* system.[54,55]

Embryo survival during the peri-implantation period when suppressor cell activity is substantially reduced may be ascribed to evasion (non-expression of target structures), by the down-regulation of natural effector cells by prosta-glandins, and by direct active suppression by the embryonic trophoblast cells.[37,49,56] Suppression by trophoblast has also been associated with release *in vitro* of a soluble immunosuppressive activity neutralised by anti-progesterone antibody.[56] Active suppression is no longer a convincing explanation for early embryo survival. Embryo tissue (that is readily rejected when grafted under the kidney capsule of immune mice) is as suppressive as trophoblast *in vitro*,[57,58] and the soluble suppressor activity is not produced to any extent until 4 days after *in vitro* "implantation" (DA Clark and J Brierley, unpublished; P Van Vlasselar and M Vandeputte, personal communication). Further, trophoblast cells adjacent to embryo tissue under the kidney capsule do not prevent rejection of the embryo.[51]

In view of the potential importance of non-specific paraimmune effector mechanisms in early pregnancy failure, the regulation of NK and macrophage activity would appear potentially more relevant to understanding early implant survival then studies of suppression of T lymphocyte function. At the implantation site, there is a local infiltration of maternal cells. We have been interested in the possibility that the reduction in suppression of T cell responses by the peri-implantation decidua might be due to the presence of cells that produce "help". We tested for anti-suppression by use of anti-Fc receptor (FcR) antibody plus complement and found that killing the FcR+ cells substantially increased suppressor activity in the suspension (DA Clark and J Brierley, unpublished). Thus suppressor cell activity may still be important in protecting the embryo. The role of these persisting suppressor cells and FcR+ helper cells in peri-implantation endometrium is currently being examined in animal models of peri-implantation pregnancy failure, and using *in vitro* assays testing regulation of non-specific paraimmunological host effector cells.

POST-IMPLANTATION SUPPRESSION AND EARLY ABORTION

Four to 5 days after implantation, net suppressor activity again develops in the uterine decidua.[46] Decidua-associated cells of both large and small size have been described, with dominant activity associated with small granulated lymphocytic cells.[50,60] Enzymatic disaggregation can destroy this activity but reveals another population of large immunosuppressive PGE_2-producing macrophages[61,62]

The dependence of recruitment of granulated small lymphocytic suppressor cells on fetal trophoblast has been described elsewhere.[46] In spontaneous abortion in the *Mus caroli-Mus musculus* and in the CBA × DBA/2 systems, suppressor cell deficiency in the decidua occurs on Days 8.5-10.5 prior to the onset of overt abortion[46,60,61] and is associated with loss of resistance to maternal anti-paternal transplantation immunity[50,55,60,61] (and see Chaouat, Clark, Wegmann, this volume). Interestingly, in mice aborting due to the action of lethal T/t locus genes, fetal death is not preceded by suppressor deficiency (DA Clark, unpublished). These findings imply that a deficiency of local suppressor activity is not just a non-specific concomitant of all types of fetal death but rather is related to certain types of abortion, i.e. "rejection" rather than genetic death. The soluble suppressor factors released by cultured decidua block the action of a variety of lymphokines known to activate non-specific cytotoxic cells (IL-2, IL-3, interferon).[44] Deficiency of local suppression therefore may be relevant to models of pregnancy failure in which non-specific maternal effector cells play a role.

STUDIES OF HUMAN POST-IMPLANTATION PREGNANCY FAILURES

Spontaneous abortion occurring in mice within the first 10 days after implantation may provide a good model for early pregnancy failure due to occult abortion in humans. The rate of development is, of course, more rapid in the mouse as a completely viable fetus must be produced within 17 days after implantation. Nevertheless, the available histological information about early human pregnancy shows a development of placenta with syncytio- and cytotrophoblast by Day 16 after implantation.[63] It is not easy to obtain specimens of the implantation site from pregnant humans for functional analysis. The closest approximation has come from the histological studies of Nebel *et al*,[64] who monitored IVF-ET recipients and performed diagnostic curettages on failing chemical pregnancies. A mononuclear cell infiltration of the failing embryo reminiscent of the infiltration seen in the *Mus caroli-Mus musculus* and CBA × DBA/2 systems was seen.[50,54,64,65]

It has been possible to obtain biopsies from the placental bed of women at 6-14 weeks of gestation either at therapeutic termination or prior to miscarriage anticipated from serial βhCG assays and/or ultrasound examination. Our studies of therapeutic termination decidua have shown the presence of suppressor cells, small in size, and release of soluble suppressor factors blocking lymphocyte proliferation.[45,66] Unlike the suppressor activity found in IVF supernatants, suppression by decidual supernatants only affects cells dependent upon lymphokines such as interleukin-2 for growth, a finding similar to that made in the mouse system.[46,66] We found that suppressor cells were deficient in the decidua of women with missed abortion at 11 weeks of gestation.[45] Using phloxine-tartrazine stained biopsies of the placental bed from women prior to completion of the abortion (either natural or therapeutic), we have made two new observations. First, there are changes in the granulated mononuclear cell populations associated with spontaneous miscarriage.[67,68] One can distinguish between mononuclear cells with large cytoplasmic granules ⩾ 1 micron in diameter (CLG) at 1000 X and those cells with small diameter granules (LGL). The ratio of CGL/LGL and percentage of granulated mononuclear cells with large-sized granules was found to be significantly reduced in women with incipient first trimester abortion (see M. Michel *et al* in discussion for details). The reduction in the ratio was found to be due to both a decrease in the CLG population and an increase in the LGL population counted per section. We were able to make supernatants by incubating biopsy fragments at 37C for 48 hours in culture medium. When aborting patients and control legal termination patients were compared, significantly less suppressive activity on *in vitro* concanavalin A-stimulated T cell proliferation was shown by the aborters.

It is worth noting that maternal lymphocytic infiltration was only occasionally seen in biopsies of placental bed decidua and in placenta and villi of women destined to abort (DA Clark and M Michel, unpublished). Recent studies in mice suggest three possible explanations for this observation. First, infiltration of the fetoplacental unit by cytotoxic T and NK cells is transient, and the target of the T cell component appears to be the fetus itself rather than the trophoblast.[50,55,66] The result is a trophoblastic sac containing a necrotic embryo, analogous to an anembryonic sac in humans. Once the fetus is destroyed, cytotoxic cells disappear.[65] Biopsies of failing human pregnancies may therefore have been done too late to detect infiltration by cytotoxic maternal effector cells. It is possible, however, that the LGL seen in our placental bed biopsies represent an NK cell infiltrate similar to that seen in the mouse.[51] Second, it is possible that fetal death in the human (and also mouse) system is not mediated by a direct effector cell rejection of the fetus but rather, by impairment of trophoblast growth resulting in poor placentation so that the fetus dies from malnutrition.[46]

It is not yet clear how trophoblast function and growth could be impaired without a cellular infiltrate. Anti-trophoblast antibodies and the soluble toxins from non-specific para-immunological effector cells might be able to produce trophoblast dysfunction.[38,40,55] Damage occurring early in pregnancy could then lead to embryo failure at a much later stage of gestation, as discussed earlier, for the mouse system. Examination of tissue at the time of abortion may therefore miss the key events.

A third possible mechanism of pregnancy failure without cellular infiltration has been suggested by the studies of Athanassakis *et al.*[70,71] Both T cell-derived and non-T cell-derived cytokines can stimulate the growth of murine placental cells *in vitro*. From these findings it has been proposed that a deficiency of factors stimulating trophoblast growth may lead to pregnancy failure. Murine trophoblast cells also bear receptors for EGF (epithelial growth factor), and mice rendered deficient in circulating EGF activity abort![46] The types of growth factors in decidua and their origin must be further investigated before their relevance to early pregnancy failure can be determined.

SUMMARY

1. The high frequency of early pregnancy wastage cannot be completely explained by lethal chromosomal and anatomical defects of the embryo.
2. It is possible to identify *in vitro*-fertilised human embryos with reduced probability of implanting by presence of proliferation stimulating factors in the culture supernatant.
3. The pre-implantation and implanting embryo interacts actively with the endometrium to reduce hormone-dependent suppressor cell activity at implantation. Suppressor cells are still present, however, but are masked by a "helper" cell population bearing Fc receptors.
4. Post-implantation, suppressor cells, recruited or activated by trophoblast, release factors blocking the action of a variety of lymphokines capable of activating cytotoxic cells. Suppressor activity is deficient in decidua in only some types of abortion and may be normal where pregnancy fails due to a lethal genetic lesion.
5. Current evidence from study of recurrent spontaneously aborting mice supports a key role for non-antigen specific non-T effectors such as natural killer (NK) cells, NC cells and macrophages acting in the peri-implantation period before the embryo expresses any MHC antigens. At this time in pregnancy, the conceptus is more analogous to a tumour than a classic allograft. Later in gestation MHC antigens are expressed by the fetus and confer susceptibility to allospecific effectors of transplantation immunity. Although specific immunity may co-operate with natural para-immune effector mechanisms in abortion, natural immunity appears to be the underlying mechanism initiating the pregnancy failure.

ACKNOWLEDGEMENTS

This work was supported by MRC Canada. I thank Mrs M. Potter for her expert preparation of this manuscript.

REFERENCES

1. Roberts CJ, Lowe CR. Where have all the conceptions gone? *Lancet* 1975; **1:** 498-499.
2. Chen C, Jones WR, Bastin F, Forde C. Monitoring embryos after *in vitro* fertilisation using early pregnancy factor. *Ann New York Acad Sci* 1985; **442:** 420-428.
3. Rolfe EE. Detection of fetal wastage. *Fertil Steril*, 1982; **37:** 655-660.
4. Smart CY, Fraser IS, Roberts TK, Clancy RL, Cripps AW. Fertilisation and early pregnancy loss in healthy women attempting conception. *Clin Reprod Fertil* 1982; **1:** 177-184.
5. Edwards RG. I.V.F.—the problems. In: *Implantation.* Eds. JG Grudzinskas, MG Chapman. Berlin: Springer-Verlag, 1987; In press.
6. Miller JF, Williamson E, Glue J, Gordon YB, Grudzinskas JG, Sykes A. Fetal loss after implantation: a prospective study. *Lancet* 1980; **2:** 554-556.
7. Wilcox AJ, Weinberg CR, Wehmann RE, Armstrong EG, Canfield RE, Nisula BC. Measuring early pregnancy loss: laboratory and field methods. *Fertil Steril* 1985; **44:** 366-374.
8. Sharp NC, Anthony F, Miller JF, Masson GM. Early conceptual loss in subfertile patients. *Br J Obstet Gynaecol* 1983; **93:** 1072-1081.
9. Whittaker PG, Taylor A, Lind T. Unsuspected pregnancy loss in healthy women. *Lancet* 1983; **1:** 1126-1127.
10. Chartier M, Roger M, Barrat J, Michelon B. Measurement of plasma human chorionic gonadotrophin (hCG) and β-hCG activities in the late luteal phase: evidence of the occurrence of spontaneous menstrual abortions in infertile women. *Fertil Steril* 1979; **31:** 134-137.
11. Fleming R, Coutts JRT, Hamilton MP. Evidence against genetic factors causing major loss of embryos. *Br Med J* 1984; **288:** 1576.
12. Hertig AT, Rock J, Adams EC, Menkin EC. Thirty-four fertilized human ova, good, bad and indifferent recovered from 210 women of normal fertility. *Paediatrics* 1959; **23:** 202-211.
13. Warburton D. Reproductive loss: How much is preventable? *N Engl J Med* 1987; **316:** 158-160.
14. Lopata A, Martin M, Oliva K, Johnston I. Embryonic development and blastocyst implantation following *in vitro* fertilization and embryo transfer. *Fertil Steril* 1982; **38:** 682-687.
15. Van der Ven H, Al-Hasani S, Diedrich K, Krebs D. Embryo wastage and frequency of abortion following in vitro fertilization and embryo transfer (IVF-ET). Fifth World Congress on In Vitro Fertilization and Embryo Transfer, April 1987, AP-623 (abstract) p.155.
16. Romeu A, Masher SJ, Acosta AA, Veeck LL, Diaz J, Jones GS, Jones HW, Rosenwaks Z. Results of *in vitro* fertilization attempts in women 30 years of age and older: The Norfolk experience. *Fertil Steril* 1987; **47:** 130-136.
17. Clark DA, Croy BA, Rossant J, Chaouat G. Immune presensitization and local intrauterine defences as determinants of success in interspecies pregnancies. *J Reprod Fertil* 1986; **72:** 633-643.
18. Luckett DC, Muckherjee AB. Embryonic characteristics in superovulated mouse strains. *J Hered* 1986; **77:** 39-42.
19. Abe Y, Rin K, Katayana S, Harumi K. The investigating factors influencing implantation of mouse embryos fertilized *in vitro* and transferred to host. In: *Handbook of Abstracts, XII World Congress on Fertility and Sterility.* Eds. TE Soon, SS Ratnam, LS Min. Singapore, October 1986; 898.
20. Papaioannou VE, Ebert KM. Development of fertilized embryos transferred to oviducts of immature mice. *J Reprod Fertil* 1986; **76:** 603-608.

21. Gidley-Baird AA, O'Neil C, Sinosich MJ, Porter RN, Pike IL, Saunders DM. Failure of implantation in human *in vitro* fertilization and embryo transfer patients: The effects of altered progesterone/estrogen ratios in humans and mice. *Fertil Steril* 1986; **45:** 69-74.

22. Shaar CJ, Smalstig EB, Bennett DR, Cochrane RL. Effects of differing absolute and relative doses of progesterone and estrone on implantation and fetal survival in ovariectomized rats. *J Endocrinol Invest* 1986; **9:** 421-425.

23. Rider V, Heap RB, Wang MY, Feinstein A. Anti-progesterone monoclonal antibody affects early cleavage and implantation in the mouse by mechanisms that are influenced by genotype. *J Reprod Fertil* 1987; **79:** 33-43.

24. Wilmut I, Sales DI, Ashworth CJ. Maternal and embryonic factors associated with prenatal loss in mammals. *J Reprod Fertil* 1986; **76:** 851-864.

25. Bayna EM, Runyan RB, Scully NF, Reichner J, Lopez LC, Shur BD. Cell surface galactosyltransferase as a recognition molecule during development. *Mol Cell Biochem* 1986; **72:** 141-151.

26. Helmer SD, Hansen RJ, Anthony RV, Thatcher WW, Bazer FW, Roberts RM. Identification of bovine trophoblast protein-1, a secretary protein immunologically related to ovine trophoblast protein-1. *J Reprod Fertil* 1987; **79:** 83-91.

27. O'Neill C, Pike IL, Porter RN, Gidley-Baird AA, Sinosich MJ, Saunders DM. Maternal recognition of pregnancy prior to implantation: methods for monitoring embryonic viability in vitro and in vivo. *Ann New York Acad Sci* 1985; **442:** 429-439.

28. Morton H. Early pregnancy factor (EPF): a link between fertilization and immuno-modulation. *Aust J Biol Sci* 1984; **37:** 393-407.

29. Bersinger NA, Germond M. Detection of SP1 in IVF culture media and predictive value of embryo implantation after transfer. In: *Implantation*. Eds. JG Grudzinskas, MG Chapman. Berlin: Springer-Verlag (abstract); In press.

30. Cocchiara R, Di Trapani G, Azzolina A, Albeggiani G, Geraci D. Isolation of an embryo-derived histamine releasing factor (EHRF) from two cell human embryo culture media. A new model for human embryo implantation. In: *Implantation*. Eds. JG Grudzinskas, MG Chapman. Berlin: Springer-Verlag (abstract); In press.

31. Smart YC, Cripps AW, Clancy RL, Roberts TK, Lopata A, Shutt DA. Detection of an immunosuppressive factor in human preimplantation embryo cultures. *Med J Australia* 1981; **1:** 78-79.

32. Fischer B. Developmental retardation in cultured preimplantation rabbit embryos. *J Reprod Fertil* 1987; **79:** 115-123.

33. Dorsman BG, Tumboh-Oeri AG, Roberts TK. Detection of cell-mediated immunity to spermatazoa in mice and man by the leukocyte adherence-inhibition test. *J Reprod Fertil* 1978; **53:** 277-283.

34. McLean JM, Saya EI, Gibb ACC. Immune response to first mating in the female rat. *J Reprod Fertil* 1980; **1:** 285-295.

35. Hamilton MS. Maternal immune response to first mating in the female rat. *J Reprod Fertil* 1983; **5:** 249-264.

36. Clark DA. Local suppressor cells and success or failure of the fetal alograft. *Ann Immunol* 1984; **135D:** 321-324.

37. Clark DA. Current concepts of immunoregulation in implantation. In: *Implantation*. Eds. JG Grudzinskas, MG Chapman. Berlin: Springer-Verlag (abstract); In press.

38. Hill J, Wickersham C, Anderson D. Supernatants of mitogen and MLC-stimulated lymphocyte cultures inhibit the development of mouse embryos *in vitro*. *J Reprod Immunol* 1986; Suppl **1:** 153.

39. Carthew P, Wood M, Kirby C. Mouse interferon produced *in vivo* does not inhibit the development of preimplantation mouse embryos. *J Reprod Fertil* 1986; **77:** 75-79.

40. Fakih H, Baggett B, Holz G, Tsang K-Y, Lee JC, Williamson HO. Interleukin 1: a possible role in the infertility associated with endometriosis. *Fertil Steril* 1987; **47:** 213-217.

41. Daya S, Clark DA. Production of immunosuppressor factor(s) by pre-implantation human embryos. *Amer J Reprod Immunol Microbiol* 1986; **11:** 98-101.
42. Daya S, Lee S, Underwood J, Mowbray J, Craft I, Clark DA. Prediction of outcome following transfer of *in vitro* fertilized human embryos by measurement of embryo-associated suppressor factor. In: *Reproductive Immunology 1986*. Eds. DAClark and BA Croy. Amsterdam: Elsevier, 1986; pp.277-285.
43. Daya S, Clark DA. Identification of two species of immunosuppressor factor of differing molecular weight released by in vitro fertilized human oocytes. *Fertil Steril* 1988; **49:** In press.
44. Brierley J, Clark DA. Characterization of hormone-dependent suppressor cells in the uteri of mated and pseudopregnant mice. *J Reprod Immunol* 1987; **10:** 201-217.
45. Day S, Clark DA, Devlin MC, Jarrell J. Preliminary characterization of two types of suppressor cells in the human uterus. *Fertil Steril* 1985; **44:** 778-785.
46. Clark DA. Maternofetal relations: a minireview. *Immunol Letters* 1985; **9:** 179-188.
47. Slapsys RM. The accumulation of a novel type of suppressor cell in the uteri of allopregnant mice during successful pregnancy. Ph.D Thesis, McMaster University 1987.
48. O'Neill CO, Quinn P. Inhibitory influence of uterine secretions on mouse blastocysts decreases at time of blastocyst activation. *J Reprod Fertil* 1983; **68:** 269-274.
49. de Fougerolles AR, Baines MG. Modulation of the natural killer cell activity in pregnant mice alters the spontaneous abortion rate. *J Reprod Immunol* 1987; **11:** 147-153.
50. Clark DA, Chaput A, Tutton D. Active suppression of host-versus-graft reaction in pregnant mice. VII. Spontaneous abortion of allogeneic CBA/J × DBA/2 fetuses in the uterus of CBA/J mice correlates with deficient non-T cell suppressor cell activity. *J Immunol* 1986; **136:** 1668-1675.
51. Chaouat G. Placental immunoregulatory factors. *J Reprod Immunol* 1987; **10:** 179-188.
52. Voth R, Storon E, Huller K, Kirchner H. Activation of cytotoxic activity in cultures of bone marrow-derived macrophages by indomethacin. *Eur J Immunol* 1987; **17:** 145-148.
53. Scodras JM, Lala PK. Reactivation of maternal killer lymphocytes in the decidua with indomethacin, IL-2 or combination therapy is associated with embryonic demise. *Amer J Reprod Immunol Microbiol* 1987; **14:** 12.
54. Croy BA, Crepeau M, Yamashiro S, Clark DA. Further studies on the transfer of *Mus Caroli* embryos to immunodeficient *Mus musculus*. In: *Reproductive Immunology: Materno-fetal relationship*. Ed. G. Chaouat. Paris: INSERM Colloque, 1987; **154:** 101-112.
55. Clark DA, Croy BA, Wegmann TG, Chaouat G. Immunologic and paraimmunologic mechanisms in spontaneous abortion: recent insights and future directions. *J Reprod Immunol* 1987; In press.
56. Van Vlasselaer P, Vandeputte M. Immunosuppressive properties of murine tropho-blast. *Cell Immunol* 1984; **83:** 422-432.
56. Croy BA, Rossant J, Clark DA, Wegmann TG. Nonspecific suppression of *in vitro* generation of cytotoxic lymphocytes by allogeneic and xenogeneic embryonic tissue. *Transplantation* 1983; **35:** 627-629.
58. Drake BL, Rodger JC. Nonspecific suppression of *in vitro* immune responses by placental and nonplacental tissue. *Transplantation Proc* 1985; **17:** 1653-1654.
59. Simmons RL, Russell PS. The histocompatibility of fertilized mouse eggs and tropho-blast. *Ann New York Acad Sci* 1966; **129:** 35-45.
60. Clark DA, Damji N, Chaput A, Daya S, Rosenthal KL, Brierley J. Decidua-associated suppressor cells and suppressor factors regulating interleukin 2: Their role in the survival of the "fetal allograft". In: *Prog Immunol VI*. Eds. B Cinader and RG Miller. New York: Academic Press, 1987; **6:** pp.1089-1099.

61. Clark DA, Brierley J, Slapsys RM, Daya S, Damji N, Chaput A, Rosenthal KL. Trophoblast dependent and trophoblast independent suppressor cells of maternal origin in murine and human decidua. In: *Reproductive Immunology 1986*. Eds. DA Clark, BA Croy. Amsterdam: Elsevier, 1986; pp.219-226.
62. Wood G. Decidua-associated immunoregulatory cells and factors. In: *Reproductive Immunology 1986*. Eds. DA Clark, BA Croy. Amsterdam: Elsevier, 1986; pp.296-297.
63. Boyd JD, Hamilton W. *The human placenta*. Cambridge: James Dixon, Heffer, 1970.
64. Nebel L, Rudak E, Mashiah S, Dor J, Goldman B. Malimplantation caused by trophoblastic insufficiency resulting in failure of gestation following *in vitro* fertilization-embryo transfer. In: *Contributions to Obstetrics and Gynecology*. Eds. V Toder, AE Beer. Basel: Karger, 1985; **14**: 170-175.
65. Croy BA, Rossant J, Clark DA. Histologic and immunological studies of post-implantation death of *Mus caroli* embryos in the *Mus musculus* uterus. *J Reprod Immunol* 1982; **4**: 277-293.
66. Daya S, Rosenthal KL, Clark DA. Immunosuppressor factor produced by decidua-associated suppressor cells,—a proposed mechanism for fetal allograft survival. *Amer J Obstet Gynecol* 1987; **156**: 344-350.
67. Clark DA, Mowbray J, Underwood J, Liddell H. Histopathologic alterations in the decidua of human spontaneous abortion: loss of cells with large cytoplasmic granules. *Amer J Reprod Immunol Microbiol* 1987; **13**: 19-22.
68. Clark DA, Underwood J, Mowbray J, Michel M. Letter to editor. *Amer J Reprod Immunol Microbiol* 1987. In press.
69. Croy BA, Rossant J, Clark DA. Recruitment of cytotoxic cells by ectopic grafts of xenogeneic but not allogeneic trophoblast. *Transplantation* 1984; **37**: 84-90.
70. Athanassakis I, Wegmann TG. The immunotrophic interaction between maternal T cells and fetal trophoblast-macrophages during gestation. In: *Reproductive Immunology 1986*. Eds. DA Clark, BA Croy. 1986; pp.99-105.
71. Athanassakis I, Bleachley RC, Paetkau V, Guilbert L, Barr PJ, Wegmann TG. The immunotrophic effect of T cells and T cell lymphokines on murine fetally derived placental cells. *J Immunol* 1987; **138**: 37-44.

Discussion

Chairman: Dr. W. D. Billington

Professor BEER: Recently at the Society for the Study of Reproduction meeting, Ken Beaman and Roger Hoversland presented some very interesting data regarding antigen-specific suppressor T cell factor described by Dick Gershon, produced by stimulated leucocytes. They have found a hundred-fold increase in this antigen-specific suppressor factor in the uterus and its draining lymph nodes of Balb/C mice mated to strain A male. They haven't separately studied the decidua and myometrium. *In vivo* administration of specific monoclonal antibody against this suppressor factor at the time it is first being stimulated in the uterus, totally prevents implantation. If they wait to allow the suppressor factor to be produced and implantation to occur before giving the antibody, the pregnancies go on perfectly well. So, here is data that really supports what you are saying about a role for suppressor T cells in very early pregnancy.

Professor CLARK: That is very interesting. I haven't seen the details of those particular experiments. I think that I would say that any phenomenon where the successful pregnancy is altered by a defined reagent is definitely worthy of further analysis. Before we impute any type of mechanism as underlying the results, I think we really have to take the system apart and measure what has happened with administration of the antibody. There are many models of pregnancy failure produced using antibodies. The specificity of the effect with anti-suppressor factor antibody must also be tested.

Professor BEER: I agree. I want to make one other comment about the trophoblast proliferation experiments. Every one that is claiming immunotropism (i.e. immunologic stimulation of trophoblast) should clean up their act in terms of purifying the trophoblast cells before culturing with growth factors. One must absorb out the macrophages and/or the trophoblast with protein-A columns linked to specific monoclonals, or at least antibody-coated sheep erythrocytes to rosette out the macrophages, because there is at least 25% lymphoid cells contaminating placental cell preparations. You can't claim immunotropism for trophoblast from data obtained using a mixture of different cells.

Professor CLARK: I agree. It is also important to show that soluble factors in decidua that stimulate *in vitro* are T cell-derived. Our data using decidua from

229

allopregnant T cell-deficient mice raises further concerns about the immunotropism hypothesis.

Professor KENNEDY: A question about the suppressor activity in the IVF supernatants. Was there any correlation between the rate of cleavage of those embryos and the suppressor activity? The reason for asking is that David Armstrong's laboratory has recently demonstrated using rats that you can avoid the deleterious effect of *in vitro* culture if you allow the embryos additional time to mature before putting them back in the recipient uterus. There is a case, I think, to be made that the deleterious effects of culture may be due to a slowing down in the rate of growth of the embryos so that its development is retarded and out of synchrony with the uterus. Perhaps suppressor activity predicts success because the rate of cleavage of the embryos is faster?

Professor CLARK: In our initial study, there was a trend to greater supression with 8 cell vs 2 or 4 cell embryos. I have yet to review this issue using the data obtained via our collaborators who were kind enough to send supernatants. In the human system, we have certainly seen both suppression and pregnancy after transfer of 2 cell embryos. We have been able to duplicate the human findings using mouse IVF, and we have mouse IVF embryos which either have suppression or do not. So we will, I think, be able to look at a variety of correlates including cleavage rate in that system. Perhaps Dr. Daya has some comments?

Dr DAYA: Yes. The cleavage rates in our IVF studies are the same as those reported by others. However, only 40% of cleaving embryos produced suppression supernatants.

Professor GILL: I wouldn't be too quick to dispense with the allograft model. The conceptual framework of an organism's response to a foreign tissue, be it a fetus, a tumour, or an organ graft—provides a model with which we can deal experimentally with the issue. Mechanisms might be somewhat different in different cases, but I think the same basic ground rules apply. So I wouldn't be too quick to dispense with the model.

Professor CLARK: I agree that we must continue to pay attention to specific immune responses to alloantigens expressed by the fetus and fetal trophoblast. However, at implantation and for the first few days thereafter, the conceptus does not express alloantigens. It is during this period that the processes initiating pregnancy failure occurs in models of allopregnancy failure such as the CBA/J-DBA/2 system and in the *Mus caroli-Mus musculus* system. Current evidence indicates asialo GM1+ non-specific killer cells play a key role in the CBA/J-DBA/2 system. We know from studies of tumours that susceptibility to rejection by natural non-specific effector cell mechanisms (such as NK cells) increases with loss of alloantigen expression. Trophoblast is also notoriously resistant to allospecific rejection mechanisms but may be sensitive to non-specific effector mechanisms, particularly in the pre-implantation phase of pregnancy. In trying to understand what might compromise function that allows allospecific immunity to subsequently affect the fetus, we need to pay attention to the non-specific para-immunologic effector systems. Therefore I would suggest that we "partially reject" and free ourselves from the conceptual straight jacket imposed by the classical allograft model.

Dr PAGE FAULK: I would like to remind you that if you transfer IVF supernatants into splenectomised mice, you get a profound drop in the platelet count of those mice due to a platelet-activating-factor-like molecule in the supernatant that has been isolated and fairly well characterised. Now, one characteristic of activated platelets is that they release platelet growth factor (PDGF). I wonder if platelet growth factor would give you the same inhibition of proliferation *in vitro* which you observed?

Professor CLARK: That is a good question. One of my graduate students is testing PDGF in blastocyst cultures to find out whether there will be any effects. We will also test PAF. I should mention that Dr. Daya and I tried to reproduce the splenectomised mouse assay using C3H/HeJ mice and observed an increase in platelet count following injection of suppressive IVF supernatants. Subsequently, in discussion with Chris O'Neill, I learned that you only get a drop in platelet count in strains of mice that have high platelet counts such as random bred Swiss mice of the Quackenbush strain. Indeed, when you study humans with low platelet counts, there appears to be no significant drop.

Dr PAGE FAULK: Well, I must say that in the absence of Quackenbush strain mice in Indianapolis, we have instituted O'Neill's system in John MacIntyre's laboratory, and have recreated those data precisely.

Professor CLARK: What strain did you use?

Dr PAGE FAULK: Just a Swiss white. They must be splenectomised; this is one reason why it doesn't work with humans.

Dr ALLEN: I just wanted to put a general question, to you Mr Chairman, rather than the speaker. Could you remind us in the allograft model as to your original findings when you transplanted mouse eggs or whole embryos into kidneys and testes etc., in terms of the cell-mediated response particularly.

Dr BILLINGTON: Yes. Those experiments involved the transplantation of the blastocysts and immediate post-implantation embryos. If you do that using a pre-sensitised recipient, the trophoblast cells will proliferate and the embryonic cells will succumb. Therefore, the tissues obviously mature and MHC antigens as well as non-MHC transplantation antigens presumably will have the opportunity to become expressed on the embryonic cell component in the post-transplantation period. The result doesn't say that the antigens were present at the time when you transplanted the embryo, only that they will be recognisable on the embryo at some later stage.

Dr ALLEN: But you do get a cell-mediated response?

Dr BILLINGTON: In pre-sensitised animals you deliberately generate one and the embryo is susceptible.

Dr ALLEN: And if they are not pre-sensitised, no response?

Dr BILLINGTON: It takes a long time to develop, but yes you can get it.

Professor CLARK: There are a few cells which infiltrate at the lateral areas of the trophoblast-decidual junction in some successful allopregnancies, and in grafts to ectopic sites (such as the kidney), even in unimmunised animals. In the context of the embryo within its trophoblast in the uterus, when the trophoblast is failing and when trophoblast-dependent suppressor cell activity is deficient, the lymphocytes and cytotoxic cells which infiltrate don't appear to damage the trophoblast, but rather they migrate across into the embryo which then collapses to produce an anembryonic pregnancy. Haemorrhage at the trophoblast-decidual junction and polymorphonuclear infiltrate is associated with the placental death that follows. So, the fetus within the trophoblast may act as an allograft, as David Billington has indicated, but what is outside that is protecting the fetus, i.e. the trophoblast appears to act much more like a tumour in its biologic relationship to the host.

Interplay of oestrogens, progesterone and polypeptide growth factors at about the time of implantation

R. B. Heap

INTRODUCTION

Comparative studies of the factors involved in the establishment of pregnancy highlight the importance of endocrine, paracrine and possibly autocrine mechanisms in the interactions between embryo and mother. Such studies frequently though not invariably presage those concerned with regulatory factors in human pregnancy. Species differences, however, need to be taken into account and this is particularly true with respect to the various forms of implantation and placentation that are found, ranging from the non-invasive epithelio-chorial type at one extreme (as in the pig), to that of the invasive haemochorial type at the other, as in man.[1] Among the species to be considered here, implantation in the sheep is associated with invasion of the uterine epithelium by specialised granulated binucleate cells of the fetal epithelium which subsequently contribute towards the formation of a syncytium in localised regions of the uterine wall referred to as placentomes (Figure I). This migration of fetal cells which is initiated at about the time of attachment, continues throughout gestation.[2,3] Implantation in the mouse involves trophoblast invasion of the uterine epithelium and stromal cells, decidualisation of stromal cells followed by formation of the haemochorial placenta with blood released from maternal vessels to circulate through channels within the trophoblast before returning to maternal circulation. When considering the factors which contribute to the maintenance of pregnancy at and immediately after implantation it is apparent that oestrogens and progesterone are among the key components not only in the endocrinology of implantation but also in the maternal recognition of pregnancy, whereas polypeptide growth factors have an emerging role in the processes of uterine growth, vascularisation and embryo development, and it is to these events we shall now turn.

RECOGNITION

The maternal recognition of pregnancy relates to the time when prolongation of luteal function is first initiated by the presence of an embryo in the reproductive tract.[4,5] This event occurs in several species including the human female before the stage of definitive implantation and consists of the production of a chemical

Figure I

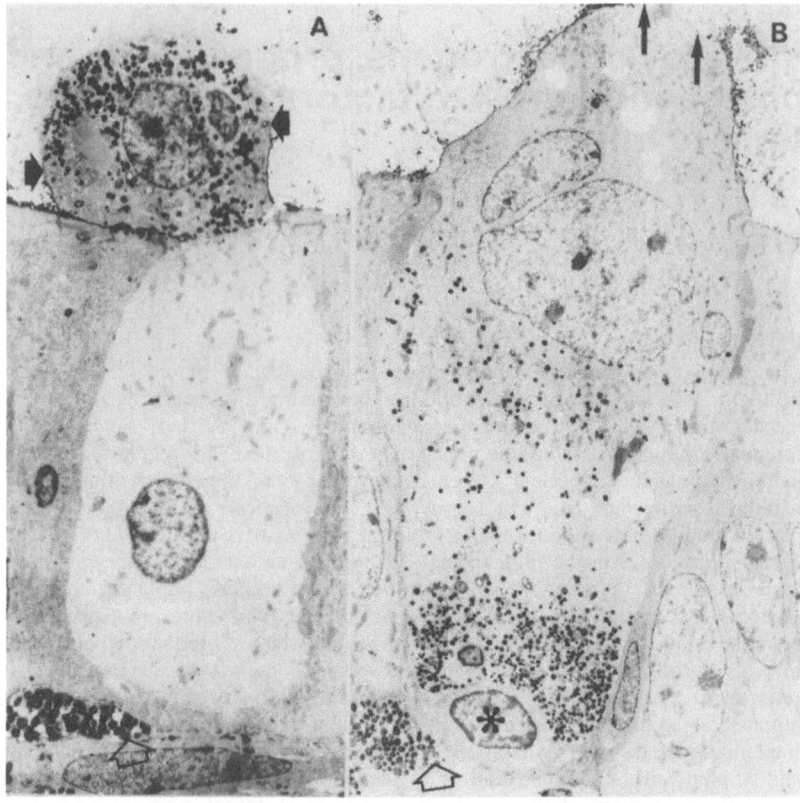

Attachment of the fetal epithelium (upper) to the maternal uterine epithelium (lower) at Day 16 of pregnancy in the sheep. Early (A) and late (B) stages in the formation of a trinucleate cell formed by fusion of a granulated binucleate cell from the fetal epithelium with a uninucleate uterine epithelial cell. During migration the granules that originate from the binucleate cell change position. In (B) they have accumulated at the base of the fused cell, which also contains two of the small lymphocyte-like cells (*) characteristically found among the columnar uterine epithelial cells. In (A) and (B), the position of the tight junctions that link the binucleate cells into the trophectodermal apical seal are marked by solid arrows. Below the uterine epithelium basement membrane, cell processes containing pigment-cell granules can be seen (open arrows). The pigment-cell granules can easily be distinguished from binucleate cell granules at higher magnifications. Pigment cells are found only below the uterine epithelium basement membrane. Figure (A) × 2,800; Figure (B) × 2,700. (By kind permission of Dr F.B.P. Wooding and the *American Journal of Anatomy*, see ref. 2).

signal which stimulates and prolongs the life-span of luteal cells in the ovary. In women the production of hCG by the embryo at about the time of implantation is considered to provide an important luteotrophic stimulus for sustained progesterone secretion prior to placental progesterone production (Figure II).[6]

Figure II

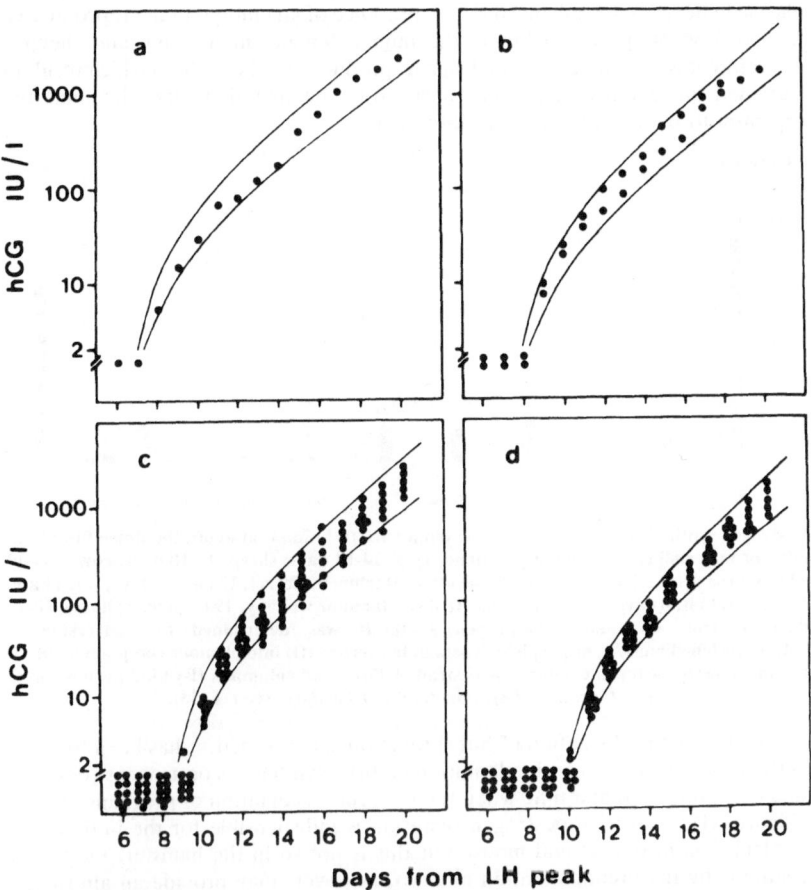

Days from LH peak

Individual plasma concentrations of hCG in 19 normal pregnancies grouped according to the day after the LH surge when the first detected increase in hCG occurred. This was on Day 8 in one cycle (a); Day 9 in two cycles (b), Day 10 in nine cycles (c), Day 11 in seven cycles (d). The sharp increase in plasma hCG values was closely associated with the expected time of implantation. (From Lenton EA, Neal LM, Sulaiman R. Plasma concentrations of human chorionic gonadotrophin from the time of implantation until the second week of pregnancy. *Fertil Steril* 1982; 37: 773. Reproduced with permission of the publisher, The American Fertility Society.)

Before this, however, there is an even earlier reaction to the presence of a fertilised egg, namely a mild thrombocytopenia seen in circulation.[7] In the mouse the reduction in platelet count has been attributed to the production by the fertilised egg of a compound resembling platelet-activating factor (PAF-acether).[8] When injected into sexually mature non-pregnant mice, PAF induces another component, early pregnancy factor (EPF), an activity in peripheral plasma believed to be enhanced by the presence of an embryo in the reproductive tract of several species including the human female, mouse, pig and sheep.[9] Therefore it is becoming clear that signals produced by the embryo which result in sustained luteal function are not necessarily the first that alert the maternal organism to the presence of a fertilised egg.

Figure III

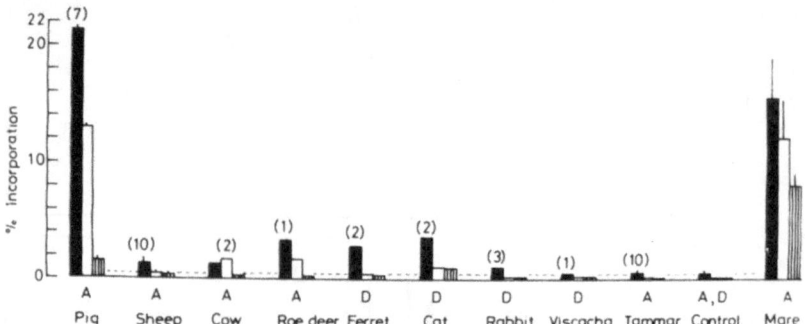

Oestrogen synthesis in trophoblast tissue from various animals at about the time of implantation or maternal recognition of pregnancy (pig, 14-18 days; sheep, 15-18 days; cow, 16 and 22 days; roe deer, allantochorionic tissue after attachment; ferret, 13 and 15 days; cat, 11 and 13 days; rabbit, 6 days; plains viscacha, 18 days; tammar wallaby, 19 to 25 days; horse, 18-27 days; control, no tissue). Oestrogen synthesis was determined by conversion of [³H]androstenedione (A), or [³H]dehydroepiandrosterone (D) into phenolic compounds (black columns), oestrone (open columns) or oestradiol-17β (lined columns). (By kind permission of the *Journal of Reproduction and Fertility*, see ref. 53).

So far as the prolongation of luteal function is concerned, it has been found in certain species that the preimplantation embryo synthesises oestrogens (oestrone and oestradiol-17β) at a time when the maternal recognition of pregnancy occurs (Figure III).[10] Ovarian oestrogen secretion is indispensible for the initiation of implantation in the rat and mouse but this is not so in the hamster. Oestrogen synthesis by the preimplantation embryo, however, may provide an alternative source of oestrogen if its action on the endometrium is obligatory for the onset of implantation. In the pig, oestrogens are luteotrophic but this is not true in all species studied, and alternative mechanisms need to be considered. Ovine trophoblast protein-1 (oTP-1) is an acidic protein (M_r approximately 18000) which represents a major secretory product of the blastocyst between days 13 and 21 of pregnancy. First produced after blastocyst expansion but before attachment to the endometrium, oTP-1 has the ability to prevent luteolysis possibly because it blocks and redirects endometrial prostaglandin $F_{2\alpha}$ ($PGF_{2\alpha}$) secretion. In this way $PGF_{2\alpha}$ is secreted predominantly into the uterine lumen rather than the venous drainage.[11] Recently it has been reported that oTP-1 has structural similarities with the interferon-α family of antiviral proteins.[12] Human α-interferon has been shown to compete with oTP-1 for endometrial binding.[13] If oTP-1 is shown to possess anti-viral properties, blastocyst production of such a protein may also be important in the prevention of infection during the preimplantation period. Scofield, Clegg and Lamming[14] found that the incidence of early embryonic wastage was closely correlated with the positive identification of intra-uterine infections, an observation substantiated by studies referred to by Wrathall[15] also in pigs.

Thus, among the factors that are produced during the preimplantation period attention continues to be focused on those that are known to promote the function of the *corpus luteum* such as chorionic gonadotrophins which are produced to a greater or lesser degree by trophoblast of many, if not all mammals; oestrogens which are luteotrophic in some, but not all species; and anti-luteolytic polypeptides whose synthesis and release is confined to crucial periods of early pregnancy when neutralisation of endogenous luteolytic compounds such as $PGF_{2\alpha}$ is a priority. Clearly the relative importance of these compounds in the establishment of pregnancy will differ between various species. Little is known about the physiological importance of compounds such as that which resembles PAF, a potent chemical mediator, or trophoblast proteins other than oTP-1 produced by the preimplantation blastocyst prior to the onset of implantation in species other than the domestic animals.

IMPLANTATION

The hormonal requirements of implantation have been extensively documented and studies show that progesterone is indispensible and that oestradiol-17β may also exert a key role. Recent studies in the mouse, rat and ferret further emphasise that perturbation of the secretion or availability of progesterone by passive immunisation seriously impairs the establishment of pregnancy.[16] The effect is particularly pronounced when antibody is administered shortly after the time of fertilisation.[5] Passive immunisation at this time does not act by modification of tubal transport, and there is no evidence from *in vitro* experiments that the antibody itself is embryotoxic, nor from *in vivo* experiments that the anti-implantation effect is due to a non-specific action of immunoglobulins. The anti-implantation effect is demonstrable only when antibodies are used that have a high affinity for progesterone.[17] There is substantial alteration in the lectin-binding properties of the oviducal epithelium and in the pattern of soluble proteins separated from uterine homogenates by two-dimensional gel electro-phoresis in pregnant animals treated with antibody compared to that found in control animals.[5] In addition the increase in uterine permeability (Figure IV) and the decidual reaction normally induced by intra-luminal oil installation are suppressed.[18]

Passive immunisation against progesterone therefore effectively blocks the establishment of pregnancy only when antibody is administered during a critical

Figure IV

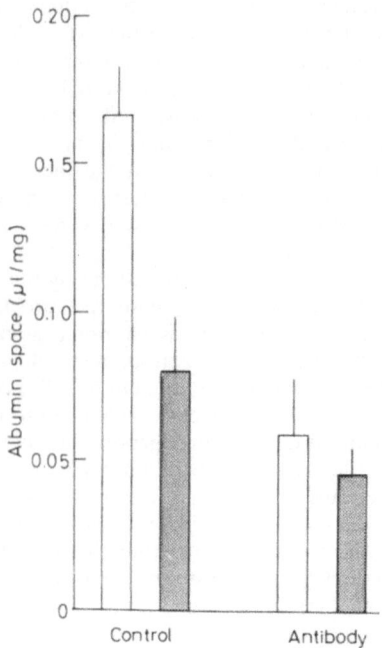

Anti-progesterone monoclonal antibody blocks the increase in uterine sensitivity expected after intra-uterine installation of oil in mice. Sesame oil (10 μl) was injected into one uterine horn of antibody- or saline-treated pseudopregnant mice 15 minutes after an i. v. injection of ¹²⁵I-labelled human serum albumin. Autopsies were carried out 6 hours after the intra-uterine injection. The open bar represents the injected horn and the stippled bar the non-injected horn. (By kind permission of the *Journal of Endocrinology*, see ref. 18).

stage shortly after fertilisation, emphasising the importance of progesterone secretion during this phase of early embryo development. Supplementation with progesterone during early pregnancy does not produce a consistent improvement in fertility in all species studied.[19] Moreover, preliminary findings in marmosets treated with the same anti-progesterone monclonal antibody indicate a lack of anti-implantation efficacy (PTK Saunders, JP Hearn and RB Heap, unpublished) implying that preimplantation progesterone secretion and endometrial preparation for nidation is of greater importance in some species than in others. The endocrinology of the preimplantation period in the marmoset is characterised by a particularly sharp rise in systemic concentrations of progesterone immediately after fertilisation which probably means that the steeply rising secretion of ovarian progesterone is difficult to neutralise by passive immunisation.[20,21]

UTERINE GROWTH AND VASCULARITY

Growth of the uterus undergoes pronounced changes during the course of the reproductive cycle. After ovulation and fertilisation in the mouse there is a decrease in uterine size due to removal of intraluminal fluid, luminal epithelial cells die and the lumen of the uterus becomes slit-shaped and closed. This is followed by a wave of mitosis in the uterine glands with increased mucopolysaccharide secretion into the glandular lumen and by endometrial stroma growth with fibroblast and blood vessel proliferation and fibroblast differentiation into decidual cells. This latter development depends on the presence of an embryo in rodents but occurs both during the menstrual cycle and during pregnancy in women. Endometrial stroma growth, along with further vascular changes, result in increased uterine weight and is influenced by ovarian hormones and by progesterone in particular acting after oestrogenic stimulation.[22] During pregnancy endometrial growth depends on a continuous supply of progesterone which stimulates the production of secretory proteins from endometrial glands,[23,24] proteolytic enzymes involved in the dissolution of blastocyst coverings—arylamidase 1[25] and neuraminidase[26]—other uterine enzymes including ornithine decarboxylase[27], glucosamine 6-phosphate synthetase[28] and oestrogen sulphotransferase,[29] and of an inhibitor of plasminogen activator.[30,31]

The mechanisms involved in the proliferative response of the uterus to ovarian hormones remain incompletely understood. Oestrogens fail to produce a proliferative response of uterine cells in culture which has led to the idea that their effect is mediated by circulating oestromedins[32] or by autocrine or paracrine growth factors.[33,34] Epidermal growth factor (EGF) stimulates the growth of uterine epithelial cells in culture[35] and EGF receptors are stimulated by oestrogen,[36] so that local growth factor production may have an important part to play in uterine growth regulation. However, the ability of oestrogen when injected directly into one uterine horn to stimulate DNA synthesis in that horn alone[37] implies that circulating oestromedins have a limited importance in the proliferative response.

In order to study this question further, Murphy et al[38] have examined the expression of c-myc and a closely related proto-oncogene, N-myc, in the rat uterus after oestradiol-17β treatment. Uterine c-myc mRNA levels were stimulated by oestradiol compared to those found in control ovariectomised animals but there was no difference in levels at various stages of the oestrous cycle. The N-myc mRNA levels increased rapidly within 15 minutes after oestradiol treatment, and there was evidence that c-myc and N-myc proto-oncogenes were restricted to different cell and tissue types. The rapidity of the N-myc response was attributed to a direct effect of oestradiol whereas the protracted c-myc response was considered to be mediated by autocrine, paracrine or circulating oestrogen-mediated growth factors.

Rothchild[39] summarised the role of progesterone in the maintenance of gestation in terms of its inhibition of myometrial contractibility, immunological protection of the embryo, inhibition of endometrial prostaglandin synthesis and the promotion of uterine growth and plasticity. Clear evidence for progesterone-induced endometrial proteins has emerged (for instance, PAPP-A,[40,41] placental protein 12 uteroglobins,[42,43] but it is only recently the idea has developed that progesterone, as with oestradiol-17β, may also act by the stimulation of local growth factor production.

The increased vascular permeability that occurs at the site of implantation is associated with a significantly higher blood flow than that which occurs in regions adjacent to implantation sites in the rat.[46] Takemori *et al*[47] have reported that angiogenesis first appears in implantation sites on Day 7, one day after the time that the blastocyst has become firmly attached to the endometrium in the rat. This process of angiogenesis may be a function of locally produced growth factors among which those of the fibroblast growth factor (FGF) family are predominant. Acidic and basic forms of FGF bind strongly to heparin[48,49] and recently, uterine derived growth factors have been identified in the pig uterus that bind to heparin-Sepharose affinity columns and stimulate proliferation of Swiss mouse 3T3 cells in culture.[50,51] Three oncogenes have been identified that encode for proteins structurally similar to the fibroblast growth factors, one of which is *int-2*, an oncogene originally detected in mouse mammary cancer cells caused by the mouse mammary tumour virus. In the human the site of the mammary oncogene *int-2* is chromosome band 11q13, now discovered to be the location of the progesterone receptor gene.[52] This finding raises the intriguing question of whether progesterone exerts a regulatory effect on the production of putative angiogenic molecules in organs such as the uterus and to what extent uterine growth and vascularity are influenced by this means.

The interplay of the classical ovarian hormones, oestrogens and progesterone, in the maternal recognition of pregnancy and implantation has entered a new phase of investigation. The possibility that hormonal effects are mediated through locally produced polypeptide growth factors emphasises the importance of new studies on defined sub-populations of uterine cells in order to elucidate the signalling processes within the endometrium that are initiated by the developing embryo.

REFERENCES
1. Perry JS. The mammalian fetal membranes. *J Reprod Fert* 1981; **62:** 321-335.,
2. Wooding FB. Role of binucleate cells in fetomaternal cell fusion at implantation in the sheep. *Am J Anat* 1984; **170:** 233-250.
3. Wooding FB, Flint AP, Heap RB, Morgan G, Buttle HL, Young IR. Control of binucleate cell migration in the placenta of sheep and goats. *J Reprod Fert* 1986; **76:** 499-512.
4. Short RV. Implantation and the maternal recognition of pregnancy. In: *Foetal Anatomy*. (Ciba Foundation Symposium No. 23). London: Churchill Livingstone, 1969; pp.2-26.
5. Heap RB, Fleet IR, Fin C, Yang C-B, Whyte A. Maternal reactions affecting early embryogenesis and implantation. *J Reprod Fert Suppl*; In press.
6. Lenton EA, Neal LM, Sulaiman R. Plasma concentrations of human chorionic gonadotrophin from the time of implantation until the second week of pregnancy. *Fertil Steril* 1982; **37:** 773-778.
7. O'Neill C. Thrombocytopenia is an initial maternal response to fertilization in mice. *J Reprod Fertil* 1985; **73:** 559-566.
8. O'Neill C. Partial characterization of the embryo-derived platelet-activating factor in mice. *J Reprod Fertil* 1985; **75:** 375-380.

9. Orozco C, Perkins T, Clarke FM. Platelet-activating factor induces the expression of early pregnancy factor activity in female mice. *J Reprod Fertil* 1986; **78**: 549-555.
10. Gadsby JE, Heap RB, Burton RD. Oestrogen production by blastocyst and early embryonic tissue of various species. *J Reprod Fertil* 1980; **60**: 409-417.
11. Bazer FW, Vallet JL, Roberts RM, Sharp DC, Thatcher WW. Role of conceptus secretory products in establishment of pregnancy. *J Reprod Fertil* 1986; **76**: 841-850.
12. Imakawa K, Anthony RV, Kazemi M, Marotti KR, Polites HG, Roberts RM. Interferon-like sequence of ovine trophoblast protein secreted by embryonic trophectoderm. *Nature* 1987; **330**: 377-378.
13. Stewart HJ, McCann SHE, Barker PJ, Lee KE, Lamming GE, Flint APF. Interferon sequence homology and receptor binding activity of ovine trophoblast antiluteolytic protein. *J Endocrinol* 1987; **115**: R13-R15.
14. Scofield AM, Clegg FG, Lamming GE. Embryonic mortality and uterine infection in the pig. *J Reprod Fertil* 1974; **36**: 353-361.
15. Wrathall AE. *Reproductive disorders in pigs*. Commonwealth Agricultural Bureaux, 1975.
16. Rider V, Wang M-Y, Finn C, Heap RB, Feinstein A. Anti-fertility effect of passive immunization against progesterone is influenced by genotype. *J Endocrinol* 1986; **108**: 117-121.
17. Ellis ST, Heap RB, Butchart AR, Rider V, Richardson NE, Wang M-Y, Taussig MJ. Efficacy and specificity of anti-progesterone monoclonal antibodies in preventing the establishment of pregnancy in the mouse. *J Endocrinol*; In press.
18. Rider V, McRae A, Heap RB, Feinstein A. Passive immunisation against progesterone inhibits endometrial sensitization in pseudopregnant mice and has antifertility effects in pregnant mice which are reversible by steroid treatment. *J Endocrinol* 1985; **104**: 153-158.
19. Flint APF, Saunders PTK, Ziecek AJ. Blastocyst-endometrial interactions and their significance in embryonic mortality. In: *Control of pig production*. Eds: DJA Cole, GR Foxcroft. London: Butterworth, 1982; pp.253-276.
20. Chambers PL, Hearn JP. Peripheral plasma levels of progesterone, oestradiol-17β oestrone, testosterone, androstenedione and chorionic gonadotrophin during pregnancy in the marmoset monkey, *Callithrix jacchus*. *J Reprod Fertil* 1979; **56**: 23-32.
21. Hodges JK, Henderson C, Hearn JP. Relationship between ovarian and placental steroid production during early pregnancy in the marmoset monkey (*Callithrix jacchus*). *J Reprod Fertil* 1983; **69**: 613-621.
22. Finn CA. Growth of the uterus. *Res Reprod* 1987; **19**: 3-4.
23. McLaughlin DT, Sylvan PE, Richardson GS. The search for progesterone-dependent proteins secreted by human endometrium. *Adv Exp Med Biol* 1981; **138**: 113-131.
24. Salamonsen LA, O WS, Doughton B, Findlay JK. The effects of oestrogen and progesterone *in vivo* on protein synthesis and secretion by cultured epithelial cells from sheep endometrium. *Endocrinology* 1985; **117**: 2148-2159.
25. Denker HW. Proteases of the blastocyst and of uterus. In: *Proteins and steroids in early pregnancy*. Eds: IIM Beier, P Karlson. Berlin: Springer-Verlag, 1982; pp.183-208.
26. Srivastava PN, Farooqui AA. Studies on neuraminidase activity of the rabbit endometrium. *Biol Reprod* 1980; **22**: 858-863.
27. Levy C, Glikman P, Vegh I, Mester J, Baulieu EE, Suto R. Oestradiol, progesterone and tamoxifen regulation of ornithine decarboxylase (ODC) in rat uterus and chick oviducts. *Prog Clin Biol Res* 1984; **142**: 133-144.
28. Rukmini V, Reddy PR. Effect of estradiol and progesterone on glucosamine 6-phosphate synthetase in the uterus of rat. *Steroids* 1981; **37**: 573-579.

29. Meyers SA, Lozon MM, Corombos JD, Saunders DE, Hunter K, Christensen C, Brooks SC. Induction of porcine uterine estrogen sulfotransferase activity by progesterone. *Biol Reprod* 1983; **28**: 1119-1128.
30. Mullins DE, Bazer FW, Roberts RM. Secretion of a progesterone induced-inhibitor of plasminogen activator by the porcine uterus. *Cell* 1980; **20**: 865-872.
31. Savouret JF, Misrahi M, Milgrom E. Molecular action of progesterone. In: *Oxford reviews of reproductive biology.* Ed: JR Clarke. Oxford: Clarendon Press; In press.
32. Sirbasku DA, Benson RH. Estrogen-inducible growth factors that may act as mediators (estromedins) of estrogen-promoted tumor cell growth. In: *Hormones and cell culture.* Eds: GH Sato, R Ross. New York: Cold Spring Harbor, 1979; pp.477-497.
33. Ikeda T, Lin QF, Daneilpour D, Officer JB, Ho M, Leland FE, Sirbasku DA. Identification of estrogen-inducible growth factors (estromedins) for rat and human mammary tumor cells in culture. *In Vitro* 1982; **18**: 961-979.
34. Imai Y. Epidermal growth factor in the rat uterine luminal fluid. *64th Annual Meeting, The Endocrine Society* (Abstract 331), San Francisco, California, 1982; 162.
35. Tomooka Y, DiAugustine RP, McLachlan JA. Proliferation of mouse epithelial cells *in vitro. Endocrinology* 1986; **118**: 1011-1018.
36. Mukku VR, Stancel GM. Regulation of epidermal growth factor receptor by estrogen. *J Biol Chem* 1985; **260**: 9820-9824.
37. Stack G, Gorski J. Direct mitogenic effect of estrogen on the prepubertal rat uterus: studies on isolated nuclei. *Endocrinology* 1984; **114**: 1141-1150.
38. Murphy LJ, Murphy LC, Friesen HG. Estrogen induction of N-myc and c-myc proto-oncogene expression in the rat utëus. *Endocrinology* 1987; **120**: 1882-1888.
39. Rothchild I. Role of progesterone in initiating and maintaining pregnancy. In: *Progesterone and progestins.* Eds: CW Bardin, E Milgrom, P Mauvais-Jarvis. New York: Raven Press, 1983; pp.219-229.
40. Bischof P, Duberg S, Schindler AM, Obradovic D, Weil A, Faigaux R, Herrmann WL, Sizonenko PC. Endometrial and plasma concentrations of pregnancy-associated plasma protein-A (PAPP-A). *Br J Obstet Gynaecol* 1982; **89**: 701-703.
41. Sjoberg J, Wahlstrom T, Seppala M. Pregnancy associated plasma protein A in the human endometrium is dependent on the effect of progesterone. *J Clin Endocrinol Metab* 1984; **58**: 359-362.
42. Wahlstrom T, Seppala M. Placental protein 12 (PP12) is induced in the endometrium by progesterone. *Fertil Steril* 1984; **41**: 781-786.
43. Koistinen R, Kalkkinen N, Huhtala MJ, Seppala M, Bohn H, Rutanen E-M. Placental protein 12 is a decidual protein that binds somatomedin and has an identical N-terminal amino-acid sequence with somatomedin-binding protein from human amniotic fluid. *Endocrinology* 1986; **118**: 1375-1378.
44. Kumar NM, Chandra T, Woo SLC, Bullock DW. Transcriptional activity of the uteroglobin gene in rabbit endometrial nuclei during early pregnancy. *Endocrinology* 1982; **111**: 1115-1120.
45. Savouret JF, Guiochon-Mantel A, Milgrom E. The uteroglobulin gene, structure and interaction with the progesterone-receptor. In: *Oxford survey of eucaryotic genes.* Ed: N McLean. Oxford: Oxford University Press, 1984; pp.192-214.
46. McRae A, Heap RB. Uterine vascular permeability, blood flow and extracellular fluid space during implantation in rats. *J Reprod Fertil*; In press.
47. Takemori K, Okamura H, Kanzaki H, Koshida M, Konishi I. Scanning electro-microscopy study on corrosion cast of rat uterine vasculature during the first half of pregnancy. *J Anat* 1984; **138**: 163-173.
48. Lobb RR, Fett JW. Purification of two distinct growth factors from bovine neural tissue by heparin affinity chromatography. *Biochemistry* 1984; **23**: 6295-6299.
49. Gospadarowicz D, Cheng J, Lui G-M, Baird A, Bohlen P. Isolation of brain fibroblast growth factor by heparin-sepharose affinity chromatography: identity with pituitary fibroblast growth factor. *Proc Natl Acad Sci USA* 1984; **81**: 6963-6967.

50. Brigstock DR, Brown KD, Heap RB, Laurie MS. Cell growth-promoting polypeptides in the uterus of the pig. *J Physiol (Lond)* 1983; **343:** 126P.
51. Brigstock DR, Laurie MS, Heap RB, Brown KD. Characterization of an acidic heparin-binding growth factor from pig uterus. *Biol Reprod* 1986; **34: Suppl No 1:** 133 (Abstract).
52. Law ML, Kao FT, Wei Q, Hartz JA, Greene GL, Zarucki-Schulz T, Conneely OM, Jones C, Puck TT, O'Malley BW, Horwitz KB. The progesterone receptor gene maps to human chromosome band 11q13, the site of the mammary oncogene *int-2*. *Proc Natl Acad Sci USA* 1987; **84:** 2977-2881.
53. Heap RB, Hamon Maureen, Allen WR. Studies of oestrogen synthesis by the preimplantation equine conceptus. *J Reprod Fertil* 1982; **Suppl 32:** 343-352.

Discussion

Chairman: Professor D. A. Clark

Professor GRUDZINSKAS: A question for Dr. Heap. Can he make some comment on any possible function of the ovary other than the production of progesterone and oestrogen? New information indicates that women previously castrated can have successful pregnancies after embryo donation if synthetic progesterone and oestrogen are given. So does the ovary have any role to play at all in pregnancy other than the production of these two hormones?

Dr HEAP: That is quite a big question. I think the point that comes to mind immediately would take us back to the issue of the production of early pregnancy factor. Whether in fact there is a role for early pregnancy factor in the establishment and maintenance of gestation, I think is a question that certainly hasn't been answered adequately as yet. We can't exclude the possibility that there may be ovarian factors that influence the probability of success in the very early stages. As far as the later stages are concerned, I would agree with you that there is strong evidence that the ovary probably has very little additional function other than producing oestrogen and progesterone. There might be those who would also say that the other is important in the production of relaxin, but that is another story.

Professor GILL: Do I correctly infer that you are trying to make a relationship between the production of progesterone and the control of growth factors, and the influence of growth factors on vascularity?

Dr HEAP: I am trying to draw attention to the fact that at the moment this could be a profitable line of future research. There is certainly no direct link yet shown, but one should not ignore the fact that one of the growth factors that has now been specifically identified from the uterus is related to a group of proteins that are also being synthesised and coded by genes that can function as oncogenes, and there is a possibility that there is a link between one of these and progesterone and the regulation of progesterone receptor. I think those are the facts that we have at the moment. How we link those together in our minds is going to be obviously dependent on further experimentation.

Dr LOKE: May I just clarify the information on your 2D gels? Are you saying that anti-progesterone removes three molecules from the uterus which are not progesterone?

Dr HEAP: Yes.

Dr LOKE: What are these molecules?

Dr HEAP: Those molecules on the 2D gels were polypeptides. They were stained by Coumassie blue and they were molecules that appeared when the animal was not treated with progesterone antibody. One interpretation of these results would be that, in spite of the data that I showed on circulating levels of progesterone where there appears to be an increase in the amount of free progesterone which is present in the circulation, the antibody is preventing locally the steroid gaining entrance to the target cells. Now if that is the case, then I think it must mean that those target cells are being deprived of progesterone and therefore they are not switching on the synthesis of these polypeptides in early pregnancy.

Dr BILLINGTON: What are your current views on the role of blastocyst oestrogen as a signal for implantation in the different species in which you are interested?

Dr HEAP: To summarise a lot of data from many laboratories including our own, the picture that is emerging is that there are certain species in which the quantity of oestrogen produced by the pre-implantation blastocyst is substantial and can be chemically demonstrated and chemically quantified. The pig and the mare are the two most outstanding examples of species in terms of the quantity that is produced. The difficulty comes with the other species where the quantities are not so great, although I can say that in the sheep and the cow there is very much less oestrogen produced. I think it may turn out that the oestrogen production by the pre-implantation blastocyst is common to quite a number of species, and might also occur in the rodent. Thus, it may not simply be maternal oestrogen that is required for implantation, but also a local production of oestrogen.

Dr BILLINGTON: Is there any evidence that failure of adequate amounts of oestrogen is actually a part of the failure of implantation?

Dr HEAP: That is a question asked by many. The difficulty is that when people have used antioestrogens to try to answer that question, such as in the rabbit for example, and then administer an antioestrogen at the appropriate time hoping to block the action of oestrogen on oestrogen receptors in the uterus, surely it can be shown that there is an effect, and the pregnancy is lost. But the problem is that many of these drugs are themselves embryotoxic and it is extremely difficult to interpret the results. I would hold back on saying that the question has been settled.

Professor BEER: I am interested in your levels of progesterone being higher following the administration of the antibody. Is the antibody specific for progesterone, or might it be interfering with the steroid binding globulins altering their levels and/or the interaction of progesterone with this carrier.

Dr HEAP: We have measured the amount of the steroid binding globulins at that point. Fortunately, in the pre-implantation phase, the steroid binding globulins are present at a rather low concentration. They have not started to rise. I think the evidence does suggest that the difference that we see is not due to an interaction with the steroid binding globulin.

Professor CLARK: We have heard a lot about granulated cells from this meeting. I am sure that we are going to hear more about them, but I was intrigued by the granules that seemed to be in those trophoblast cells. What is in those granules?

Dr HEAP: Certainly now I need to quote Peter Wooding. His work shows very clearly that placental lactogen is synthesised and stored within those granules. There are a number of other molecules that are stored in those granules and work that he has done with Lee in Melbourne has identified a monoclonal antibody that is very specific for these granules. As yet they don't know what the antigen is.

Prostaglandins and other non-steroidal mediators at and immediately after implantation

T.G. Kennedy

INTRODUCTION

Implantation is arguably the most crucial stage in the establishment of pregnancy. In order for implantation to be successful, synchronisation of the development of the embryo and endometrium is required;[1] the embryo must be at the blastocyst stage of development and hormone-dependent changes resulting in the development of a "receptive" endometrium must have occurred. Lack of synchronisation results in the failure, or less commonly the postponement, of implantation.

There are considerable differences between species in the reactions which occur during implantation, especially in the extent of trophoblastic invasion of the endometrium.[2,3] At one extreme of the spectrum are species with central implantation in which there is no trophoblastic invasion of the endometrium. Contact between the conceptus and endometrium is made as a consequence of blastocyst enlargement; the luminal epithelium of the endometrium generally remains intact. Changes in the underlying endometrial stroma are usually limited in these species. By contrast, in species with eccentric or interstitial implantation, the blastocyst remains small and the trophoblastic cells break through the luminal epithelium as a consequence of apoptosis of the epithelial cells, or alternatively by separating the epithelial cells, and invade the endometrial stroma. Changes in the underlying endometrial stroma are generally extensive in these species. The endometrial stromal cells proliferate and differentiate to decidual cells which ultimately give rise to the maternal component of the placenta.

In many species in which invasive implantation occurs, changes in the endometrial stroma similar to those obtained in response to an implanting conceptus can be obtained in the absence of a conceptus if an appropriate stimulus is applied to the uterus at the time when implantation would normally occur.[1,3] This uterine response, referred to as the decidual cell reaction or decidualisation, has been used extensively as a model for the study of implantation.

249

In virtually all species investigated, the earliest macroscopically-observable indication of blastocyst implantation is an increase in endometrial vascular permeability which is restricted to the areas immediately adjacent to the blastocysts.[1] The increase in permeability is usually taken as defining the initiation of implantation; in the rat, for example, the increase in permeability can be first observed some 20-24 hours before trophoblastic invasion or differentiation of decidual cells.[1] In those species in which decidualisation occurs in response to artificial stimuli, an increase in endometrial vascular permeability precedes the growth and differentiation of decidual cells. Psychoyos[1] has proposed that the increase in permeability is requisite for implantation and decidualisation.

The localised nature of the permeability change at implantation suggests that it occurs in response to a signal from the blastocyst. In women, however, there is no need to involve a local-acting embryonic signal because during each menstrual cycle there is a generalised increase in endometrial vascular permeability followed by differentiation within the stroma of the pre-decidual cells.[1] These changes presumably are a consequence of a systematic stimulus. In the species in which an embryonic signal seems to be involved, the nature of the signal is uncertain, but there is now considerable evidence for a number of species that eicosanoids, particularly prostaglandins (PGs), have an obligatory role in the permeability changes and subsequent decidualisation. The PGs may not be the primary embryonic signal and probably act not alone but in concert with other vasoactive substances.

This contribution primarily reviews the evidence for the involvement of PGs in implantation and decidualisation, and briefly touches on the possible involvement of other non-steroidal mediators. Because little work has been done in our own species or in primates, most of the data are derived from non-primate species. The involvement of PGs in the decidual cell reaction is also reviewed because this reaction has been used widely and profitably as a model for implantation.

EVIDENCE FOR THE INVOLVEMENT OF PROSTAGLANDINS

In pregnant animals, treatment with indomethacin, an inhibitor of PG synthesis,[4] has been reported to delay or inhibit the localised increase in endometrial vascular permeability[5-9] and implantation[10-17] in a number of species. The intrauterine administration of PG antagonists at the expected time of implantation reduces the number of implantation sites.[18] In addition, the concentrations of PGs are elevated in the areas of increased endometrial vascular permeability,[5,7,19-21] and exogenous PGs can reverse, at least partially, the effects of inhibitors of PG synthesis on implantation.[12,14,15,22] These data are consistent with the notion that PGs are involved in the implantation process.

In non-pregnant animals with uteri sensitised for the decidual cell reaction, the endometrial vascular permeability increase[23] which precedes decidualisation, the increase in endometrial alkaline phosphatase activity[24] which accompanies the differentiation of decidual cells, and decidualisation itself[25-32] are reduced by indomethacin. Uterine PG concentrations are elevated by artificial deciduogenic stimuli[23,28,33,34] with a time-course which is consistent with the interpretation that the increased concentrations are a cause, rather than a consequence, of the permeability change. Prostaglandins administered into the uterine lumen of animals in which endogenous PG production has been inhibited increase endometrial vascular permeability,[23,31] endometrial alkaline phosphatase activity[24] and bring about decidualisation.[31,32,35,36] The PGs are probably involved not only in the initiation of the endometrial vascular permeability changes but also in the growth and differentiation of decidual cells.[32]

SOURCE OF PROSTAGLANDINS

If the blastocysts are the source of the PGs which are involved in implantation, then the localised nature of the endometrial permeability response could readily be explained as being the consequence of PGs diffusing from the blastocysts into the endometrium to act, directly or indirectly, on the microvasculature. There is evidence for PG synthesis by blastocysts of a number of species.[21,37-46] Initially these reports were confined to blastocysts which undergo marked expansion prior to implantation, and attempts to demonstrate PG synthesis by rat[47] and mouse[45] blastocysts, which remain small prior to implantation, were unsuccessful. Recently, using an immunohistochemical technique, Niimura and Ishida[46] have reported evidence of PGE_2 production by mouse blastocysts. These data are complemented by indirect evidence for PG production by mouse blastocysts: inhibitors of PG synthesis prevent the hatching of mouse blastocysts *in vitro*.[48-50] However, these data by themselves are insufficient to implicate the blastocyst as the source of the PGs which are important for implantation; before such a conclusion can be reached, it will be necessary to demonstrate that the blastocyst-produced PGs act on the endometrium. Blastocyst-produced PGs may have function within the blastocyst.[48]

The results of embryo transfer studies in rabbits in which blastocysts from control or indomethacin-treated donors were transferred to control or indomethacin-treated recipients suggested that the endometrium was the source of the PGs involved in implantation.[52] An endometrial source of PGs is potentially capable of explaining the PG-dependent increase in endometrial vascular permeability induced by blastocysts and by artificial stimuli. Perhaps blastocysts, as a consequence of their interactions with the luminal epithelium, and artificial deciduogenic stimuli have the common property of "traumatising" the endometrium, thereby stimulating PG production.

If the endometrium is the source of the PGs, then the cells within the endometrium which produce them are of obvious interest. If the luminal epithelium is not the site of production, it would be necessary for the primary signal, whether it be from a blastocyst or an artificial deciduogenic stimulus, to be transferred across the epithelium to act within the underlying stroma; this may involve the transformation of the original signal to a chemical signal capable of stimulating stromal cell PG production.[53]

Possibly of relevance to these considerations is the localised depletion of neutral lipids which occurs in the epithelium surrounding rat blastocysts[54] and also in the caruncular epithelium of the ewe in proximity with trophoblastic tissue.[55] This depletion may represent mobilisation of stored precursors for PG synthesis. Rat uterine luminal epithelial cells are capable of PG production[56] and, as indicated by histochemistry, PG synthase activity in the sensitised rat uterus is confined to the luminal and glandular epithelium of the endometrium.[57] Thus at implantation the PGs may be produced within the luminal epithelium in response to a physical or chemical signal from the blastocyst, and then diffuse into the endometrial stroma to produce their effects.

TYPE OF PROSTAGLANDIN

The identity of the PGs involved in implantation and decidualisation is uncertain. PGE_2, $PGF_{2\alpha}$, PGI_2 and 6-oxo-PGE_1 have all been proposed as potential mediators. In rats, the concentrations of PGE, PGF and PGI_2 (measured as 6-oxo-$PGF_{1\alpha}$) are elevated at implantation sites[5,19] and in the uterus following the application of an artificial deciduogenic stimulus,[23,33] consistent with a possible role for these PGs. By contrast, uterine concentrations of 6-oxo-PGE_1 are not changed by a deciduogenic stimulus. Blastocyst implantation in ovariectomised, progesterone-treated rats can be initiated by exogenous $PGF_{2\alpha}$.[22]

The intrauterine administration of PGE_2, $PGF_{2\alpha}$ or 6-oxo-PGE_1, but not PGI_2, results in increased endometrial vascular permeability and/or decidualisation.[27,29,31,32,35,58] These data suggest that, at least for the rat, PGE_2 and $PGF_{2\alpha}$ are the PGs most likely involved in the decidual cell reaction.

The ability of $PGF_{2\alpha}$ to produce decidualisation in the rat is perplexing because, while endometrial binding sites, presumably representing receptors, have been reported for the E-series PGs,[59,60] equivalent binding sites have not been found for $PGF_{2\alpha}$. [61] It is also of interest to note that human endometrium contains PGE_2, but not $PGF_{2\alpha}$, binding sites.[62,63] Kennedy and Doktorcik[64] have suggested that $PGF_{2\alpha}$ is converted within the uterus to PGE_2 which then acts via the presumptive PGE_2 receptors. When analogues of PGE_2 and $PGF_{2\alpha}$, used on the assumption that they could not readily be converted to a corresponding F- or E-type analogue, respectively, were infused into the uterine lumen, decidualisation was only obtained in response to the E-analogue.[64] The $PGF_{2\alpha}$ analogue was inhibitory. These data suggest that PGE_2 mediates the decidual cell reaction, and that the decidualisation obtained in response to $PGF_{2\alpha}$ may have involved its conversion within the uterus to PGE_2. This proposal is supported by observations that, in general, PGE_2 is more effective than $PGF_{2\alpha}$ in bringing about implantation and decidualisation.[14,36,65]

MODE OF ACTION OF PROSTAGLANDINS

The mechanisms by which PGs produce increased endometrial vascular permeability and subsequent decidualisation are poorly understood. Prostaglandins are probably involved not only in the permeability response but also throughout the transformation of stromal cells to decidual cells. This suggestion is based on observations that inhibition of PG synthesis by the administration of indomethacin 12 hours[26] or even 48 hours[32] after the application of a deciduogenic stimulus reduces the extent of the decidual cell reaction.

Kennedy and Armstrong[47] have argued that, by analogy with the inflammatory response, there may be two mediators of the endometrial vascular permeability response: one, a PG may cause vasodilation; the other, possibly histamine (although there are other possible candidates) may alter endothelial cell function to increase vascular permeability. In support of this proposal are observations that an increase in uterine blood volume, presumably indicative of vasodilation, accompanies the endometrial permeability response to an artificial deciduogenic stimulus.[66] However, an increase in uterine blood volume was not observed by Milligan and Mirembe [67] in the mouse. The evidence for the involvement of histamine is indirect, and not very convincing. Rabbit and mouse blastocysts are purportedly capable of histamine synthesis[68,69] and in rabbits the intrauterine injection of an inhibitor of histidine decarboxylase interrupts implantation.[68,70] Rabbit endometrium and blastocysts have histamine H_1- and H_2-receptors, respectively.[71] However, the initiation of implantation in rats was not affected when the animals were treated with both histamine H_1- and H_2-receptor antagonists.[72] Thus the possibility that PGs interact with histamine to mediate the endometrial vascular permeability changes remains uncertain and requires further investigation.

Recently there has been interest in the possibility that PGs may interact within the uterus with leukotrienes or platelet-activating factor. Because both classes of compounds have very potent effect on the microvasculature,[73,74] they may be involved in mediating the endometrial vascular changes. The rat uterus produces leukotrienes[75] and the intrauterine infusion of FPL 55712, an antagonist of leukotrienes, combined with indomethacin, inhibits decidualisation to a greater extent than does indomethacin by itself.[76] Platelet-activating factor has been detected in rat and rabbit uteri.[77,78]

The mode of action of PGs at the cellular level within the endometrium is poorly understood. In a number of cell types, cAMP acts as a second messenger for PGs of the E-series.[79-81] The available data for the involvement of cAMP in implantation and decidualisation are paradoxical. In favour of a role are observations that uterine concentrations of cAMP are elevated at implanation sites in the rat,[82] and that in ovariectomised progesterone-treated mice, blastocysts implant in response to the intraluminal injection of cAMP or its dibutyryl analogue.[83,84] In animals sensitised for the decidual cell reaction, artificial deciduogenic stimuli rapidly increase uterine cAMP concentrations,[28,85-87] and this increase can be inhibited by indomethacin,[28,87] suggesting that the response is mediated by PGs. The intrauterine injection of PGE_2 in rats pretreated with indomethacin increases uterine cAMP concentrations.[87] By contrast, observations which raise questions about the role of cAMP include reports that in the rat analogues of cAMP do not mimic the effects of PGE_2 on endometrial vascular permeability.[87] In addition, in mice, rats and rabbits, the intrauterine administration of cAMP or its analogues does not induce decidualisation.[65,85,86,88] It is possible, therefore, that PGs have their effects within the endometrium by mechanisms not involving cAMP as a second messenger. Presumably activation of protein kinase C and calcium mobilisation are not involved because the intrauterine administration of a tumour-promoting phorbol ester or a synthetic diacylglycerol together with a calcium ionophore inhibited, rather than stimulated, decidualisation.[89]

The endometrial cells which respond to PGs during implantation and decidualisation are not known. If E-series PGs are the mediators, then the responding cells are presumably within the endometrial stroma because high-affinity binding sites have been detected in the stroma but not in the epithelium.[60] In agreement with this suggestion are the observations of a PGE-dependent adenylate cyclase in rabbit endometrial stromal, but not epithelial, cells.[90] Using autoradiography, Chegini *et al.*[63] have demonstrated that ^{3}H-PGE$_2$ binds to stromal cells, glandular epithelium, arterioles and erythrocytes of the human endometrium. Prostaglandin E$_2$ can act directly on rat endometrial stromal cells as indicated by measurements of alkaline phosphatase activity in cultured cells.[91] Taken together, these observations suggest that PGs may potentially act directly on the endometrial vascular system to modify its permeability, and may also act directly on stromal cells to induce their differentiation into decidual cells. The observations also indicate that interactions between endometrial cell types are also possible as a consequence of exposure to elevated levels of PGE$_2$.

CONCLUSIONS

While considerable experimental evidence indicates that PGs have an important role in the initiation of implantation as well as decidualisation, relatively little is known about the types of PG involved, their site of production or mode of action. It is likely that the PGs do not act alone, but interact with other vasoactive compounds, the identity of which are presently unknown. The extent to which these findings in animals are relevant to our own species is unknown.

REFERENCES
1. Psychoyos A. Endocrine control of egg implantation. In: *Handbook of physiology*. Section 7, Vol II, Part 2. Eds. RO Greep, EB Astwood, SR Geiger. Bethesda: American Physiological Society, 1973; pp.187-215.
2. Amoroso EC. Placentation. In: *Marshall's physiology of reproduction*. Vol II. Ed. AS Parker. London: Longmans, Green and Co, 1952; pp.127-311.
3. Finn CA, Porter DG. *The uterus*. Acton: Publishing Sciences Group, 1975.
4. Vane JR. Inhibition of prostaglandin synthesis as a mechanism of action of aspirin-like drugs. *Nature New Biol* 1971; **231**: 232-235.
5. Kennedy TG. Evidence for a role for prostaglandins in the initiation of blastocyst implantation in the rat. *Biol Reprod* 1977; **16**: 286-291.
6. Hoffman LH, DiPietro DL, McKenna TJ. Effects of indomethacin on uterine capillary permeability and blastocyst development in rabbits. *Prostaglandins* 1978; **15**: 823-828.
7. Evans CA, Kennedy TG. The importance of prostaglandin synthesis for the initiation of blastocyst implantation in the hamster. *J Reprod Fertil* 1978; **54**: 255-261.
8. Lundkvist Ö, Nilsson BO. Ultrastructural changes of the trophoblast-epithelial complex in mice subjected to implantation blocking treatment with indomethacin. *Biol Reprod* 1980; **22**: 719-726.
9. Phillips CA, Poyser NL. Studies on the involvement of prostaglandins in implantation in the rat. *J Reprod Fertil* 1981; **62**: 73-81.

10. Lau IF, Saksena SK, Chang MC. Pregnancy blockade by indomethacin, an inhibitor of prostaglandin synthesis: its reversal by prostaglandins and progesterone in mice. *Prostaglandins* 1973; **4**: 795-803.
11. Gavin MA, Dominguez Fernandez-Tejerina JC, Montañes de las Heras MF, Vigil Maeso E. Efectos de un inhibidor de la biosíntesis de las prostaglandinas (indo-metacina) sobre la implantación en la rata. *Reproduccion* 1974; **1**: 177-183.
12. Saksena SK, Lau IF, Chang MC. Relationship between oestrogen, prostaglandin F_{2x} and histamine in delayed implantation in the mouse. *Acta Endocrinol* 1976; **81**: 801-807.
13. El-Banna AA. The degenerative effect on rabbit implantation sites by indomethacin. I. Timing of indomethacin action, possible effect on uterine proteins and the effect of replacement doses of $PGF_{2\alpha}$. *Prostaglandins* 1980; **20**: 587-599.
14. Holmes PV, Gordashko BJ. Evidence of prostaglandin involvement in blastocyst implantation. *J Embryol Exp Morphol* 1980; **55**: 109-122.
15. Garg SK, Chandhury RR. Evidence for a possible role of prostaglandins in implanta-tion in rats. *Arch Int Pharmacodyn* 1983; **262**: 299-307.
16. Cao Z-D, Jones MA, Harper MJK. Progesterone and oestradiol receptor concentra-tion and translocation in uterine tissue of rabbits treated with indomethacin. *J Endocrinol* 1985; **107**: 197-203.
17. Kraeling RR, Rampacek GB, Fiorello NA. Inhibition of pregnancy with indomethacin in mature gilts and prepuberal gilts induced to ovulate. *Biol Reprod* 1985; **32**: 105-110.
18. Biggers JD, Baskar JF, Torchiana DF. Reduction of fertility of mice by the intra-uterine injection of prostaglandin antagonists. *J Reprod Fertil* 1981; **63**: 365-372.
19. Kennedy TG, Zamecnik J. The concentration of 6-keto-prostaglandin F_{1x} is markedly elevated at the site of blastocyst implantation in the rat. *Prostaglandins* 1978; **16**: 599-605.
20. Sharma SC. Temporal changes in PGE, PGF_x oestradiol 17β and progesterone in uterine venous plasma and endometrium of rabbits during early pregnancy. *INSERM Symp* 1979; **91**: 243-264.
21. Kasamo M, Ishikawa M, Yamashita K, Sengoku K, Shimizu T. Possible role of prostaglandin F in blastocyst implantation. *Prostaglandins* 1986; **31**: 321-336.
22. Oettel M, Kock M, Kurischko A, Schubert K. A direct evidence for the involvement of prostaglandin F_{2x} in the first step of estrone-induced blastocyst implantation in the spayed rat. *Steroids* 1979; **33**: 1-8.
23. Kennedy TG. Prostaglandins and increased endometrial vascular permeability result-ing from the application of an artificial stimulus to the uterus of the rat sensitized for the decidual cell reaction. *Biol Reprod* 1979; **20**: 560-566.
24. Yee GM, Kennedy TG. Stimulatory effects of prostaglandins (PGs) upon uterine alkaline phosphatase (ALP) during the decidual cell reaction (DCR) in the rat. *Biol Reprod* 1987; **36 Suppl 1**: 66 (Abstract).
25. Castracane VD, Saksena SK, Shaikh AA. Effect of IUDs prostaglandins and indo-methacin on decidual cell reaction in the rat. *Prostaglandins* 1974; **6**: 397-404.
26. Tobert JA. A study of the possible role of prostaglandins in decidualization using a non-surgical method for the instillation of fluids into the rat uterine lumen. *J Reprod Fertil* 1976; **47**: 391-393.
27. Sananes N, Baulieu E-E, Le Goascogne C. Prostaglandin(s) as inductive factor of decidualization in the rat uterus. *Mol Cell Endocrinol* 1976; **6**: 153-158.
28. Rankin JC, Ledford BE, Jonsson HT, Baggett B. Prostaglandins, indomethacin and the decidual cell reaction in the mouse uterus. *Biol Reprod* 1979; **20**: 399-404.
29. Sananès N, Baulieu E-E, Le Goascogne C. A role for prostaglandins in decidualiza-tion of the rat uterus. *J Endocrinol* 1981; **89**: 25-33.
30. Buxton LE, Murdoch RN. Lectins, calcium ionophore A23187, and peanut oil as deciduogenic agents in the uterus of pseudopregnant mice: effects of tranycypromine, indomethacin, iproniazid and propranolol. *Aust J Biol Sci* 1982; **35**: 63-72.

31. Kennedy TG, Lukash LA. Induction of decidualization in rats by the intrauterine infusion of prostaglandins. *Biol Reprod* 1982; **27:** 253-260.
32. Kennedy TG. Evidence for the involvement of prostaglandins throughout the decidual cell reaction in the rat. *Biol Reprod* 1985; **33:** 140-146.
33. Kennedy TG, Barbe GJ, Evans CA. Prostaglandin I_2 and increased endometrial vascular permeability preceding the decidual cell reaction. In: *The endometrium*. Ed. FA Kimball. New York: Spectrum Publications, 1980; pp.331-342.
34. Milligan SR, Lytton FDC. Changes in prostaglandin levels in the sensitized and non-sensitized uterus of the mouse after the intrauterine instillation of oil or saline. *J Reprod Fertil* 1983; **67:** 373-377.
35. Miller MM, O'Morchoe CCC. Inhibition of artificially induced decidual cell reaction by indomethacin in the mature oophorectomized rat. *Anat Rec* 1982; **204:** 223-230.
36. Kennedy TG. Intrauterine infusion of prostaglandins and decidualization in rats with uteri differentially sensitized for the decidual cell reaction. *Biol Reprod* 1986; **34:** 327-335.
37. Shemesh M, Milaguir F, Ayalon N, Hansel W. Steroidogenesis and prostaglandin synthesis by cultured blastocysts. *J Reprod Fertil* 1979; **56:** 181-185.
38. Watson J, Patek CE. Steroid and prostaglandin secretion by the corpus luteum, endometrium and embryos of cyclic and pregnant pigs. *J Endocrinol* 1979; **82:** 425-428.
39. Dey SK, Chien SM, Cox CL, Crist RD. Prostaglandin synthesis in the rabbit blasto-cyst. *Prostaglandins* 1980; **19:** 449-453.
40. Marcus GJ. Prostaglandin formation by the sheep embryo and endometrium as an indication of maternal recognition of pregnancy. *Biol Reprod* 1981; **25:** 56-64.
41. Lewis GS, Thatcher WW, Bazer FW, Curl JS. Metabolism of arachidonic arachidonic acid *in vitro* by bovine blastocysts and endometrium. *Biol Reprod* 1982; **27:** 431-439.
42. Hyland JH, Manns JG, Humphrey WD. Prostaglandin production by ovine embryos and endometrium *in vitro*. *J Reprod Fertil* 1982; **65:** 299-304.
43. Harper MJK, Norris CJ, Rajkumar K. Prostaglandin release by zygotes and endo-metria of pregnant rabbits. *Biol Reprod* 1983; **28:** 350-362.
44. Lacroix MC, Kann G. Comparative studies of prostaglandin $F_{2\alpha}$ and E_2 in late cyclic and early pregnant sheep: *in vitro* synthesis by endometrium and conceptus-effect of *in vivo* indomethacin treatment on establishment of pregnancy. *Prostaglandins* 1982; **23:** 507-526.
45. Racowsky C, Biggers JD. Are blastocyst prostaglandins produced endogenously? *Biol Reprod* 1983; **29:** 379-388.
46. Niimura S, Ishida K. Immunohistochemical demonstration of prostaglandin E-2 in preimplantation mouse embryos. *J Reprod Fertil* 1987; **80:** 505-508.
47. Kennedy TG, Armstrong DT. The role of prostaglandins in endometrial vascular changes at implantation. In: *Cellular and molecular aspects of implantation*. Eds. SR Glasser, DW Bullock. New York: Plenum Press, 1981; pp.349-3.
48. Biggers JD, Leonov BV, Baskar JF, Fried J. Inhibition of hatching of mouse blasto-cysts *in vitro* by prostaglandin antagonists. *Biol Reprod* 1978; **19:** 519-533.
49. Baskar JF, Torchiana DF, Biggers JD, Corey EJ, Andersen NH, Subramanian N. Inhibition of hatching of mouse blastocysts *in vitro* by various prostaglandin antagonists. *J Reprod Fertil* 1981; **63:** 359-363.
50. Hurst PR, MacFarlane DW. Further effects of nonsteroidal anti-inflammatory com-pounds on blastocyst hatching *in vitro* and implantation rates in the mouse. *Biol Reprod* 1981; **25:** 777-784.
51. Chida S, Uehara S, Hoshiai H, Yajima A. Effects of indomethacin, prostaglandin E_2, prostaglandin $F_{2\alpha}$ and 6-keto-prostaglandin $F_{1\alpha}$ on hatching of mouse blastocysts. *Prostaglandins* 1986; **31:** 337-342.
52. Snabes MC, Harper MJK. Site of action of indomethacin on implantation in the rabbit. *J Reprod Fertil* 1984; **71:** 559-565.

53. Kennedy TG. Interactions of eicosanoids and other factors in blastocyst implantation. In: *Eicosanoids and reproduction.* Ed. K Hillier. Lancaster: MTP Press, 1987; In press.
54. Boshier DP. Effects of the rat blastocyst on neutral lipids and non-specific esterases in the uterine luminal epithelium at the implantation area. *J Reprod Fertil* 1976; **46:** 245-247.
55. Boshier DP, Fairclough RJ, Holloway H. Assessment of sheep blastocyst effects on neutral lipids in the uterine caruncular epithelium. *J Reprod Fertil* 1987; **79:** 569-573.
56. Moulton BC. Epithelial cell function during blastocyst implantation. *J Biosci* 1984; **6:** Suppl 2: 11-21.
57. Ohta Y. Histochemical localization of prostaglandin synthetase in the rat endometrium with reference to decidual cell reaction. *Proc Jpn Acad* 1985; **61:** Ser B: 467-470.
58. Doktorcik PE, Kennedy TG. 6-Keto-prostaglandin E_1 and the decidual cell reaction in rats. *Prostaglandins* 1986; **32:** 679-689.
59. Kennedy TG, Martel D, Psychoyos A. Endometrial prostaglandin E_2 binding: characterization in rats sensitized for the decidual cell reaction and changes during pseudopregnancy. *Biol Reprod* 1983; 29: 556-564.
60. Kennedy TG, Martel D, Psychoyos A. Endometrial prostaglandin E_2 binding during the estrous cycle and its hormonal control in ovariectomized rats. *Biol Reprod* 1983; **29:** 565-571.
61. Martel D, Kennedy TG, Monier MN, Psychoyos A. Failure to detect specific binding sites for prostaglandin $F_{2\alpha}$ in membrane preparations from rat endometrium. *J Reprod Fertil* 1985; **75:** 265-274.
62. Hofmann, GE, Rao ChV, DeLeon FD, Toledo AA, Sanfilippo JS. Human endometrial prostaglandin E_2 binding sites and their profiles during the menstrual cycle and in pathologic cases. *Am J Obstet Gynecol* 1985; **151:** 369-375.
63. Chegini N, Rao ChV, Wakim N, Sanfilippo J. Prostaglandin binding to different cell types of human uterus: quantitative light microscope autoradiographic study. *Prostaglandins Leukotrienes Med* 1986; **22:** 129-138.
64. Kennedy TG, Doktorcik PE. Effects of analogues of prostaglandin E_2 and $F_{2\alpha}$ on the decidual cell reaction in the rat. *Prostaglandins* 1987; In press.
65. Hoffman LH, Strong GB, Davenport GR, Frölich JC. Deciduogenic effects of prostaglandins in the pseudopregnant rabbit. *J Reprod Fertil* 1977; **50:** 231-237.
66. Bitton V, Vassent G, Psychoyos A. Réponse vasculaire de l'utérus au traumatisme, au cours de la pseudogestation chez la ratte. *CR Seances Acad Sci (III)* 1965; **261:** 3474-3477.
67. Milligan SR, Mirembe FM. Time course of the changes in uterine vascular permeability associated with the development of the decidual cell reaction in ovariectomized steroid-treated rats. *J Reprod Fertil* 1984; **70:** 1-6.
68. Dey SK, Johnson DC, Santos JG. Is histamine production by the blastocyst required for implantation in the rabbit? *Biol Reprod* 1979; **21:** 1169-1173.
69. Dey SK, Johnson DC. Histamine formation by mouse preimplantation embryos. *J Reprod Fertil* 1980; **60:** 457-460.
70. Dey SK. Role of histamine in implantation: inhibition of histidine decarboxylase induces delayed implantation in the rabbit. *Biol Reprod* 1981; **24:** 867-869.
71. Dey SK, Villanueva C, Abdou NI. Histamine receptors on rabbit blastocyst and endometrial cell membranes. *Nature* 1979; **278:** 648-649.
72. Brandon JM, Raval PJ. Interaction of estrogen and histamine during ovum implantation in the rat. *Eur J Pharmacol* 1979; **57:** 171-177.
73. Samuelsson B. Leukotrienes: mediators of immediate hypersensitivity reactions and inflammation. *Science* 1983; **220:** 568-575.
74. Braquet P, Touqui L, Shen TY, Vargaftig BB. Perspectives in platelet-activating factor research. *Pharmacol Rev* 1987; **39:** 97-145.

75. Malathy PV, Cheng HC, Dey SK. Production of leukotrienes and prostaglandins in the rat uterus during periimplantation period. *Prostaglandins* 1986; **32:** 605-614.
76. Sagrillo C, Tawfik OW, Johnson DC, Dey SK. Leukotrienes are necessary for decidualization in the rat. *Biol Reprod* 1987; **36 Suppl 1:** 156 (Abstract).
77. Angle MJ, Jones MA, Pinckard RN, McManus LM, Harper MJK. Platelet-activating factor (PAF) in the rabbit uterus during early pregnancy. *Biol Reprod* 1985; **32 Suppl 1:** 143 (Abstract).
78. Yasuda K, Satouchi K, Saito K. Platelet-activating factor in normal rat uterus. *Biochem Biophys Res Comm* 1986; **138:** 1231-1236.
79. Kuehl FS, Cirillo VJ, Zanetti ME, Beveridge GC, Ham EA. The effect of estrogen upon cyclic nucleotide and prostaglandin levels in the rat uterus. *Adv Prostagl Thromb Res* 1976; **1:** 313-323.
80. Lazarus SC, Basbaum CB, Gold WM. Prostaglandins and intracellular cyclic AMP in respiratory secretory cells. *Am Rev Respir Dis* 1984; **130:** 262-266.
81. Biddulph DM, Sawyer LM, Smales WP. Chondrogenesis of chick limb mesenchyme in vitro. Effects of prostaglandins on cyclic AMP. *Exp Cell Res* 1984; **153:** 270-274.
82. Vilar-Rojas C, Castro-Osuna G, Hicks JJ. Cyclic AMP and cyclic GMP in the implantation site of the rat. *Int J Fertil* 1982; **27:** 56-59.
83. Holmes PV, Bergstrom S. Induction of blastocyst implantation in mice by cyclic AMP. *J Reprod Fertil* 1975; **43:** 329-332.
84. Webb FTB. Implantation in ovariectomized mice treated with dibutyryladenosine 3',5'-monophosphate (dibutyryl cyclic AMP). *J Reprod Fertil* 1975; **42:** 511-517.
85. Leroy F, Vansande J, Shetgen G, Brasseur D. Cyclic AMP and the triggering of the decidual reaction. *J Reprod Fertil* 1974; **29:** 207-211.
86. Rankin JC, Ledford BE, Baggett B. Early involvement of cyclic nucleotides in the artificially stimulated decidual cell reaction of the mouse uterus. *Biol Reprod* 1977; **17:** 549-554.
87. Kennedy TG. Prostaglandin E$_2$, adenosine 3':5'-cyclic monophosphate and changes in endometrial vascular permeability in rat uteri sensitized for the decidual cell reaction. *Biol Reprod* 1983; **29:** 1069-1076.
88. Webb FTG. The inability of dibutyryl adenosine 3':5'-monophosphate to induce the decidual reaction in intact pseudopregnant mice. *J Reprod Fertil* 1975; **42:** 1987-1988.
89. Feyles V, Kennedy TG. Inhibitory effect of the intrauterine infusion of phorbol 12-myristate 13-acetate and 1-oleoyl-2-acetylglycerol on the decidual cell reaction in rats. *Biol Reprod* 1987; **37:** 96-104.
90. Fortier MA, Boulanger M, Boulet AP, Lambert RD. Cell-specific localization of prostaglandin E$_2$-sensitive adenylate cyclase in rabbit endometrium. *Biol Reprod* 1987; **36:** 1025-1033.
91. Daniel SAJ, Kennedy TG. Prostaglandin E$_2$ enhances uterine stromal cell alkaline phosphatase activity *in vitro*. *Prostaglandins* 1987; **33:** 241-252.

Discussion

Chairman: Professor D. A. Clark

Dr DAYA: Just a comment in response to your two models. I have assayed both immunosuppressive and non-suppressive IVF supernatants for prostaglandin, and have not been able to demonstrate the presence of prostaglandin. This would be in agreement with findings in other species.

Professor KENNEDY: The only demonstration of prostaglandin synthesis in the pre-implantation rodent blastocysts is that of Niimura and Ishida in 1987. They had to use an immunohistochemical technique to demonstrate the presence of PGE_2 within the blastocyst, that is, by using indomethacin, they showed that during the culture period, there was a difference in the amount of immuno-histochemical material there, suggesting that the embryo could indeed synthesise it.

Professor GILL: Your talk on prostaglandins seems to implicate the importance of vascularity in the implantation process. Has anyone tried to enhance the implantation of an embryo or maybe to treat a spontaneous aborting system by simply inducing an inflammatory response in the uterus with some non-specific stimulus such as croton oil?

Professor KENNEDY: That raises a very interesting point that I didn't have time to go into . The only time you can get an increase in vascular permeability within the uterus is at the time when implantation would occur. You can traumatise the uterus at other times, and not get an increase in individual vascular permeability. This raises the possibility that, except at the time of implantation, the uterus is producing something which inhibits its ability to undergo a vascular permeability response. An alternative explanation is that one of the elements required for a permeability response may be missing. I have heard of experiments which testify that what we are really missing is the prostaglandin, but that is not simply the case. The onset of the receptivity is correlated with the appearance of binding sites for PGE_2. In the earlier stages of pregnancy, when you can't get a vascular permeability response, it may be because there are no receptors within the endometrium for PGE_2

Professor BEARD: You started your talk by distinguishing between an increase in vascularity and an increase in permeability. Now you talk about an increased vascular permeability. Are they two distinct phenomena, or in this particular example, do they have to be distinguished from more general vascular changes that may occur without a change in permeability?

Professor KENNEDY: This has been inadequately studied.

Dr HEAP: I am very interested in the effect you showed of growth hormone and thyroxin. There is evidence, of course, that there is substantial increase in uterine blood flow prior to implantation which is related to the ovarian hormone secretion rather than the presence of the embryonic cells.

Professor KENNEDY: You raise a very complex issue in separating changes in endometrial blood flow, vascularity, and endometrial vascular permeability which determine the concentration of radioactivity in the stimulated and non-stimulated uterine horn 15 minutes after the intravenous injection of iodinated albumen. There are suggestions of a greater blood volume in the treated animals, but concerning the increased radioactivity in stimulated uterine horns—whether it is vasodilation or greater permeability—we don't have the data at the present time.

Professor CLARK: Dr Michael Chapman has a few comments about endometrial proteins in the human.

Dr CHAPMAN: A series of secretory proteins of the endometrium/decidua have been characterised over the last decade. Their biological significance is beginning to emerge. A 28KD molecular weight glycoprotein with 2 electrophoretic mobility (PP14, PEP, $_2$EG) has been shown to be the principal secretory product of the late luteal phase endometrium and early decidua. Radiolabelled aminoacid incorporation experiments confirm protein synthesis in tissue explant studies. Immunohistochemical evidence localises the protein to the endometrial glandular epithelium. Serum levels show a biphasic pattern in the normal menstrual cycle being highest just prior to menstruation in the ovulatory cycles. In pregnancy serum levels rise in the days following implantation and peak at the 8th week of gestation in a pattern similar to hCG. The biological significance remains uncertain. N terminal sequence data from purified material reveals partial momology with lactoglobulin from other species. A known biological role for lactoglobulins is as a retinol binding protein. *In vitro* studies utilising the M.L.R. with purified PP14 have suggested an immunosuppressive activity which can be blocked by addition of monoclonal antibody (Bolton *et al*, 1987).

A 34KD molecular weight glycoprotein with electrophoretic mobility (PP12, PEG) has been shown to be secreted by the stromal cells of the decidua. N terminal sequence data from purified material shows 100% homology with small molecular weight somatomedin binding protein (or IGF-BP). Serum levels rise through the first trimester reaching a plateau in mid-pregnancy. Very high concentrations are present in amniotic fluid. Its role in the modulation of IGF activity in pregnancy remains to be elucidated.

That two secretory proteins have relationships with the factors that may modify fetal and placental growth would suggest they have an important role in the implantation and maintenance of early pregnancy.

Professor CLARK: What do we know about the significance of these early proteins?

Professor KENNEDY: Could I ask the question of whether or not these proteins are there early enough to be really involved in mediating the events of early pregnancy?

Dr CHAPMAN: They are present in the endometrium and rise during the pseudo-decidualisation that takes place toward the end of the cycle. So they are there and can be detected immunochemically post-ovulation.

Professor KENNEDY: What happens to them if you just continue with the administration of progesterone so that you do get a decidualisation of the uterus? In other words, is there any difference between the pseudo-pregnant and the pregnant situation?

Dr CHAPMAN: We have only looked in the short term.

Dr BELL: We have shown that this product is actually made from secretory glandular epithelium. In pregnancy, the glandular epithelium involutes so eventually the glands disappear. In situations where we have had patients on long-term progesterone, the proteins seem to be still present, and actually the glandular structures turn into a sort of micro-tubular gland. As far as synthesis is concerned, you can detect it by day 19 to 21 of the menstrual cycle, perhaps even post-ovulation, by histology, by *in vitro* synthesis secretion, and also by flushing from the uterus. I think that probably it is produced too late to affect any pre-implantation embryonic development. Thus it is a situation of a carrier protein capable of providing a link between the endometrium and the trophoblast, which I think was mentioned yesterday.

Professor KENNEDY: The only difficulty with this idea I think is that this binding protein is not stimulated by growth hormone in contrast to the high molecular weight IGF-binding protein in serum.

Professor CLARK: As Anne Croy pointed out yesterday with her three intersecting circles diagram, those of us who are concerned about the mechanisms of success or failure of early pregnancy really need to keep in mind that there may be more than one interaction which could be responsible and could be triggering a sequence of events leading to failure. It is pleasing to see a dialogue between those studying patients and those attempting to apply observations made in animal systems to human reproduction. In an earlier session, Dr Bulmer discussed cell types in human endometrium and decidua of successful pregnant females. Mr Magdi Michel from the Department of Obstetrics and Gynaecology of St Mary's Hospital wishes to give you a short presentation now based on applying information from animal studies to women with failing (i.e. aborting) pregnancies.

Mr MICHEL: The background of this study derived from studies from mice showing that there is a deficiency or reduction in proportion of the granulated lymphocytic cells and a reduced local suppressor activity in the decidua of recurrent aborters. Suppressor cell activity was also deficient in the decidua of women who were suffering from missed abortion. In both the human and mouse, decidual cultures generate a soluble suppressor activity. A preliminary study published in the *American Journal of Reproductive Immunology* in January 1987[1] reported data from ten patients having placental bed biopsies prior to miscarriage. There was a reduction in the proportion of mononuclear cells with large granules (CLG) in their decidua. Because these data were qualitative, we initiated a study to quantitate the granulated cells in the decidua and to measure the release of soluble suppressor activity from this biopsy tissue. The work was done in collaboration with Professors Clark, Mowbray, Beard and Jenny Underwood. Three groups of patients have been evaluated: Group A patients came to the hospital for elective terminations of an intact pregnancy, Group B were patients who were recurrent miscarriers whose pregnancies had become anembryonic, and Group C were patients who did not have any history of recurrent miscarriage but were diagnosed as missed abortion by ultrasound. All pregnancies were 7-14 weeks gestation, and none of the aborters had any heavy bleeding or pain that had precipitated their attendance at our hospital. On the day of the evacuation of the uterus, using continuous ultrasound monitoring to locate the placenta, a chorion biopsy instrument was passed through the cervical canal and a biopsy was taken from the placenta and adjacent decidual bed at the thickest part of the placenta. I took three samples from each patient; the first set was sent for histological staining by phloxine-tartrazine to identify granulated cells, the second was sent for preparation of the supernatant, and the third sample was sent for chromosomal analysis. The slides were coded in the histology

Figure I

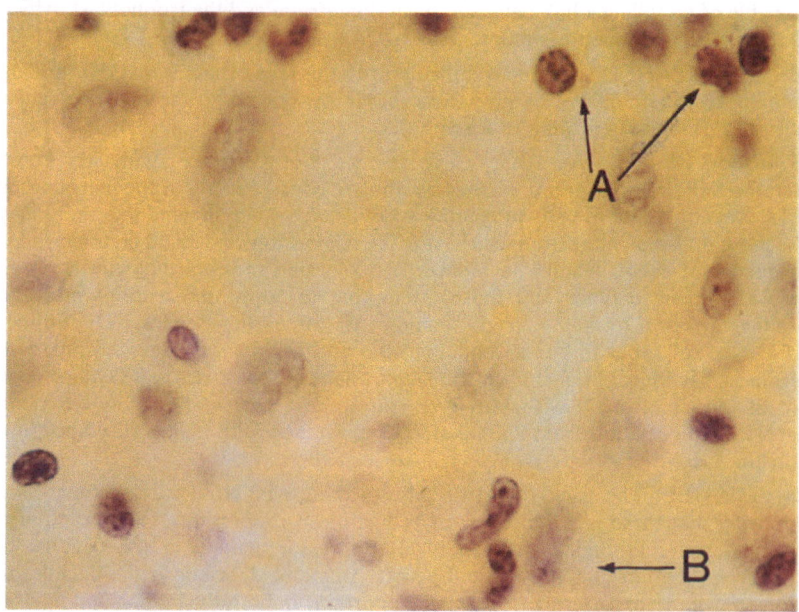

Photomicrograph of phloxine-tartrazine stained biopsy of human decidua illustrating two types (A, B) of mononuclear cells containing cytoplasmic granules. 1000 × magnification.

department so we did not know which slide belonged to whom, and have been examined independently by myself and by Professor Clark. In Figure I, "A" identifies mononuclear cells with large granules (CLG) (at least 1 granule ≥1 um in size); morphologically, it looks like a lymphocyte because it has a small nucleus. "B" identifies a second-cell type that is a mononuclear cell with a large nucleus and very small granules,—usually more than one. These are similar to LGL (large granular lymphocytes). We enumerated the number of CLG and LGL separately on each slide without knowledge of the clinical status of the

Figure II

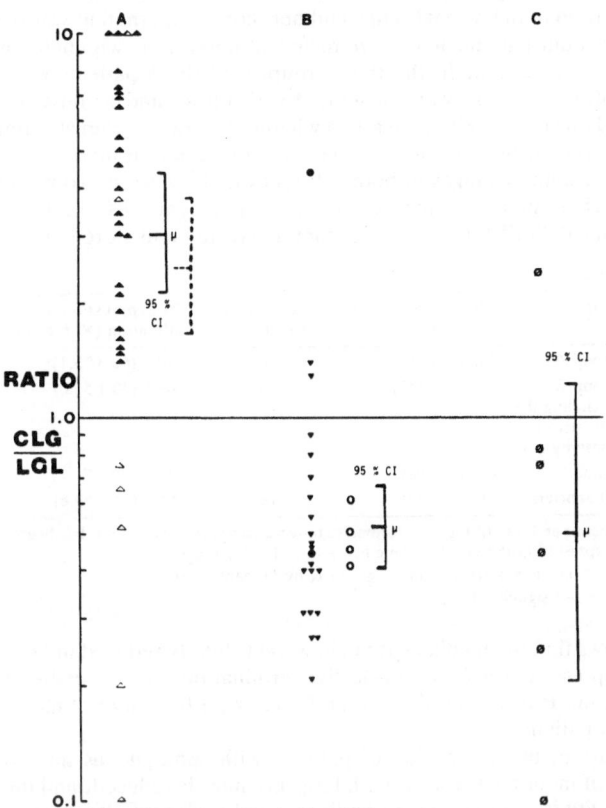

Ratio of cells with large granules—CLG (i.e. 1 or more granules > 1 um) to large granulated lymphocytes—LGL (i.e. 1 or more granules < 1 um). Group A controls (n=27) (▲). (△) were of six blocks from three patients where areas of necrosis and significant increase in the number of polymorphs suggestive of early spontaneous abortion. Group B recurrent miscarriers (i.e. > 3 miscarriages) who had received no immunotherapy (○) or paternal lymphocyte immunotherapy (▼).(●) chromosomally abnormal abortuses. Group C, sporadic aborters (∅).

patient. Figure II shows the ratio of CLG to LGL. We can see there that most of the samples from elective terminations (Group A) had a ratio > 1. Of 5 samples which were below the line it was interesting to note that there was necrosis and polymorphonuclear infiltration in the slide. It is possible that some of these women would have aborted spontaneously. Of Group B women who were recurrent aborters and had been found on ultrasound to have an anembryonic sac, the ratio of CLG/LGL was reduced compared to Group A. Many were recurrent miscarriers who had been immunised with their paternal lymphocytes, but unfortunately failed. Two patients here showed chromosomally abnormal biopsies, one trisomy 20 and the other trisomy 22. The latter patient had a CLG/LGL ratio in the normal range and her biopsy supernatant was quite highly suppressive. Four patients here were recurrent miscarriers who had not received immunisation treatment. In the third group, 5 of the 6 patients who were not recurrent miscarriers but were diagnosed with ultrasound as missed abortions, also showed low ratios. When we asked whether low ratios from aborting patients meant a decreased number of CLG per slide or rather an increase in LGL, we found that absolute changes in both cell types had occurred. To prepare supernatants, each sample was incubated for 48 hours at 37°C in RPMI culture medium, and 10% FBS for 48 hours, then harvested and stored at 4°C.

Table 1

Patient Group	Specimen Weight mg ($\times \pm$ sem)	Number of supernatants	% Suppression of Proliferation ($\times \pm$ sem)
Group A	128 (115-142)[a]	16	70.6 (66.3-75.1)[a]
Group B (excluding the patient with trimsomy 22)	127 (109-147)	13	48.6 (40.1-59.0)[b]
Group C	83 (63-108)	5	59.5 (49.7-71.2)[c]
All aborters	112 (97-129)	18	51.4 (44.3-59.6)[b]

[a] means and sem of log transformed data were computed. The result has been expressed arithmetically as median and $\pm$ 1 SEM range.
[b] $p < 0.05$ compared to control group A by Student's test.
[c] p = not significant.

Table 1 shows that the median specimen weight slightly reduced in Group C. The median suppression was 70.6% in elective terminations of "successful pregnancy" while in Group B it was 48.6%. Group C was slightly greater at 60%, but there were only 5 patients.

In conclusion, in the decidua of patients with spontaneous miscarriage, the proportion of mononuclear cells with large granules is reduced, and immunosuppressor activity is reduced. These findings could represent alterations associated with the process of miscarriage, such as inflammation. Since granulated suppressor cells and suppressor factor in the pregnant mouse is trophoblast dependent, our findings in aborting women could also be a reflection on an underlying trophoblast insufficiency. Alternatively, one could speculate there may be rejection occurring due to deficient suppressor cell activity at the fetomaternal interface.

Professor MOWBRAY: Unless there is a relationship between the small granule cells and the large granule cells, I don't really think that a diminution in the number of large granule cells is necessarily linked to an increase in the number of small ones. If they are separate populations of the kind that Judith Bulmer was suggesting yesterday with her surface markers, they are not going to change in a reciprocal manner. Have you any evidence that they are?

Professor CLARK: In the mouse decidua oen can show that natural killer (NK) cell activity is mediated by LGL which are larger than the granulated lymphocytic suppressor cell population. The suppressor cell population also lacks the asialo-GM1 marker that can be found on NK cells. I believe Dr Bell suggested that in the human, the granulated cells belonged to one population.

Professor MOWBRAY: I don't think they are. But do you think they are one population and inter-convertible?

Professor CLARK: I think that this is a very interesting question that can only be answered by further work.

Dr MICHEL: We need to separate these cells and look at the cell surface markers. Then we will know if LGL and CLG are related.

REFERENCES
1. Clark DA, Mowbray J, Underwood J, Lidell H. Histopathologic alterations in the decidua in human spontaneous abortion: loss of cells with large cytoplasmic granules. *Am J Reprod Immunol Microbiol* 1987; **13:** 19-23.

SECTION 5

GENETIC CAUSES OF EARLY PREGNANCY FAILURE

Is there a *t* complex in man?

J. Klein, V. Vincek, M. Kasahara and F. Figueroa

The *t* complex was originally discovered with the help of a mutation that appeared spontaneously in laboratory mice more than 60 years ago.[1] This brachyury (*T*) mutation caused shortening of the tail and was lethal in a homozygous state: the *T/T* embryos died at 10.5 days of gestation because of irregularities in the formation of the neural tube and notochord.[2] These irregularities are first noticeable morphologically at 8.5 days of gestation as blebs, vesicles, and deviations of the neural tube. At the time of death the notochord is either completely missing or is greatly reduced in size. By all accounts, the *T* is a point mutation in a locus that maps approximately 3 cM from the centromere on chromosome 17.[3]

When the *T/+* heterozygotes, which show no other abnormalities except for the shortening of their tails, are crossed with wild mice, a certain percentage of the crossings will produce some animals that are completely tail-less.[4] The reason for the further shortening of the tail to this extreme is the presence of an abnormal segment of chromosome 17 in wild mice; this is referred to as the *t* complex and its different forms in different wild mice as *t* haplotypes. The *t* haplotypes have been found in all wild mouse populations except certain small isolates,[5] in frequencies of up to 40%.[6] A complete *t* haplotype carries two non-overlapping inversions in the proximal segment of chromosome 17[7,8,9] arranged in tandem, with a small segment of normal chromatin separating them. The proximal inversion spans a chromosomal segment estimated to be 5 cM long which translates into some 10^4 kb of nucleotide sequence. The *T* locus is positioned approximately in the middle of this inversion (Figure I). The distal inversion is somewhat longer,

Figure I

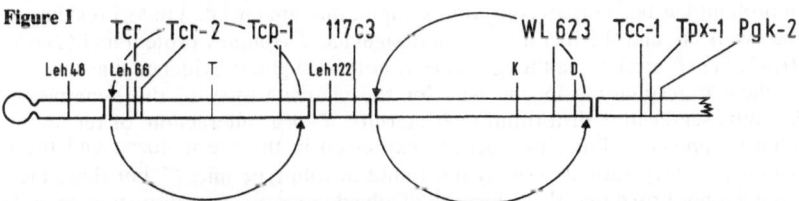

Genetic map of the proximal part of mouse chromosome 17. For references to the relevant markers see: Leh number, ref. 8; Tcr and Tcr-2, ref. 21; 117c3, ref. 19; Tcp-1, ref. 18; Tpx-1, ref. 20; WL623. T. Meo and M. Levi-Strauss, personal communication; Tcc-1 and Pgk-2, L. Silver, personal communication.

spanning about 10 cM of the chromosome and 2×10^4 kb of DNA. The *H-2* complex, the major histocompatibility complex of the mouse, is included in this inversion. As a result of the two inversions, crossing-over is severely suppressed between the wild-type and the *t*-form of chromosome 17 in this region. Rare recombinations, however, do occur within the *t* complex, producing partial *t* haplotypes which possess only part of the abnormal chromatin.

The two inversions would have long been eliminated from mouse populations had they not been associated with powerful segregation distorters responsible for the abnormally high transmission of the *t* chromosomes via male germ cells.[10,11] In many instances, almost 100% of the progeny of a *t*-haplotype-bearing male inherits the abnormal chromosome. The distortion is caused by a set of genetic elements scattered over the two inversions and divided into two classes— distorters and responders.[12-14] Complex interactions among the individual elements determine the degree of distortion, which can range from 10% (i.e., lower than expected transmission ratio) to almost 100% (i.e., high transmission ratio). The nature of the genetic elements and the mode of their action on spermatozoa are not known. It appears, however, that the same elements also cause male sterility when present in certain combinations.[14] The female gametes are unaffected by the action of the segregation distortion elements.

Virtually all complete *t* haplotypes are characterised by two other traits: they carry a mutation that interacts with the *T* mutation in such a way that it results in a complete absence of the tail in *T/t* heterozygotes; and they carry lethal genes. The T-interacting gene may be allelic with the *T* gene; the two have, at least, not been separated by genetic recombination in any of the studies carried out thus far. The lethal genes are numerous (at least 16 have been identified thus far),[15] and they are scattered over the two inversions. When present in a homozygous state, any of the genes can lead to embryonic death, the individual genes affecting different stages of embryonic and fetal development and bringing about characteristic morphological changes.[5] The earliest acting gene kills the *t/t* embryos at 3.5 days of gestation; the late acting genes cause lethality around the time of birth at 17-19 days of gestation. None of the genes have as yet been isolated and the cause of death of the *t/t* embryos is not known.

To answer the question posed in the title of this contribution, we must first ask ourselves what constitutes the *t* complex. There are two answers to this. One could say that the *t* complex is the entire DNA comprising the two inversions. This definition seems to have been adapted by some workers in the field. A series of proteins has been discovered, for example, that are encoded in loci residing in the inversion, and the loci have been designated *T*-complex protein loci (*Tcp-1*, *Tcp-2*, *Tcp-3*, etc.),[16,17] although there is not the slightest evidence that any one of them is responsible in any way for the characteristics of the *t*-complex— lethality, segregation distortion, male sterility, *T*-locus interaction, or recombination suppression. True, the loci are expressed in the spermatozoa and the *t*-haplotypes carry variants usually not found in wild-type mice,[17] but these facts alone do not prove that these loci are involved in segregation distortion or male sterility. Indeed, it appears that mouse chromosome 17 is rich in genes that are expressed in spermatozoa. Seven such genes have been cloned thus far.[18,19,20,21]

Some of these genes, however, are probably outside the *t* complex and therefore cannot be responsible for the *t*-associated phenomena. We have cloned a sperm-specific gene, *Tpx-1*, which is found near the *Pgk-2* gene (another testes-expressed gene), and both are located telemetrically from the distal inversion.[30] It may still turn out, however, that the distorters are not genuine genes but are either some sort of insertion elements,[22] or some other, as yet unidentified, genes. Designations such as "T-complex protein" have already led to confusion since in the minds of some non-experts they are what their names claim them to be—proteins responsible for the *t*-associated traits.[23] The *Tcp-1* locus in particular has been heralded as coding for just such a protein, although it will probably turn out to be one of many loci on chromosome 17 that happen to lie within one of the two inversions and happen to be expressed in testes, but otherwise have no relation to any of the *t* phenomena. By this criterion, any locus residing in one of the two inversions—*H-2*, *tufted*, *globin a*, *α-crystallin*, to name but a few—could be called a *T*-complex locus, which, of course, is absurd.

The second possible way of defining the *t* complex is to include in the complex only those loci that code for the essential characteristics of the *t* complex. We have suggested[24] that there are two such characteristics—segregation distortion (sterility) and crossing-over suppression. Without these two characteristics, the *t* phenomena could not exist: without the distortion, the inversions would have been eliminated from the populations, and without the inversions, the complex array of interacting elements responsible for the high transmission ratio could not have been assembled. The other traits that are now part of the *t* complex can be associated with the basic elements only secondarily and are of no consequence for the assembly of the true *t* elements. The various lethal genes, for example, are probably the result of mutations that gradually accumulate in the abnormal chromosomes, because in the presence of strong recombination suppression there is no efficient way of getting rid of them. The tail-interaction mutation could have also been acquired in this way in the early phase of the *t*-chromosome assembly. An indication that this was probably so is our finding of bits of *t*-chromatin in wild mice from Israel. In these animals, the *t*-chromatin does not seem to be associated either with lethal or with strong tail-shortening gene effects.[6]

If we take the first definition of the *t*-complex, then we can, of course, say that humans also possess this complex. Humans probably possess most of the genes located within the two inversions, just as they possess other genes that they share with the mouse. Some of these mouse chromosome 17 genes are undoubtedly present in a single block in the human genome (on human chromosome 6; see Figure II). There is, however, nothing unusual about this finding either: many such homology blocks exist between human and mouse chromosomes. To claim that because humans have a locus homologous to *Tcp-1*[25] and linked to *HLA*, the human major histocompatibility complex, they therefore must have a *t*-complex, is not justified. Even if *Tcp-1* were involved in segregation distortion (for which function, we emphasise again, there is no evidence), it would have to be a special mutant form of the gene that would be distorting the ratios. No evidence has been provided that such a mutant form exists in man. One can, therefore, consider

Figure II

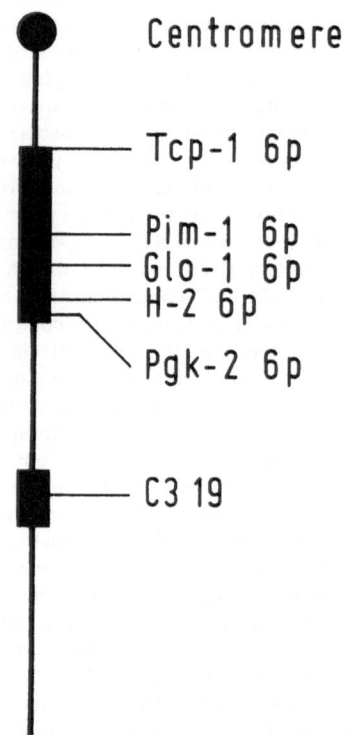

MOUSE CHROMOSOME 17

Centromere

Tcp-1 6p

Pim-1 6p
Glo-1 6p
H-2 6p

Pgk-2 6p

C3 19

Schematic representation of the proximal part of mouse chromosome 17 showing genes whose homologues have been mapped to human chromosomes 6 and 19.

Tcp-1 and similar genes to be human homologues of the *t*-complex, but such an assumption serves no useful purpose.

If we accept the second definition, we must conclude that the *t*-complex of man has not yet been discovered and probably does not even exist. No evidence for the presence of inversions on human chromosome 6 has been provided and reports of segregation distortion involving the *HLA* complex[26] have been questioned.[27] Even in the supposedly abnormal transmission ratios, the distortion has been mild, just on the border of statistical significance, and certainly nowhere near that observed in wild mice. If humans had a distorter system analogous to the mouse, there would be no difficulty demonstrating it even in small families.

We do not wish to claim that some of the distorting elements—whatever their nature—do not occasionally pop up in the human population. They do, but they never become assembled, with the necesary help of inversions, into a system of strong distorters of the type found in some 40% of wild mice. In this sense, the *t*-complex does not exist in man.

ACKNOWLEDGEMENTS

This work was supported in part by grant No. IMB 1 R01 AI23667 from the National Institutes of Health, Bethesda, Maryland. We thank Ms. Lynne Yakes for editorial assistance.

REFERENCES
1. Dobrovolskaia-Zavadskaia N. Sur la mortification spontanée de la queue chez la souris nouveau-née et sur l'existence d'un caractère (facteur) héréditaire 'non viable'. *C R Soc Biol* Paris 1927; **97:** 114-116.
2. Chesley P. Development of the short-tailed mutant in the house mouse. *J Exp Zool* 1935; **70:** 429-455.
3. Klein J. Cytological identification of the chromosome carrying the IXth linkage group (including H-2) in the house mouse. *Proc Nat Acad Sci USA* 1971; **68:** 1544-1547.
4. Dobrovolskaia-Zavadskaia N, Kobozieff N. Les souris anoures et la queue filiforme qui se reproduisent entre elle sans disjunction. *C R Soc Biol* Paris 1932; **110:** 782-784.
5. Klein J. *Biology of the Mouse Histocompatibility-2 complex.* New York: Springer-Verlag, 1975.
6. Figueroa F, Neufeld E, Ritte U, Klein J. *t*-specific DNA polymorphisms among wild mice from Israel and Spain. *Genetics*; In press.
7. Artzt K, Shin HS, Bennet D. Gene mapping within the *T/t* complex of the mouse. II Anomalous position of the *H-2* complex in *t* haplotypes. *Cell* 1982; **28:** 461-476.
8. Herrman B, Bucán M, Mains PE, Frischauf AM, Silver LM, Lehrach H. Genetic analysis of the proximal portion of the mouse *t* complex: evidence for a second inversion within t haplotypes. *Cell* 1986; **44:** 469-476.
9. Shin HS, Flaherty L, Artzt K, Bennett D, and Ravetch J. Inversion in the *H-2* complex of *t*-haplotype in mice. *Nature* 1983; **306:** 380-383.
10. Kobozieff N. Recherches morphologiques et génétiques sur l'anourie chez la souris. *Bull Biol* 1935; **69:** 265-405.
11. Chesley P, Bunn LC. The inheritance of taillessness (anury) in the house mouse. *Genetics* 1936; **21:** 525-536.
12. Styrna J, Klein J. Evidence for two regions in the mouse *t* complex controlling transmission ratios. *Genet Res Camb* 1981; **38:** 315-325.
13. Lyon MF. Transmission ratio distortion in mouse *t*-haplotypes is due to multiple distorter genes acting on a responder locus. *Cell* 1984; **37:** 621-628.
14. Lyon MF. Male sterility of the mouse *t*-complex is due to homozygosity of the distorter genes. *Cell* 1986; **44:** 357-363.
15. Klein J, Sipos P, Figueroa F. Polymorphism of *t*-complex genes in European wild mice. *Genet Res Camb* 1984; **44:** 39-46.
16. Silver LM, Artzt K, Bennet D. A major testicular cell protein specified by a mouse T/complex. *Cell* 1970; **17:** 275-284.
17. Silver LM, Uman J, Danska J, Garrels JI. A diversed set of testicular cell proteins specified by genes within the mouse *t* complex. *Cell* 1983; **35:** 35-45.
18. Willison KR, Dudley K, Potter J. Molecular cloning and sequence analysis of a haploid expressed gene encoding *t* complex polypeptide 1. *Cell* 1986; **44:** 727-738.
19. Rappold GA, Stubbs L, Labeit S, Crkvenjakov RB, Lehrach HH. Identification of a testis-specific gene from the mouse *t*-complex next to a CpG-rich island. *EMBO J* 1987; **6:** 1975-1980.
20. Kasahara M, Figueroa F, Klein J. Random cloning of genes from mouse chromosome 17. *Proc Natl Acad Sci USA* 1987; **84:** 3325-3328.

274   *Study Group: Early Pregnancy Loss*

21. Schimenti J, Cebra-Thomas J, Silver LM. A candidate gene for the mouse *t* complex responder locus responsible for haploid effects on sperm function. *Nature*; In press.
22. Klein J, Golubić M, Budimir O, Schöpfer R, Kasahara M, Figueroa F. On the origin of *t* chromosomes. *Curr Topics Microbiol Immunol* 1986; **127**: 239-246.
23. Fonatsch C, Gradl G, Ragoussis J, Ziegler A. Assignment of the Tcp-1 locus to the long arm of human chromosome 6 by in situ hybridization. *Cytogenet Cell Genet* 1987; **45**: 109-112.
24. Klein J, Nizetić D, Golubić M, Dembić Z, Figueroa F. Evolution of *H-2* genes on *t* chromosomes. *Cell biology of the Major Histocompatibility Complex*. In: Eds. B Pernis, HJ Vogel. Orlando: Academic Press, 1985: pp.97-106.
25. Willison K, Kelly A, Dudley K, Goodfellow P, Spurr N, Groves V, Gorman P, Sheer D, Trowsdale J. The human homologue of the mouse *t*-complex gene, TCP-1, is located on chromosome 6 but is not near the HLA region. *EMBO J* 1987; **7**: 1967-1974.
26. Awdeh ZL, Raum DD, Yunis EJ, Alper CA. Extended HLA/complement allele haplotypes: Evidence for T/t-like complex in man. *Proc Natl Acad Sci USA* 1983; **80**: 259-263.
27. Weitkamp LR. HLA segregation ratios. *Lancet* 1979; **2**: 745.
28. Röhme D, Fox H, Herriman B, Frischauf AM, Edström JE, Mains P, Silver LM, Lehrach H. Molecular clones of the mouse *t* complex derived from microdissected metaphase chromosomes. *Cell* 1984; **36**: 783-788.

Discussion

Chairman: Professor T J Gill

Professor BEER: Alpers and Awdeh in Boston have claimed to have evidence for a *t*-complex equivalent in humans. Might their definition be different?

Professor KLEIN: They HLA-typed families and found that there is a transmission distortion of 60%, and showed that this is statistically significant. That is no evidence for a *t*-complex. In the wild mouse population, 60% segregation distortion would not maintain the *t*-haplotype in this population. Really, it is selected for very high segregation distortion. Thus, if there were segregation distortion of the *t*-complex type in humans you would see it right away. And for this there is no evidence.

Professor GILL: Have the t-probes been shown to complex only the *t*-DNA?

Professor KLEIN: No. They hybridise with wild type as well as with the *t*, but the restriction pattern is different with the *t*. You find one or two bands that are specific for the *t*-haplotype which are absent in the wild.

Dr. HEAP: Can we press you to say a bit more about the failure of fertilisation? Is this failure of attachment or of recognition or of penetration of the zona pellucida?

Professor KLEIN: No, I don't think it is. You see, it is very difficult to study because until now there was no marker. Now we have at least the DNA, so we can do it at the population level. You still can't study it at a single cell level; you would have to be able to identify the original sperm to see which one is *t* and which one is non-*t*.

Dr BILLINGTON: There are claims in the earlier literature that some of the *t*-haplotypes encode for molecules expressed on the cell surface and that they are involved in cellular interaction during embryogenesis, and that alterations in them may be responsible for some of the lethality. Is that a view which is currently supported?

Professor KLEIN: The best thing you can do is to forget about that. Nobody can reproduce those studies.

Professor CLARK: If there is no *t* equivalent in humans, can you still have recessive lethals in humans that would be preserved and lead to problems during reproduction?

Professor KLEIN: Absolutely. I don't know how long they would be preserved, but something will be occurring, and I think that some of these lethal genes in humans will be on chromosome 6. There are several systems in other organisms that are very similar to the *t*-complex in the mouse but do not show segregation distortion.

Professor GILL: Are there any other questions?

Dr ANTCZAK: Just one final point. It seems that you have said that most of the genes in the *t*-complex are probably going to be present in other species. The critical difference is perhaps the inversion.

Professor KLEIN: And the distorters. What is special about the mouse is the combination of mutations and their fixation by the inversions? To maintain them in the population you need a strong segregation distortion which will compensate for the lethal genes.

Dr BILLINGTON: The DR3 haplotype is found commonly in diabetes and appears to be preferentially transmitted.

Professor KLEIN: Yes, but as I said this is a minor distortion.

Immunogenetic factors influencing the survival of the fetal allograft

T.J. Gill III, H.N. Ho, A. Kanbour,
T.A. Macpherson, D.N. Misra and H.W. Kunz

INTRODUCTION

The ability of the fetal allograft to avoid immune rejection presents a perplexing problem in transplantation immunology. Medawar[1] and Billingham[2] discussed a variety of potential mechanisms by which the fetal allograft might be protected, and much work has been done to examine the various possibilities.[3-8] A considerable amount of attention has been devoted to the question of whether there are Class I antigens in the placenta and, if so, where they are and what type of antigenic determinants they carry. Such antigens have been demonstrated in the placenta of the mouse,[9,10] the human[11-14] and the rat[15-17] Immunochemical studies of these placental Class I antigens showed that they carry broadly crossreactive, public antigenic determinants in both the rat[15] and the human.[18,19] There are no Class II antigens in the placenta of the mouse,[20,21] the human[11,14,15,22] and the rat.[23]

In the rat, the haplotypes of the mating combination in which the highest antipaternal antibody response is elicited is u x a (female x male).[15,16,24,25] Detailed examination of this response showed that the antibodies were directed against a placental Class I molecule, the pregnancy-associated (Pa) antigen, that carries a broadly shared antigenic determinant but not the allele-specific determinant of RT1.A^a, which is a major classical Class I transplantation antigen of the a haplotype.[26] The Pa antigen is controlled by a dialellic system, and it is present in the a, d, f, b and m haplotypes but absent in the n, c, l, u, g, k and h haplotypes. Using both alloantisera and specific monoclonal antibodies, the Pa antigen and the A^a antigen were localised to the basal—but not labyrinthine—trophoblast. Since only the Pa antigen elicited an antibody response in the pregnant female, it alone appears to be present in an immunogenetically active form in the placenta. The study described here was undertaken to test this hypothesis by exploring the presence of MHC antigens in the basal and labyrinthine trophoblast of the rat and by localising the Class I antigens in the placenta using electron microscopy and the immunogold technique.

PRESENCE OF MHC ANTIGENS IN THE PLACENTA

The very low level of polymorphism in the rat makes it possible to develop monoclonal antibodies that are unique to specific Class I antigens. Such monoclonal
antibodies have been developed against the Pa antigen (mAb 124)[24] and against
the classical Class I transplantation antigen A^u (mAb 211).[23] These antibodies
were used in the avidin-biotin complex immunoperoxidase method to localise the
Pa and A^u antigens in the placenta. The localisation in the placenta and in the
uterus is summarised in Table 1, and their localisation in other tissues in Table 2.

Table 1

Expression of the Pa and A^u antigens in the placenta and uterus
of WF rats bearing WF x DA fetuses at 12-20 days of gestational age[a,b]

Placenta	Antigen Pa	A^u	Uterus	Antigen Pa	A^u
Basal zone trophoblast:			Endovascular trophoblast lining		
basophilic and giant cells	++	++	blood vessels in metrial gland	++	++
basophilic cells in intimate contact with maternal sinus	+++	+++	Interstitial trophoblast	++	++
glycogen cells	0	0			
Labyrinthine zone trophoblast	0	0			
Reichert's membrane	+++	+++			
Yolk sac epithelium	++	++			

[a]Scale of o to +++.
[b]Reference 23.

Both antigens appear at the same time in ontogeny and have the same tissue
distribution. They are present in the basal trophoblast, except for the glycogen
cells, but are absent from the labyrinthine trophoblast. They are also present in
the endovascular and the interstitial trophoblast. The presence of Pa and A^u
antigens on the basal trophoblast, but not on the labyrinthine trophoblast, was
confirmed by electron microscopy using the immunogold technique with the
anti-Pa and anti-A^u monoclonal antibodies (Figure I).[27]

The genetics of the system being studied allowed us to explore explicitly the
presence of Class II antigens in the placenta, since monoclonal antibodies against
all of the relevant antigens were available.[23] The allogeneic mAb reacts with the
Class II molecules carried by the *a* and *k* haplotypes, and the xenogeneic monoclonal antibody OX3 reacts with the Class II antigens of the *u* haplotype.
Placentas from the WF x DA (*u* x *a*), WF x WF (*u* x *u*) and DA x DA (*a* x *a*)
mating combinations were examined, and no Class II antigens were found. These
observations show that there is constitutive tissue-specific suppression of the
synthesis of Class II antigens in the placenta.

Figure I

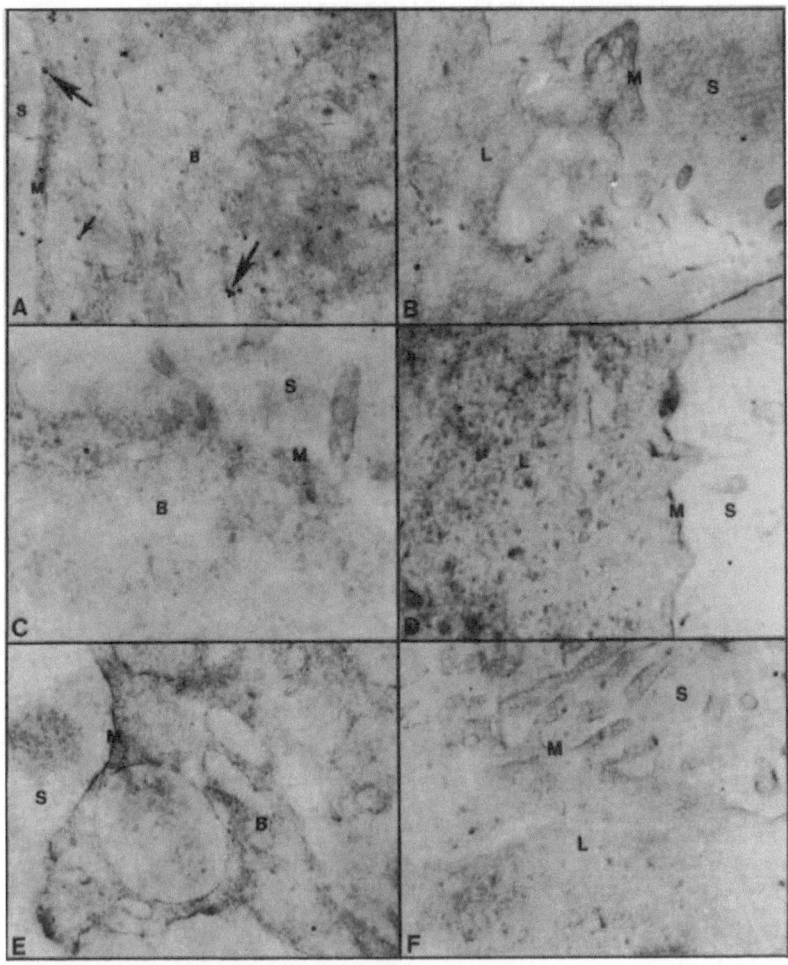

Staining of the rat placenta (Day 17 of gestation) using the double-label protein A-gold technique. B, basal trophoblast; M, cell membrane; S, maternal sinus; and L, labyrinthine trophoblast. The large arrows denote the Pa antigen (mAb 124 labelled with 20 nm gold particles), and the small arrow denotes the A^s antigen (mAb labelled with 10 nm gold particles). (A,B) WF x DA placenta: The basal trophoblast (a) has the Pa antigen only on its surface but has both the Pa and A^s antigens in its cytoplasm. The labyrinthine trophoblast (B) does not stain for either antigen. (C,D) WF x WF placenta: Neither the basal (C) nor the labyrinthine (D) trophoblast stains for the Pa or A^s antigen. (E,F) WF x DA placenta: Neither basal (E) nor the labyrinthine (F) trophoblast stains with the unrelated anti-A^n monoclonal antibody (mAb 42). x58000.

Table 2

The expression of the Pa and A* antigens on tissues other than the
placenta in WA x DA rats of different ages determined with
monoclonal antibodies 124 (anti-Pa) and 211 (anti-A*)

	Intensity of staining at different ages[a]													
	Before birth (gestational day)										After birth (day)			
	12		14		16		18		20		7		56	
Localisation	*Pa*	*A*'	*Pa*	*A*'	*Pa*	*A*'	*Pa*	*A*'	*Pa*	*A*'	*Pa*	*A*'	*Pa*	*A*'
Skin														
Epidermis	++	++	+++	+++	+++	+++	+++	+++	+++	+++	+++	+++	+++	+++
Hair follicles			+++	+++	+++	+++	+++	+++	+++	+++	+++	+++	+++	+++
Subcutaneous tissue	0	0	0	0	0	0	0	0	0	0	0	0	0	0
Brain														
Cortex	0	0	0	0	0	0	0	0	0	0	0	0	0	0
Midbrain					0	0	0	0	0	0	0	0	0	0
Cerebellum					0	0	0	0	0	0	0	0	0	0
Liver														
Hepatocytes	0	0	0	0	0	0	0	0	0	0	0	0	0	0
Kupffer cells					++	++	++	++	++	++	++	++	++	++
Lung														
Bronchial epithelium					++	++	++	++	++	++	++	++	++	++
Parenchyma					0	0	0	0	0	0	+	+	+	+
Gastrointestinal tract														
Epithelium					++	++	++	++	++	++	++	++	++	++
Lamina propria					0	0	0	0	0	0	0	0	0	0
Submucosa					0	0	0	0	0	0	0	0	0	0
Kidney														
Glomeruli and tubular cells[b]					+	+	+	+	+	+	+	+	+	+
Transitional cells of Renal pelvis and ureter													+++	+++
Medulla					0	0	0	0	0	0	0	0	0	0
Heart														
Myocardium	0	0	0	0	0	0	0	0	0	0	0	0	0	0
Endocardium					+	+	+	+	+	+	+	+	+	+
Blood vessels														
Endothelium					++	++	++	++	++	++	++	++	++	++
Thymus														
Cortex					0	0	0	0	0	0	0	0	0	0
Medulla					++	++	++	++	++	++	++	++	++	++
Spleen					++	++	++	++	++	++	++	++	++	++

[a]Scale of 0 to +++
[b]The staining of the glomeruli was variable, and most were negative.

LOCALISATION OF THE PA AND A* ANTIGENS IN THE BASAL TROPHOBLAST

As a further development of this work, two questions were asked. First, is only
the Pa antigen on the surface of the basal trophoblast cells in accordance with the
serological finding of an antibody response in the *u* x *a* pregnancy to the Pa
antigen but not to the A* antigen? Second, is the localisation of the Class I
antigens in the placenta the same in both allogeneic and syngeneic pregnancies.
This question will provide insight into the control of Class I expression on the cell
surface and whether it is constitutive or inducible. The approach to these

problems employed the immunogold technique with electron microscopy[27] and the monoclonal antibodies against the Pa antigen (mAb 124) and against the A^a antigen (mAb 211).

Figure II

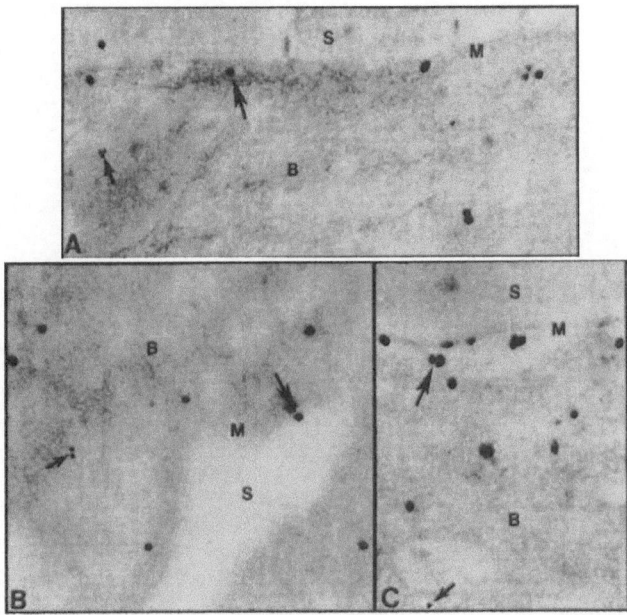

Staining of the basophilic trophoblast of the WF x DA rat placenta (Day 17 of the gestation) using the double-label protein A-gold technique. Symbols are the same as in Figure I. (A-C) are different sections of the basophilic trophoblast, and they show that only the Pa antigen (large arrows) is on the cell surface, whereas both the Pa and A^a (small arrows) antigens are present in the cell cytoplasm. x98000.

Studies in the allogeneic WF x DA pregnancy showed that only the Pa antigen was on the surface of the basal trophoblast cells, whereas both the Pa and A^a antigens were present in the cytoplasm of these cells (Figure II). By contrast, in the syngeneic DA x DA pregnancy, both the Pa and A^a antigens were on the basal trophoblast cell surface as well as in the cytoplasm (Figure III). Morphometric analysis of the electron photomicrographs (Table 3) confirmed these observations. Thus, the hypothesis developed on the basis of serological studies, i.e., that only the Pa antigen is exposed on the basal trophoblast surface, has been confirmed by morphological studies. In addition, the mechanism by which the classical Class I transplantation antigen is suppressed is an inducable one, since this antigen is absent from the basal trophoblast surface in allogeneic pregnancies but not in syngeneic pregnancies.

Figure III

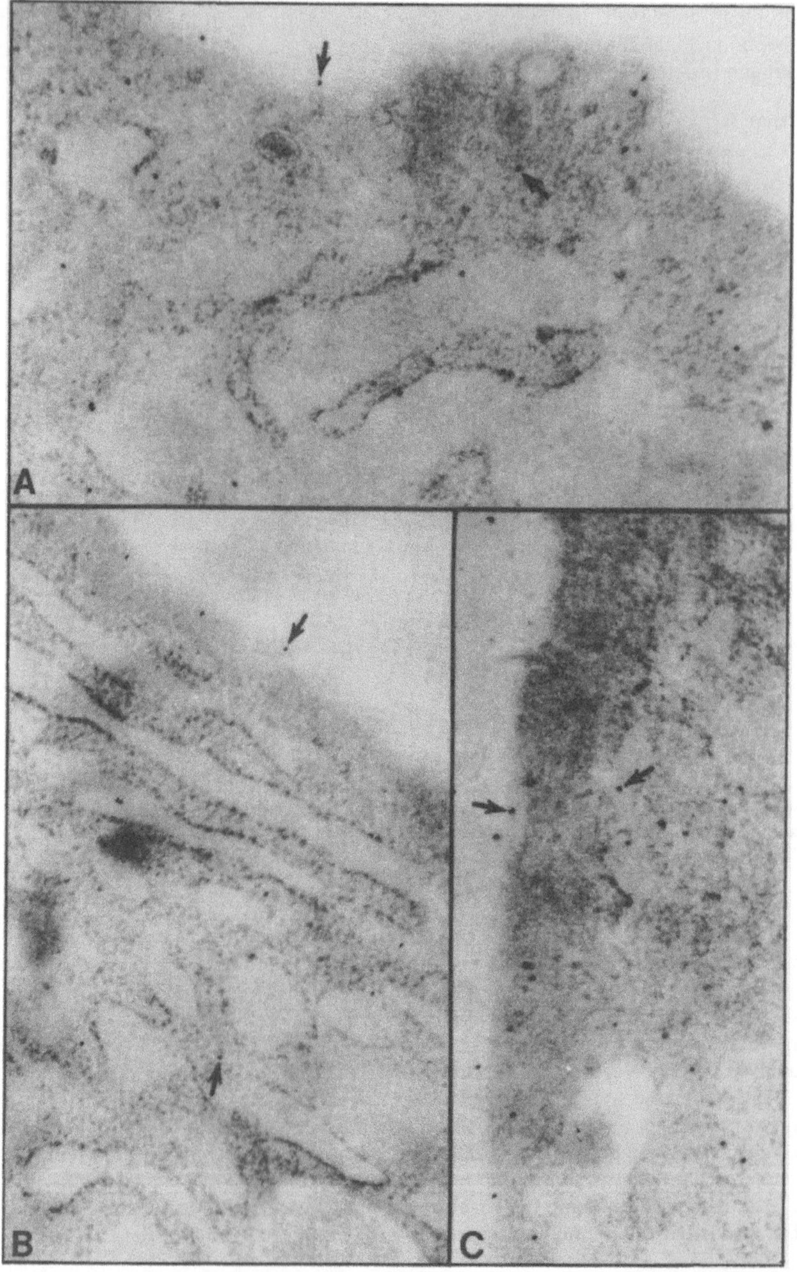

Staining of the basophilic trophoblast of the DA X DA rat placenta (Day 17 of gestation) using the single-label protein A-gold technique (10 nm gold particles). (A) Staining for the Aᵃ antigen. Both antigens are on the cell surface and in the cell cytoplasm. x 58000.

Figure IV

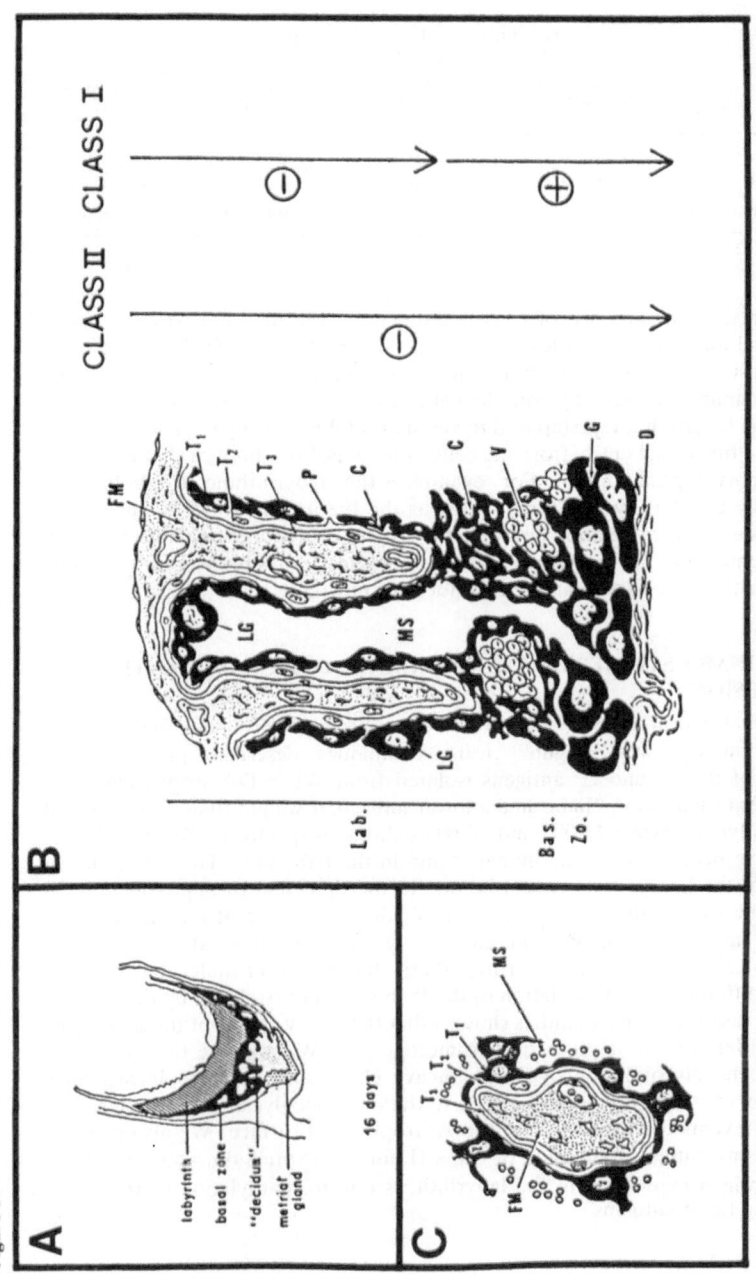

Schematic diagram of the rat placenta (from Davis and Glasser, ref 31) and the distribution of MHC Class I and Class II antigens in the placenta. (A) Schematic diagram of the placental structures at Day 16 of gestation. (B) Longitudinal section through the placenta. (C) Horizontal section through a placental villus. Lab., labyrinth; and Bas. Zo., basal zone. LG, labyrinthine giant cells; FM, vascular fetal mesenchyme; and MS, maternal sinus. The labyrinthine trophoblastic epithelium is trilaminar: layer 1 (T1) is cytotrophoblastic and periodically discontinuous (P), and layers 2 (T2) and 3 (T3) are syncytial. The basal zone trophoblast is composed of three kinds of cells: small basophilic cytotrophoblastic cells (C), giant cells (G) and vacuolated glycogen cells (V). D, uterine decidua.

284   *Study Group: Early Pregnancy Loss*

Table 3

<table>
<tr><td rowspan="3">Placenta</td><td colspan="4" align="center">Presence of the Pa and A^a antigens in the
basophilic trophoblast cells^a</td></tr>
<tr><td colspan="2" align="center">Antigen molecules/μ membrane^b</td><td colspan="2" align="center">Antigen molecules/μ₂ cytoplasm^b</td></tr>
<tr><td>Pa</td><td>A"</td><td>Pa</td><td>A"</td></tr>
<tr><td>WF x DA</td><td>1.55 ± 0.65</td><td>0.13 ± 0.07</td><td>3.27 ± 2.48</td><td>3.25 ± 0.94</td></tr>
<tr><td>DA x DA</td><td>1.14 ± 0.76</td><td>1.13 ± 0.63</td><td>3.07 ± 2.93</td><td>3.56 ± 1.96</td></tr>
<tr><td>WF x WF (control)</td><td>0.21 ± 0.14</td><td>0.19 ± 0.15</td><td>0.89 ± 0.34</td><td>0.76 ± 0.28</td></tr>
</table>

^aReference 23.
^bMean ± S.D.

The presence or absence of Class I antigens in the placenta correlates with anatomical and funtional differences in that organ (Figure IV). Both the basal trophoblast cells and the labyrinthine trophoblast cells in contact with the maternal sinuses are derived from the germinal cytotrophoblast.[31] However, the cells in the labyrinth are juxtaposed to vascular fetal mesenchyme, and they form a separate functional entity from the cells of the basal trophoblast that are of the same embryological origin. For example, the labyrinthine trophoblast is profoundly affected by fetectomy, whereas the basal trophoblast is not.[31] The significance of this correlation between the structural and functional differences in the placenta and the presence (basal trophoblast) or absence (labyrinthine trophoblast) of the Class I antigens is not yet known.

PRELIMINARY STUDIES ON THE MECHANISM OF CLASS I ANTIGEN SUPPRESSION

Biochemical and immunochemical studies on the mechanism of suppression of Class I antigens were begun[23] using techniques described previously.[28,29] Analysis of the Pa and A^a antigens isolated from WF x DA trophoblast cells showed that their heavy chains had a lower molecular weight than those isolated from DA lymphocytes: 43,000 and 46,000 daltons, respectively. Similar observations have been made in the human[30] and in the baboon.[31] This difference in the size of the heavy chains could be due to the detection of approximately 30 amino acids or to a difference in the carbohydrate structure of the heavy chain, since the molecular weight of the completely unglycosylated rat Class I heavy chain is 37,500 daltons.[29] It is our hypothesis that the lower molecular weight is due to a difference in glycosylation of the Pa and A^a heavy chains by the trophoblast, because preliminary studies showed that the heavy chains of these antigens behave differently on lentil lectin chromotography. We propose that there is a defect in the glycosylation of the A^a heavy chain such that the intracellular conversion of the high-mannose glycan to the complex glycan is incomplete and thereby prevents the expression of the A^a trophoblast surface. We also propose that the constitutive suppression of Class II antigen expression, and possibly of Class I antigen expression in the labyrinth, is due to methylation of the genes controlling these antigens.

CONCLUSION

The observations presented in this paper show that there are Class I antigens only in the basal trophoblast of the rat placenta and that Class II antigens are entirely absent from both the basal and the labyrinthine trophoblast. The mechnanism that controls the expression of Class I antigens on the placenta and thereby plays the major role in allowing the allogeneic placenta to escape immunological rejection is three-fold. First, there is constitutive and tissue-specific suppression of the synthesis of Class II antigens. Second, the synthesis of Class I antigens in the labyrinth is constitutively suppressed. Third, there is inducable suppression of the classical Class I transplantation antigens in the basal trophoblast in heterozygous matings but not in homozygous matings.

ACKNOWLEDGEMENT

This work was supported by NIH grants HD 08662 and HD 09880.

REFERENCES
1. Medawar PB. Some immunological and endocrinological problems raised by the evolution of viviparity in vertebrates. *Symp Soc Exp Biol* 1953; **7:** 320-338.
2. Billingham RE. Transplantation immunity and the maternal-fetal relation. *N Eng J Med* 1964; **270:** 667-672.
3. Gill TJ III. Immunological and genetic factors influencing pregnancy and development. *Am J Reprod Immunol* 1986; **10:** 116-120.
4. Gill TJ III. Immunological and genetic factors influencing pregnancy. In: *The Physiology of Reproduction.* Eds. E Knobil, JD Neill. New York: Raven Press; In press.
5. Hunziker RD, Wegmann TG. Placental immunoregulation. *CRC Crit Rev Immunol* 1986; **6:** 245-285.
6. Wegmann TG, Gill TJ III, editors. *Immunology of Reproduction* New York: Oxford University Press. 1983.
7. Gill TJ III, Wegmann TG, Eds. *Immunoregulation and Fetal Survival.* New York: Oxford University Press. 1987.
8. Clark DA, Croy BA Eds. *Reproductive Immunology 1986.* Amsterdam: Elsevier Science Publishers. 1986.
9. Wegmann TG, Carlson GA. Allogeneic pregnancy as immunoabsorbent. *J Immunol* 1977; **119:** 1659-1663.
10. Chatterjee-Hasrouni S, Lala PK. Localization of H-2 antigens on mouse trophoblast cells. *J Exp Med* 1979; **149:** 1238-1253.
11. Goodfellow PN, Barnstaple CJ, Bodmer WF, Snary D, Crumpton MJ Expression of HLA system antigens on placenta. *Transplantation* 1976; **22:** 595-603.
12. Faulk WP, Sanderson AR, Temple A. Distribution of MHC antigens in human placental chorionic villi. *Transplant Proc* 1977; **9:** 1379-1384.
13. Redman CWG, McMichael AJ, Stirrat GM, Sunderland CA, Ting A. Class I major histocompatibility complex antigens on human extravillous trophoblast. *Immunology* 1984; **52:** 457-468.
14. Ellis SA, Sargent IL, Redman CWG, McMichael AJ. Evidence for a novel HLA antigen found on human extravillous trophoblast and a choriocarcinoma cell line. *Immunology* 1986; **59:** 595-601.
15. Ghani AM, Gill TJ III, Kunz HW, and Misra DN Elicitation of the maternal antibody response to the fetus by a broadly shared MHC class I antigenic determinant. *Transplantation* 1984; **37:** 187-194.

16. Macpherson TA, Ho NH, Kunz HW, Gill TJ III. Localization of the Pa antigen on the placenta of the rat. *Transplantation* 1986; **41:** 392-394.
17. Billington WD, Burrows FJ. The rat placenta expresses paternal class I major histocompatibility antigens. *J Reprod Immunol* 1986; **9:** 155-160.
18. McIntyre JA, Faulk WP, Verhulst SJ, Colliver JA. Human trophoblast-lymphocyte cross-reactive (TLX) antigens define a new alloantigenic system. *Science* 1983; **222:** 1135-1137.
19. Konoeda Y, Terasaki PI, Wakasaka A, Park MS, Mickey MR. Public determinants of HLA indicated by pregnancy antibodies. *Transplantation* 1986; **41:** 253-259.
20. Raghupathy R, Singh B, Leigh JB, Wegmann TG. The ontogeny and turnover kinetics of paternal H-2K antigenic determinants on the allogeneic murine placenta. *J Immunol* 1981; **127:** 2074-2079.
21. Chatterjee-Hasrouni, S, Lala PK. MHC antigens on mouse trophoblast cells: paucity of Ia antigens despite the presence of H-2K and D. *J Immunol* 1981; **127:** 2070-2073.
22. Brami CJ, Sanyal MK, Dwyer JM, Johnson CC, Kohorn EI, Naftolin F. HLA-DDR antigen on human trophoblast. *Am J Reprod Immunol* 1983; **3:** 165-174.
23. Kanbour A, Ho N-H, Misra DN, Macpherson TA, Kunz HW, Gill TJ III. Differential expression of MHC class I antigens on the placenta of the rat: a mechanism for the survival of the fetal allograft. *J Exp Med*; In press.
24. Ghani AM, Kunz HW, Gill TJ III. Pregnancy-induced monoclonal antibody to a unique fetal antigen. *Transplantation* 1984; **37:** 503-506.
25. Smith RN, Sternlicht M, Butcher GW. The alloantibody response in the allogeneically pregnant rat. I. The primary and secondary responses and detection of Ir gene control. *J Immunol* 1982; **129:** 771-776.
26. Ho HN, Macpherson TA, Kunz HW, Gill TJ III. Ontogeny of expression of Pa and RT1.Aᵃ antigens on rat placenta and on fetal tissues. *Am J Reprod Immunol Microbiol* 1987; **13:** 51-61.
27. Bendayan M, Nanci A, Herber GH, Gregoire S, Duhr MA. A review of the study of protein secretion applying the protein A-gold immunocytochemical approach. *Am J Anat* 1986; **175:** 379-400.
28. Misra DN, Kunz HW, Gill TJ III. Analysis of class I MHC antigens in the rat by monoclonal antibodies. *J Immunol* 1985; **134:** 2520-2528.
29. Misra DN, Kunz HW, and Gill TJ III. Carbohydrate moieties of rat MHC class I antigens. *Immunogenetics*; In press.
30. Stern PL, Beresford N, Friedman CI, Stevens WC, Risk JM, Johnson PM. Class-I like MHC molecules expressed by baboon placental syncytiotrophoblast. *J Immunol* 1987; **138:** 1088-1091.
31. Davis J, Glasser SR. Histological and fine structure observations on the placenta of the rat. *Acta Anatomica* 1968; **69:** 542-608.

Discussion

Chairman: Professor T. J. Gill

Dr CHAOUAT: It is exciting to find an inducible expression of an MHC Class I. Did you try to make embryo transfer of a DA x DA embryo to a pseudopregnant WF female to see whether the Class I antigens were repressed?

Professor GILL: No, we haven't done that yet. That is a very good experiment and certainly one that we should do as soon as we can.

Professor CLARK: I think I probably missed this, but is this repression of Class I antigens seen in all heterozygous matings in rats?

Professor GILL: We have only looked at this mating in which there is the strongest immune response. In most of the other matings, there is either no immune response or very low immune response.

Professor CLARK: What was the evidence that the Pa antigen can't elicit a cytotoxic response?

Professor GILL: The antisera to Pa are essentially not cytotoxic: only a few are, and their titres are quite low. The Pa monoclonal antibodies are non-cytotoxic as well.

Dr BILLINGTON: I find it rather hard to accept this hypothesis. The matings which we commonly use are the PVG by DA, where the DA is the male, and we are therefore probing toward the RT1.A^a haplotype with our monoclonal antibody. The indications are that this is a surface-expressed Class I product. Your evidence contrary to that is based on the immunogold labelling and I frankly find that the level of immunogold labelling is very low considering the amount of expression of Class I product shown by the immunoperoxidase. I am just wondering about the technology, and whether anyone else here could comment on that level of labelling using the very sensitive immunogold assay.

Professor GILL: There are several things. First, there is no way that you can equate immunoperoxidase labelling with electron microscopic data—that simply can't be done. Secondly, we counted 500-1000 microns or square microns to get these data: hence they are fairly tight. With the immunogold technique you are looking at the molecular level. Thirdly, in the PVG x DA system there is a very low antibody response; it is essentially a non-responding system. Finally, there is just no way that you can tell whether an antigen is on the cell surface or in the cytoplasm at the light electron microscopic level. It just can't be done.

Dr LOKE: Maybe if I could follow on from what David Billington was saying, I am inclined to side, sadly, with David, in the sense that if you are using 15-20 nm immunogold to detect cytoplasmic antigens, there is no way that the gold will get inside. You can only demonstrate outside antigens with immunogold of that molecular size.

Professor GILL: But if you take a slice through the cell, you are surely going to slice through the middle of the cell exposing both the cytoplasm and the cell membrane. So you would be able to stain both. The gold doesn't have to get inside.

Dr LOKE: I would also agree with David that maybe you should expect the section to be covered with "dots".

Professor GILL: Not necessarily. I think that in the placenta there is probably a much lower synthesis rate for Class I antigens than in lymphocytes. Nonetheless, there are differences in the number of "dots" on the surface of the trophoblast cells in the different matings.

Professor MOWBRAY: How many of your antibody molecules had gold on them?

Professor GILL: We didn't quantitate that, but probably most antibody molecules were labelled. Let me stress that the A^a and Pa antibodies themselves were labelled with the immunogold and used as primary antibodies. No amplification techniques were used when the tissues were stained. Also, the magnification of the electron photomicrographs was quite high.

Dr CHAOUAT: There is a question which fascinates me; by what mechanism would you have repression in one case and expression in the other?

Professor GILL: It probably involves the recognition of foreign paternal antigens by the mother, and the subsequent immune response.

Dr PAGE FAULK: It would be very simple if you just used colloidal gold with the light and electron microscopes, which can be amplified with silver chloride.

Professor BEER: The question I have also relates to the immunogold binding. Are there other transplantation systems where you can see cytoplasmic localisation of the Class I antigen, or is this a new finding, as far as you are concerned?

Professor GILL: We have looked at no other system, except the placenta, and in the DA x DA mating which is basically homozygous mating, we see the antigen in the cytoplasm. I imagine that in any system in which Class I antigens are synthesised they would be in the cytoplasm.

Dr ANTCZAK: Have you been able to do sequential immunoprecipitation of these two molecules from lymphocytes?

Professor GILL: These studies are in progress.

Dr LOKE: Can I clarify the last bit of the slide: "inducible repression of A^a in heterozygous matings." Have you any idea what is inducing the repression of A^a?

Professor GILL: We can't tell yet, but it may be an immunological mechanism.

Dr BILLINGTON: I understand from observations by the Aberdeen group that they have been able by immunisation to produce antibodies which map in a similar way to your Pa antigen. That would mean that it is not pregnancy-associated in the sense that it appears to be generated also by immunisation. Do you know of this unpublished work?

Professor GILL: As I said, the Pa and the A^a antigens are on all tissues, so that if you immunise with any tissue I suspect that you would get antibodies to A^a and to Pa. The key point is that we have two monoclonal antibodies that are characterised properly so that we can differentiate between the two molecules. In that part of the MHC there is evidence for a number of Class I antigens. The model I propose would be that some Class I antigens cause tissue rejection—the transplantation antigens—and others such as the Pa antigen do not. The evidence that I showed in the blocking studies indicates that they are separate molecules.

Dr ANTCZAK: Is Pa a transplantation antigen?

Professor GILL: It does not cause the rejection of tissues.

Dr CARP: Could I ask you, and possibly also Dr Klein, a couple of clinical questions? If we are to assume that in most of our habitual aborters that the problem may well be a lethal gene or some chromosomal anomaly, would it be reasonable to assume that there should be a carrier state in the parents in a large number of cases? As you well know, this is not the case. When the standard karyotype techniques are used on the parents, chromosomal anomalies are found in about 4-6%; our own figures are 8 of 300 patients, and we find that they are mainly reciprocal translocations.

Professor GILL: In the kinds of abortions that we are talking about, I think that there are two factors operative. One is the control of Class I antigens on the surface of the placenta, and that is what I have been talking about. I think that when the control mechanism goes awry, the classical Class I antigens are expressed and can elicit and anti-paternal immune response, leading to abortions caused by cytotoxic anti-MHC antibodies. The second mechanism is that there are recessive lethal genes linked to the major histocompatibility complex that can cause abortions without eliciting an immune response. I postulate that these MHC-linked genes can cause a variety of developmental abnormalities ranging from embryonic death to susceptibility to carcinogens in adult life. There is substantial evidence in the literature that there are populations of aborters who share HLA antigens, and I think that this sharing is just a marker for the sharing of MHC-linked recessive lethal genes.

Dr CARP: May I just make a couple of comments on that? The types of translocation which I am talking about are not translocations which related to chromosome 6 or to the MHC complex. We had one patient who had a reciprocal translocation of chromosomes 2 and 7; another patient, with translocations involving chromosomes 13 and 15. We have a third patient who has a chromosome 7 to 8 translocation.

Professor GILL: That is quite a different set of causes of spontaneous abortion.

Dr CARP: These are all patients who presented to us without lymphocytotoxic antibodies.

Professor GILL: That is a separate set of mechanisms from the ones that I am talking about. In the experimental systems, there is no evidence for chromosomal anomalies. So the mechanism that you are talking about—chromosomal abnormalities—is very different.

Professor BEARD: It seems to me that we haven't discussed the reality of what is being found as against the theoretical aspects that you are putting forward for the mechanisms. Our experience, and that others who are treating women with recurrent miscarriage, is that with a success rate of around 80% by whatever method you use, you are getting normal babies that are not growth retarded, and that do not show any evidence of a genetic cause for abortion. It is possible that the 20% who miscarry are part of this group, but certainly the great majority are not showing a tendency toward such a cause.

Professor KLEIN: I would like to go on the record and say that the genetic cause of abortion is a fact, whether it is a chromosomal abnormality or the inactivation of a gene, be it on chromosome 6 or some other chromosome, that is a fact. But during this whole meeting I have not heard any evidence that would convince me that there is an immunologic cause.

Professor MOWBRAY: When we are talking about women who abort all of their pregnancies, it is extremely difficult to find a genetic cause. A balanced translocation is a possibility, and we have seen one example in 1500 couples. It is not a common cause of what locally seems to be called primary abortion. You need another cause than the genetic one. It is in that group that I think we can look to the immunologists.

Professor KLEIN: There is something more than immunology. There is physiology; there is biochemistry; there are a lot of other things.

Professor MOWBRAY: I agree that just because we modify the immunology to produce a successful pregnancy, it does not prove that there is an immunological cause. Pneumonia is treated with penicillin; it is not a deficiency of penicillin that is the disease.

Professor GILL: Having come into this field from immunogenetics and transplantation, I have tried to organise the literature in reproduction into a conceptual framework that would at least allow us to ask focussed questions. These questions have led to the studies that I have just showed you about the expression of transplantation antigens on the placenta, and to another set of genetic studies. If it is shown that there are immunological causes of abortion, fine. If not, that is fine too. But at least, clearly defined questions will lead to clearly defined answers.

Dr ALEXANDER: I would like to go back to Dr Carp's question. Would the geneticists here tell us whether they think that it is good practice or not in cases where we find a translocation—that should be between 2 and 6% of the recurrent abortions—should we say to those patients: "Awfully sorry. Go home. You don't have a chance". Or should be we say, "Okay. Go further"?

Professor GILL: You are asking a clinically relevant question that probably Dr Creasy, who is our next speaker would be better qualified to answer than either Dr Klein or I.

The cytogenetics of spontaneous abortion in humans

R. Creasy

INTRODUCTION

Human spontaneous abortions have been the subject of many cytogenetic investigations because they are a source of a large number and variety of abnormal chromosome complements (karyotypes). For the same reason, they can be very informative material for the epidemiologist, as Professor Alberman has already demonstrated.[1]

A chromosomally abnormal abortus was first reported in 1961, only five years after the human chromosome number had been accurately determined.[2] A number of mostly small surveys followed and soon established that chromosome abnormality was a major cause of fetal loss.[3] The development of differential staining techniques for chromosomes—"banding techniques"—in the late sixties permitted a much more detailed identification of these chromosome abnormalities than had been previously possible. This increased our understanding of the natural history of human chromosome abnormalities.

Fetal chromosomal abnormalities acquired a more immediate practical significance for the clinician in the early sixties with the development of techniques for sampling amniotic fluid in the second trimester and for examining the chromosome constitution of the fetal cells it contains. This led to a great expansion of the diagnostic cytogenetic services in Europe and North America which continues today. However, this remains largely an area of secondary prevention. A better understanding of the biology relating to the origin of chromosomal abnormality may help towards the ultimate goal of primary prevention. It may also help us to focus precious health care resources where they will have most impact.

METHODS

Population studies of abortuses are more difficult than those of babies or adults for a number of reasons. The fetal or embryonic parts may have already been expelled before medical treatment is received, so that only curettings of decidua can be obtained. These are of no use for fetal chromosome analysis. In some cases the curettings will contain pieces of placenta or fetal membrane which can be cultured. Particular care must be taken in such circumstances to avoid contamination with maternal tissue, especially when culturing placental tissue. Even when the fetus is obtained it may have died *in utero* some time before expulsion, and hence the tissues will have undergone varying degrees of autolysis or maceration. In such cases there may not be sufficient viable cells to culture. Fetal membranes and placenta may, however, culture successfully even when the fetal tissues are no longer viable.

Spontaneous abortions occurring at early stages of gestation are less likely to result in medical treatment being sought than those occurring later in pregnancy. Loss of the fetus or the sac before medical attention is received is also much more likely at early gestational stages.[4] Thus, even in unselected series of miscarriages, later abortions will be overrepresented, particularly in those cases where chromosome analysis is possible.

It is very difficult to determine what proportion of the abortions might have been deliberately induced. This has probably become less of a problem as legislation relating to abortion has become more liberal. In the Parisian study[5] many specimens were collected at home and brought to the laboratory by the husband or a relative. Those who had endeavoured to induce the abortion would be unlikely to participate. However, this method of collection will bias the sample towards couples who are highly motivated to cooperate with such research, such as those of higher social class, advanced parental age and poor obstetric history. In the London studies[6] patients were interviewed by a social worker. The proportion of chromosomal abnormalities was no different in the group who had conceived intentionally, in those who had conceived in spite of taking contraceptive precautions, or in those who professed no strong intention either way.

THE PREVALENCE OF CHROMOSOME ABNORMALITIES

The early work of Carr showed that at least 20% of spontaneous abortions were due to chromosomal abnormalities.[3] Later surveys have found rates up to 60%.[5] The findings of 12 large studies, which each karyotyped more than 100 abortuses, are summarised in Table 1. The overall proportion of abnormalities in more than 6000 karyotyped abortuses is 43%, ranging from 22 to 61%, except for one study with only 8%.

The early studies revealed that the highest rates of chromosomal abnormality were found in early gestation, and later studies mainly tended to concentrate on early abortion, Five studies attempted to collect all pregnancy losses up to between 24 and 27 weeks, corresponding to the legal definition of miscarriage, and found between 22 and 39% chromosomal abnormalities.[3,8,9,10,14] A further 5 studies, which found between 46 and 54% abnormal, collected fetuses up to about 16 or 18 weeks of gestation, or used a developmental limit.[7,11,12,13,15] One collected fetuses up to 100mm in length,[12] and another excluded fetuses over 500gm,[7] corresponding to a normal development of about 16 and 21 weeks. The study of the Boués[5] was carried out over many years. As the study progressed, the emphasis shifted towards epidemiology, and a greater effort was made to collect early abortions. The cut-off point was eventually set at a developmental age of 12 weeks. Fetuses of greater gestational age were still included, but they would be increasingly selected for growth retardation at greater gestational ages.

Table 1

Twelve Cytogenetic Surveys of Spontaneous Abortions

Ref.	Authors	Location	No. Karyo-typed	No. Abnor-mal	% Abnor-mal
5	Boué *et al.*, 1975	Paris, France	1498	921	61
7	Hassold *et al.*, 1980	Honolulu, Hawaii	1000	463	46
8	Creasy *et al.*, 1976	London, UK	986	289	29
9	Warburton *et al.*, 1980	New York, USA	967	312	32
10	Dhadial *et al.*, 1970	London, UK	547	128	23
11	Takahara *et al.*, 1977*	Hiroshima, Japan	505	237	47
12	Kajii *et al.*, 1980	Geneva, Switzerland	402	215	54
13	Therkelsen *et al.*, 1977	Aarhus, Denmark	254	139	54
3	Carr, 1967	London, Canada	227	50	22
14	Geisler & Kleinebrecht, 1978	Frankfurt, FRG	166	65	39
15	Arakaki & Waxman, 1970	Honolulu, Hawaii	127	63	50
16	Strenchever *et al.*, 1967	Cleveland, USA	101	8	8
			6780	2890	43

*plus some data quoted in Reference 9.

Their study had the greatest proportion of early abortions and the highest proportion of chromosomal abnormalities, 61%.

The London and New York studies[8-10] included a greater proportion of specimens of more than 16 weeks gestation than the other studies which attempted to collect later abortions, such as those in Hawaii and Japan.[7,11] This may reflect a differing miscarriage rate at different stages of pregnancy, a difference in the tendency to seek hospital treatment for early abortion, or selection of larger products of conception by hospital staff for inclusion in the study. The London studies did not culture placental tissue to avoid the danger of maternal contamination, and this meant that fewer of the earlier abortuses could be investigated. There is also a tendency for the abnormality rate to be higher in more recent studies, which may suggest an increasing effort to include early abortions. Medical care for threatened miscarriage has also improved with time, so that fewer normal fetuses are lost.

The very low proportion of abnormalities in the Cleveland study[16] is difficult to explain. It may be partly due to a large proportion of induced abortions. Possibly also the attempt to exclude septic abortions, on the grounds that they might have been deliberately induced, may have led to exclusion of many macerated, chromosomally abnormal abortuses. Technical factors, such as the selection of tissue for culture, may also have played a part.

Thus, the principal factor influencing the proportion of chromosomal abnormalities is the gestational age distribution of the abortuses studied. Those studies collecting abortuses expelled up to the end of the second trimester find about 30% abnormal, while those concentrating on earlier gestation, up to about 16 weeks, find about 50% abnormal.

GESTATIONAL AGE

In our own study,[8] 30% of the abortions occurring between week 9 and 27 were chromosomally abnormal. This figure rose to 38% if weeks 9 to 19 only were considered, and to 50% for weeks 9 to 11. While this trend has been reported by most studies, Warburton[9] has pointed out that many candidates show fewer chromosomal abnormalities in the abortuses expelled before week 8: between 14% and 16%.[7,9,11,12] The numbers in individual studies are small, and most authors have felt that the findings were unreliable. In our own study there were less than 50 specimens with a reported gestation of less than 9 weeks but in a significant proportion of these specimens this was clearly incorrect from the development of the specimen. Thus, these figures must be treated with caution. The data from the Boués' study, when analysed by gestation, suggest that the proportion of chromosomal abnormalities is highest between weeks 4 and 8.[17]

Using the data from studies of spontaneous abortion in conjunction with life tables of fetal mortality, it is possible to estimate that about 50% of clinically recognisable spontaneous abortions are chromosomally abnormal. At the end of the second month of pregnancy, one fetus in fifteen is chromosomally abnormal. By the seventeenth week, this prevalence has dropped to one in a hundred, and by week 21 the prevalence is only slightly greater than at term. Including data for weeks 5 to 8[17] suggests that at the end of the first month of pregnancy one fetus in eight has an abnormal chromosome complement.[18]

THE TYPES OF CHROMOSOMAL ABNORMALITIES

There is good agreement between the various studies with regard to the relative frequency of the different types of abnormality (Table 2). About half of the

Table 2

Types of Chromosomal Abnormality in Abortions

Type	No.	%
Autosomal Monosomy	6	0.2
Sex Chromosome Monosomy	538	19.6
Autosomal Trisomy	1355	49.4
Sex Chromosome Trisomy	9	0.3
Double & Triple Trisomy	47	1.7
Triploidy	425	15.5
Hypo & Hypertriploidy	14	0.5
Tetraploidy	149	3.8
Structural Abormality	104	3.8
Mixoploidy	89	3.2
Other	7	0.3
	2743	100.0

Same sources as Table 1 (without extra data of 11 quoted in Reference 9)

chromosomally abnormal abortuses have an extra chromosome (trisomy). In the vast majority of these, the extra chromosome is an autosome (i.e., not a sex chromosome). Very few are missing an autosome (autosomal monosomy), but about a fifth have only a single sex chromosome (sex chromosomal monosomy—"XO"). About 15% have a complete extra haploid set of chromosomes (triploidy, with 69 chromosomes), while about 5% have two extra haploid sets (tetraploidy, with 92 chromosomes). The remainder are mostly structural chromosomal abnormalities (mainly translocations) or mosaics (having two different cell lines). Most of the latter have normal and trisomic cells. Some abortuses have two, or even three, independent chromosomal abnormalities. These include double and triple trisomies and missing or extra chromosomes in addition to triploidy (hypo- and hypertriploidy, with 68 or 70 chromosomes).

Table 3

Relative Frequency of Differing Trisomies.
848 Cases Identified by Banding

Chromosome	%	Chromosome	%	Chromosome	%
1	60.0	9	22.8	17	0.6
2	4.6	10	2.0	18	4.7
3	1.2	11	0.2	19	0.1
4	2.9	12	0.9	20	2.5
5	0.2	13	5.5	21	9.2
6	0.5	14	4.6	22	10.8
7	4.5	15	7.1	X	1.3
8	3.7	16	30.0	Y	0.0

From References 7, 8, 9, 11, 12, 13, 20, 21, 22

Trisomy has been described for all chromosomes except number 1 and the Y chromosome but with greatly differing frequency (Table 3). Nearly one-third of all trisomies have an extra chromosome 16, while extra chromosomes 2, 7, 13, 14, 15, 21 and 22 each account for between 5 and 10% of trisomies. Trisomies 5, 6, 11, 12, 17 and 19 each comprise less than 1% of all such abnormalities. Trisomy 1 has not been described in a spontaneous abortion, but one case has been detected in a blastula produced by *in vitro* fertilisation.[19] The sex chromosome trisomies are more than twice as often XXY and XXX. We do not know to what extent this represents variation in the incidence of these anomalies and to what extent selection in the earliest stages of development is responsible for these widely differing frequencies.

The relative proportions of sex chromosome monosomy (15-28%) and triploidy (10-20%) vary more between studies. The studies with the highest proportion of sex chromosome monosomies tend to have the lowest proportions of triploidy and vice versa. The proportion of mosaics is difficult to compare, because the proba- bility of detecting mosaicism depends upon methodology. Mosaicism may also be tissue specific, and may be more frequent in the placenta.[23]

THE EFFECT OF MATERNAL AGE

The one aetiological factor which is clearly related to the prevalence of chromo- somal abnormality is maternal age. Increasing maternal age increases the risk of a trisomic conception. Autosomal trisomies account for about a quarter of the abnormalities in younger mothers, but this rises to three-quarters in those over thirty-five. The proportion of chromosomal abnormalities excluding trisomies remains nearly constant at about 15%. The acrocentric chromosomes (those bearing nucleolar organiser regions: 13, 14, 15, 21 and 22) together with most of the other small chromosomes (17, 18, 19 and 20) show this maternal age effect most markedly (Table 4). Trisomy 16, the most common trisomy, shows very little age effect, suggesting that there are special factors causing this condition.

Table 4

Effect of Maternal Age

Maternal Age	No. Karyotyped	% Abnormal	% Non Trisomy	% Trisomy	% Acrocentric Trisomy
20	104	18.3	13.5	4.8	10.5
20-24	256	28.5	16.4	12.1	11.0
25-29	339	26.3	15.6	10.6	10.1
30-34	161	32.3	13.0	19.3	21.2
35-39	99	34.3	9.0	25.3	29.4
40+	32	65.6	15.6	50.0	42.9

From Reference 8

Some studies have reported an inverse maternal age effect for sex chromosome monosomy,[24,25] but others have found no effect in this condition.[5,7,8,13]

Hassold has suggested that paternal age may be reduced in triploidy, especially when the extra set of chromosomes was of paternal origin.[7]

FETAL DEVELOPMENT

Different studies have used very different criteria to describe the morbid anatomy of abortuses, and many cytogenetic studies have not given details. Many specimens are incomplete and so only a limited examination is possible. The highest proportion of chromosomal abnormalities is found in abortuses which are often described as "blighted ova". These include intact sacs with no embryo or very small embryos, which are often grossly abnormal. Larger fetuses are rarely associated with chromosomal abnormalities (Table 5).[26] These categories

Table 5

Prevalence of Chromosomal Abnormality by Morbid Anatomy of Abortus

Abortus	% Chromosomally Abnormal
Incomplete specimen, no embryo	47.3
Incomplete embryo/fetus	40.0
Intact empty sac	64.3
Severely disorganised embryo	68.6
Normal embryo	54.1
Embryo with focal abnormalities	55.0
Normal fetus	3.3
Fetus with malformation	18.2

From Reference 8

obviously correlate closely with the gestational age of the abortus. Trisomic abortions are predominantly empty sacs or very stunted embryos less than 5mm long. Very little embryonic development seems possible in most autosomal trisomies. The few exceptions are trisomy 13, 14, 18, 21 and 22, which, except for trisomy 14, are all described in livebirths as non-mosaic trisomies. Larger embryos with trisomy 13 or 14 may exhibit characteristic malformations, such as facial clefts, cyclopia or polydactyly. Sex chromosome trisomy (XXX and XXY) is also compatible with more advanced embryonic or fetal development. Although trisomy 16 is so abundant, it inhibits all but the most rudimentary stages of embryogenesis, which rarely exceeds 2mm.

Sex chromosome monosomy is rarely found in the absence of an embryo, and embryonic development often proceeds normally at the gross level, although focal abnormalities, such as encephalocoeles, may develop. Larger fetuses with gross oedema and the characteristic cervical hygromata are also seen at later stages of pregnancy. These are usually so macerated that they often cannot be cultured.

Triploid abortuses show a very variable morphology, ranging from empty sacs through embryos with major anomalies to large fetuses. Many malformations can be seen in the larger embryos and fetuses, including neural tube defects, facial clefts and syndactyly.

Tetraploidy permits very little embryonic development, the majority of tetraploids being empty sacs or grossly abnormal embryos less than 5mm long. Nearly all the tetraploids and trisomics, including those with potentially viable trisomies, are expelled by the 14th week of gestation. A small proportion of fetuses with trisomy 13, 18, 21, 22, and a larger proportion of those with trisomy X, survive until after the twentieth week. Similarly, most sex chromosome monosomics are expelled by the sixteenth week, but again a small proportion survive in the third trimester. Triploids show less of a peak in time of expulsion, with a much greater proportion aborting between weeks 16 and 20. Again only a small proportion survive into the third trimester.[8,12,26]

SEX RATIO

Interpretation of the data on sex ratio is difficult. Most studies show an excess of female abortuses. Those that have reported a male predominance have been those with the largest proportion of later abortions. It thus seems likely that late abortions after about the twentieth week, probably include a slight excess of males, as is seen in stillbirths and infants at term. Earlier abortuses show more females than males in most studies, but this may in part be due to maternal contamination, particularly when cultures are derived from placental or fetal membranes. The sex ratio of chromosomally normal abortuses prior to week 20 does not show a great deviation from unity, but there is probably a slight bias towards females.

There are more female chromosomally abnormal abortuses because of the large number of XO's. The situation in trisomic abortuses is even more difficult to determine. Most studies found a preponderance of males. Two of the largest studies, however, recorded an excess of females. One of these included a large proportion of early abortuses,[5] while the other contained large number of late abortions and found an excess of males in the chromosomally normal specimens.[8] There may, in fact, be differences in the sex ratio between different trisomies.

Trisomies 21 and 18 both show an excess of males in abortuses (sex ratios 1.7 and 1.8 respectively), although at term trisomy 21 shows a slight male preponderance while trisomy 18 is heavily biased towards females. Trisomy 9 shows a marked excess of females in abortuses. Nearly 200 cases of trisomy 16 reveal a small male predominance (1.18).[7]

PREGNANCY WASTAGE

One of the surprising findings to emerge from the early studies of spontaneous abortion was the high prenatal mortality of sex chromosome monosomy in spite of the relatively mild problems experienced by survivors with Turner's syndrome.[27] Later the application of banding techniques to abortion material revealed that at least two-thirds of fetuses with trisomy 21 are aborted spontaneously.[28]

We now have sufficient information to begin to look at the natural history of all chromosome abnormalities. We still do not know whether very early abortions include a large number of chromosomal abnormalities. It is possible that autosomal monosomies and some of the rarer trisomies are lost at this stage, possibly around the time of implantation. Studies of mice with translocations have shown that autosomal monosomies and some trisomies do cease development very early in gestation and that different trisomies survive for different periods.[29,30] Indeed some mouse trisomies show certain similarities to human trisomies: in particular murine trisomy 16 and human trisomy 21.[31] However, this does not necessarily mean that non-translocation monosomies occur in significant numbers in man, although meiotic non-disjunction should produce equal numbers of nullisomic and disomic gametes. Such considerations have led to speculation that 50% of human conceptions may be chromosomally abnormal.[32] It has, however, been suggested that the lower frequency of abnormal karyotypes found in early gestation is real and that all chromosomally aberrant conceptions are retained for several weeks before expulsion. This would imply that aberrant, but chromosomally normal, conceptions that fail at this stage are not retained *in utero* for some reason.

Whichever idea is correct, it is still possible to estimate prenatal mortality after the earliest stages. If we consider a cohort of 1000 clinically recognisable pregnancies, then at a conservative estimate 15% of these will be lost as spontaneous abortions, of which approximately 50% will be chromosomally abnormal. We can derive estimates of the prenatal mortality of the various abnormalities. Chromosomally normal conceptions, and those with balanced translocations, have a mortality of about 15%. Sex chromosome trisomies will suffer a 25% loss, but this will be greater for XXY than for XXX. Autosomal trisomies will be diminished by about 80% for trisomy 21, over 95% for trisomies 8, 13, 18 and 22, and 100% for the remainder. About 99% of diploids and sex chromosome monosomics will also be lost to spontaneous abortion. There is no obvious explanation why fetuses with sex chromosome monosomy or with trisomy 21 survive so long when the majority of them die in early pregnancy.

REPEATED ABORTION

Most individuals with sex chromosome abnormalities are infertile, with the main exception of XXX females. The unbalanced autosomal complements usually result in such severe mental and physical handicap that reproduction does not occur even if possible. Thus, structural chromosomal abnormalities (translocations, inversions) are the only abnormalities likely to be passed on to the next generation directly.

Comparing different studies of repeated or habitual abortion is not easy because different criteria may be used. Many studies include couples who have had two miscarriages and any number of successful pregnancies, but some have more stringent definitions. In some studies only those who have no other demonstrable reason for pregnancy loss in spite of other investigations are included. Nine studies of over 1200 couples have shown that in 7.2% one partner had a structural chromosomal abnormality, which is twenty times the rate in the newborn population.[30]

Analysis of consecutive abortions from couples show that trisomic abortions tend to recur more often than expected.[9,33] Women who have trisomic abortuses also have a higher prevalence of trisomic offspring in their previous pregnancies.[34] Thus trisomy, though often of different chromosomes, seems to recur in certain couples.

ORIGIN OF CHROMOSOMAL ABNORMALITIES

With the exception of a small proportion of translocations which have been inherited, nearly all the abnormalities seen in abortuses arise *de novo* either during meiosis (trisomy, monosomy, triploidy), during fertilisation (triploidy) or during the first cleavage division (tetraploidy). Mosaics arise during an abnormal mitotic division sometime after fertilisation. However, many of these are trisomic zygotes in which the normal cell line arises mitotically.

Studies of regions of certain chromosomes which show variation between individuals can identify the origin of the extra chromosome in informative cases. Most trisomies arise from maternal non-disjunction. 88% of abortuses with an extra acrocentric chromosome and 80% of those with trisomy 16 are due to maternal errors. Similar studies in livebirths have shown that 79% of cases of trisomy 21 are maternal in origin. The great majority of these errors occur in the first meiotic division.[30,35,36]

Similar studies of triploids have shown that 73% have two paternal sets of chromosomes, and the great majority of these result from dispermy. The remaining 37% are derived from diploid oocytes.[30,35]

It is not possible to demonstrate the origin of the X chromosome in sex chromosome monosomy in abortuses by such methods. Thus, we cannot compare abortuses with survivors, in whom 75% have a maternal X chromosome. This should now be possible using restriction fragment length polymorphisms.

SUMMARY

Cytogenetic studies of spontaneous abortion have shown that there is a high level of chromosomal abnormality in human zygotes. The vast majority of these are lost during the early stages of pregnancy, and all types of aberration have a high prenatal mortality. In some abnormalities a small proportion survive to be born alive.

Improvements in general health and in obstetric care mean that an increasing proportion of pregnancies survive to term. Thus, chromosomal abnormalities must account for an increasing proportion of those that are lost. We know little about the predisposing factors, but maternal age is the best documented.

Such high levels of chromosomal abnormalities are not found in other mammals.[37] However, all other species investigated have been selectively bred for many generations, either as laboratory animals or as livestock. Aneuploidy does increase with age slightly in the mouse,[38] and it may well be the long lifespan of human beings and their unfertilised oocytes that is responsible for the high level of aneuploidy in man. Studies of other non-inbred mammals would be interesting.

At present our ability to detect abnormal features *in utero* by amniocentesis and chorionic villus sampling is the only method of preventing these births. Amniocentesis at 16 weeks has shown a higher level of abnormalities than is seen at term, as would be predicted from our knowledge of spontaneous abortions. The level should be even higher in chorion biopsies taken at eight weeks. However, as so many abnormal conceptuses are "blighted ova", they will probably be detected by the obstetrician and not be sampled. Thus, the rate of chromosomal abnormality will not be as great as predicted for all pregnancies at eight weeks by demographic studies.

We have learned a great deal from studies of spontaneous abortion. We need to know more about the mechanisms which cause these abnormalities. We still need to know more about the very earliest losses. We may learn from *in vitro* fertilisation programmes. An experimental approach using animal models may also be of increasing use as we begin to approach the greatest challenges: how to prevent chromosome abnormalities from occurring.

REFERENCES

1. Alberman ED. The epidemiology of repeated abortion. In: *Early pregnancy loss—mechanisms and treatment*. Eds. RW Beard, F Sharp. London: Royal College of Obstetricians and Gynaecologists, 1988. pp.9-17.
2. Penrose LS, Delhanty JDS. Triploid cell culture from a macerated fetus. *Lancet* 1961; 1: 1261-1262.
3. Carr DH. Chromosome anomalies as a cause of spontaneous abortion. *Amer J Obstet Gynec* 1967; 97: 283-293.
4. Stevenson AC, Dudgeon MY, McClure H. I. Observations on the results of pregnancies in women resident in Belfast II. Abortions, hydatidiform moles and ectopic pregnancies. *Ann Hum Genet* 1959; 23: 395-411.
5. Boué J, Boué A, Lazar P. The epidemiology of human spontaneous abortions with chromosomal anomalies. In: *Aging Gametes*. Ed. RJ Blandu. Basel: Karger, 1975; pp.330-348.
6. Alberman E, Creasy M, Elliott M, Spicer C. Maternal factors associated with fetal chromosomal anomalies in spontaneous abortions. *Brit J Obstet Gynaecol* 1976; 83: 621-627.
7. Hassold T, Chen N, Funkhouser J, Jooss T, Manuel B, Matsuura J, Matsuyama A, Wilson C, Yamana JA, Jacobs PA. A cytogenetic study of 1000 spontaneous abortions. *Ann Hum Genet* 1980; 44: 151-178.

8. Creasy MR, Crolla JA, Alberman ED. A cytogenetic study of human spontaneous abortions using banding techniques. *Hum Genet* 1976; **31:** 177-196.
9. Warburton D, Stein Z, Kline J, Susser M. Chromosome abnormalities in spontaneous abortions: Data from the New York City study. In: *Human Embryonic and Fetal Death.* Eds. IH Porter, EB Hook. New York: Academic Press, 1980; 261-287.
10. Dhadial RK, Machin AM, Tait SM. Chromosomal anomalies in spontaneously aborted human fetuses. *Lancet* 1970; **2:** 20-21.
11. Takahara H, Ohama K, Fujiwara A. Cytogenetic study in early spontaneous abortion. *Hiroshima J Med Sci* 1977; **26:** 291-296.
12. Kajii T, Ferrier A, Niikawa N, Takahara H, Ohama K, Avirachan S. Anatomic and chromosomal anomalies in 639 spontaneous abortuses. *Hum Genet* 1980; **55:** 87-98.
13. Therkelsen AJ, Grunnet N, Hjort T, Myre Jansen O, Jonasson J, Lauritsen JG, Lindsten J, Bruun Petersen G. Studies on spontaneous abortion. In: *Chromosomal Errors in Relation to Reproductive Failure.* Eds. A Boué, C. Thibault. Paris: INSERM, 1973; pp.81-93.
14. Geisler M, Kleinebrecht J. Cytogenetic and histologic analyses of spontaneous abortions. *Hum Genet* 1978; **45:** 239-251.
15. Arakaki DT, Waxman SH. Chromosomal abnormalities in early spontaneous abortions. *J Med Genet* 1970; **7:** 118-124.
16. Stenchever MA, Hempel JM, McIntyre MN. Cytogenetics of spontaneously aborted human fetuses. *Obstet Gynec* 1967; **30:** 683-691.
17. Leridon H, Boué J. La mortalité intra-utérine d'origine chromosomique. *Population* 1971; **26:** 113-138.
18. Alberman ED, Creasy MR. Frequency of chromosomal abnormalities in miscarriages and perinatal deaths. *J Med Genet* 1977; **14:** 313-315.
19. Watt JL, Templeton AA, Messinis I, Bell L, Cunningham P, Duncan RO. Trisomy 1 in an eight cell human pre-embryo. *J Med Genet* 1987; **24:** 60-64.
20. Carr DH, Gedeon M. Population cytogenetics of human abortuses. In: *Population Cytogenetics. Studies in Humans.* Eds. EB Hook, IH Porter. New York: Academic Press 1977; 1-9.
21. Ikeuchi T, Sasaki M, Fujimoto S. Chromosome studies on spontaneous and theatened abortions. *Jap J Hum Genet* 1975; **20:** 245-246.
22. Meulenbroek GH, Geraedts JP. Parental origin of chromosome abnormalities in spontaneous abortions. *Hum Genet* 1982; **62:** 129-133.
23. Warburton D, Yu CY, Kline J, Stein Z. Mosaic autosomal trisomy in cultures from spontaneous abortions. *Amer J Hum Genet* 1978; **30:** 609-617.
24. Kajii T, Omaha K. Inverse maternal age effect in monosomy X. *Hum Genet* 1979; **51:** 147-151.
25. Warburton D, Stein Z, Kline J, Susser M. Monosomy X: a chromosomal anomaly associated with young maternal age. *Lancet* 1980; **1:** 167-169.
26. Creasy MR. Chromosome aberrations as a cause of prenatal death. In: *Paediatric Research. A Genetic Approach.* Eds. M Adinolfi, P Benson, F Gianelli, M Seller London: Spastics International Medical Publications 1982; pp.122-135.
27. Polani PE. The incidence of chromosomal malformations. *Proc Roy Soc Med* 1970; *63:* 50-52.
28. Creasy MR, Crolla JA. Prenatal mortality of trisomy 21 (Down's syndrome) *Lancet* 1974; **1:** 473-474.
29. Gropp A, Putz B, Zimmerman U. Autosomal monosomy and trisomy causing development failure. In: *Developmental Biology and Pathology. Current Topics in Pathology 62.* Eds. E Grundmann, WH Kirsten. Berlin: Springer 1976; pp.177-192.
30. Boué A, Boué J, Gropp A. Cytogenetics of pregnancy wastage. *Adv Hum Genet* 1985; **14:** 1-57.
31. Polani PE, Adinolfi M. Chromosome 21 of man, 22 of the great apes and 16 of the mouse. *Dev Med Child Neurol* 1980; **22:** 223-225.

32. Boué A, Boué J. Evaluation des erreurs chromosomique au moment du conception. *Bioméd* 1973; **18:** 372-374.
33. Hassold TJ. A cytogenetic study of repeated spontaneous abortion. *Am J Hum Genet* 1980; **32:** 723-730.
34. Alberman E, Elliott M, Creasy M, Dhadial R. Previous reproductive history in mothers presenting with spontaneous abortions. *Brit J Obstet Gynaec* 1975; **82:** 366-373.
35. Jacobs PA, Hassold TJ. The origin of chromosome abnormalities in spontaneous abortion. In: *Human Embryonic and Fetal Death.* Eds. IH Porter, EB Hook. New York: Academic Press 1980; pp.289-298.
36. Mikkelsen M. Down syndrome. Current state of epidemiology. In: *Human Genetics.* Part B. Ed. B Bonne-Tamir. New York: Alan R Liss 1982; pp.297-307.
37. Ford CE. The time in development at which gross genome imbalance is expressed. In: *The Early Development of Mammals.* Eds. M Balls, AE Wild. London University Press 1975; pp.285-304.
38. Maudlin I, Fraser LR. Maternal age and the incidence of aneuploidy in first-cleavage mouse embryos. *J Reprod Fert* 1978; **54:** 423-426.

Discussion

Chairman: Professor T.J. Gill

Professor JENKINS: Just allowing for the possibility that the fetus makes some contribution to the survival of itself as an allograft, is there any chance that the abnormal fetus is incapable of making that contribution?

Dr CREASY: I think there is a very good possibility, yes.

Professor JENKINS: Is there any evidence?

Dr CREASY: I don't know of any evidence. The placenta is obviously, exceedingly important in the early stages of life, and the placenta is pathologic in many chromosomally abnormal aborters. Trisomic and monosomic embryos in the mouse do manage to implant, but many of them die very soon after implantation. I don't think that really answers your question, but it is probably as far as I can go.

Dr UNANDER: I have a comment to make on that. If you believe in fetal suppressor cells—and there is substantial evidence of their existence—it may be questioned whether they would be there if they weren't important. They may play a role in the sorting out of these chromosomally abnormal fetuses.

Dr ALLEN: Can I just make a comment and also ask a question? I am intrigued to see your figures that as many as 97% of XO Turner's syndrome fetuses don't make it to term, because we recognise that condition in horses, particularly in Thoroughbreds. Unfortunately, we are totally unable to do a study like this because we can never get the aborted material. It is mostly resorbed *in utero;* the cervix remains closed and we can never get it to culture. We suspect that a significant proportion of early pregnancy losses in horses, particularly in Thoroughbreds have a chromosomal basis, as you show here. In addition, we get XXX, and occasional XY horses with female habitus that are perfectly normal horses. Again, in our Turner's syndrome, there are no structural abnormalities whatsoever. Is there any indication in the human studies that there is an increased incidence of chromosomal abnormalities that lead to abortion with any degree of inbreeding, line-breeding or family-breeding—or whatever you would like to call it?

Dr CREASY: There is certainly some evidence that an unsuccessful outcome of pregnancy is higher with inbreeding. For chromosomal abnormalities, the major

305

finding of interest is that women who are trisomic aborters are at greater risk of having another trisomic pregnancy. That is not necessarily true for horses, but women who have had a trisomic pregnancy seem to be at greater risk of having another trisomic conception. This works both where we have looked at two spontaneous abortions from the same woman, and when we look at the previous reproductive history of women who are trisomic aborters and the incidence of Down's syndrome in their children. So there seems to be a predisposition to nondisjunction in certain couples, whereby having had one trisomic conceptus, there is probably something in the order of a 1% risk of having another trisomic conceptus. You would expect translocations to recur by segregation. There does seem to be a risk of recurrence for trisomies—not necessarily the same trisomy, however. We don't really know why that should be, but it seems to be found in all the studies which have managed to look at consecutive abortuses.

Dr ALLEN: You have not looked into family pedigrees for inbreeding?

Dr CREASY: No. That has been done more in relation to single gene defects rather than chromosomal abnormalities. You would expect that translocations and structural chromosome abnormalities would run in families. I know that this is important in relation to IVF with cattle. There was one bull with a translocation which he has managed to spread through a very large proportion of a certain breed because his semen was particularly successful.

Professor KLEIN: Can you give us an explanation why trisomy, and why not monosomy?

Dr CREASY: It was originally suggested that all trisomies occurred with equal frequency and that all monosomies were being lost very early. And from those considerations, it was calculated that about 50% of all human conceptions were chromosomally abnormal. As I say, there are no reasons for doubting that, trisomy 16 seems to be peculiar. We would expect equal numbers of monosomic and disomic gametes to occur, and the evidence from mice shows that when you are using the translocation system for producing monosomies, some of them are capable of fertilisation. So, it may well be that even in the best spontaneous abortion experiments we are still missing a lot of chromosomal abnormalities at early stages. Perhaps they can't implant or they die very early after implantation. As far as I am aware, there isn't much evidence that there is selection at the gamete level.

Professor MOWBRAY: I was interested in something you said about recurrent trisomies just now. Do you know of evidence that recurrent trisomy is actually partner-specific?

Dr CREASY: I was trying to avoid putting the blame on the woman all the time. We perhaps do that because, obviously, trisomies are more often maternal in origin.

Professor MOWBRAY: There has been a suggestion that the gene, or genes responsible for the synthesis of spindle protein may be defective.

Dr CREASY: Part of the reason I hesitated was that I was thinking about polyploids and triploids. It is a different story, although they are mostly due to dispermy. What you are looking at here is again probably a problem of the ova; aging of the ova has been suggested as being important in these cases.

Professor MOWBRAY: If they are dispermy?

Dr CREASY: Yes.

Professor MOWBRAY: And not due to diploid sperm, which is the other possibility.

Dr CREASY: That is right. But the limited evidence that is available suggests that dispermy is by far the most important mechanism.

Professor HARRIS: A fairly obvious point, but it is an interesting one—the enormous selection against chromosomally abnormal embryos early on; if it were immunological, then presumably the product would look histologically a bit like a rejected kidney. As far as I know, that is not true.

Dr RUSHTON: This is what I was saying yesterday. I think that the conceptus determines its own rejection, using rejection in the sense that it gets out of the womb, not in the immunological sense. Most of these, in fact, have abnormal placentas without an embryo. Vascularity, as I said yesterday, is important; my hypothesis is that there is a disturbed metabolic gradient across the trophoblast. Because the trophoblast is pumping into the embryonic or fetal side, they could accumulate at levels at which they are toxic to the trophoblast. The trophoblast would then fail, and abortion would occur. I think that this is the self-destruct process rather than something that is happening from the outside. Certainly, there is no evidence in the very large number of chromosomal abnormalities that I have seen of any immunological changes in the placenta or in the embryo.

Professor CLARK: There is an issue which hasn't been brought up, and I think that it is potentially important. I would like to hear it discussed. It arises from the fact that the percentage of chromosomal abnormalities has to be calculated from studies on the tissue that will grow. That means that the data we have is based only on those embryos which grow, and they are only a small proportion of the embryos that actually abort. We are making extrapolations from this group that will grow to the much larger proportion of embryos that are macerated, and do not grow. Now, do we have any information about the frequency of chromosomal abnormalities from tissue which is obtained earlier in the pregnancy, before the fetus is completely destroyed and expelled, for example, by chorionic villus biopsy? Is there any information about tissue obtained earlier that would tell us whether our sense of the proportion about the prevalence of chromosomal abnormalities is likely to be correct for the majority of aborted fetuses?

Dr CREASY: It would be nice to think that by doing chorionic villus biopsies at eight weeks, we could get a nice cross-section of all pregnancies at that time, but I don't think that is the situation. My experience is that, when obstetricians come to do a chorionic villus biopsy (CVS) they reject those in which the pregnancy is no longer viable. Now, you have to remember that many of these chromosomally abnormal aborfuses don't simply die and are expelled. Their development halts, and they are actually retained in the uterus for approximately four to six weeks. And so many of these blighted ova, as they used to be called, with a developmental age of about three or four weeks are not expelled until about sixteen weeks. and so CVS sampling isn't giving you a representative sample, of a cohort of pregnancies at eight weeks. It is useful information, but it isn't a representative sample, which is what we really want.

Professor SZULMAN: You don't have to grow the macerated fetus. As a matter of fact, most of the work that some of us have done has been on placenta or on chorionic villus biopsies.

Professor STIRRAT: There is another factor which I think we might have to take into consideration and which I would like your comments on. We make the assumption that the fetus and its placenta have the same pattern of chromosomes derived equally from the same source. Is that true?

Dr B STRAY-PEDERSON: I have a similar question on the role of mosaicism in the screening of the couples with habitual recurrent abortion.

Dr CREASY: Of course, mosaicism will always be a problem in the science of genetics. There seem to be real and artificial problems. If you go on looking at enough cells, eventually you are going to find some abnormal cells. That is one of the big problems when you are looking at Turner's syndrome cases. If you look long enough you are going to find some XO Turner cells in almost any female. Most of the structural abnormalities that we see in habitual aborters are going to be straightforward translocations. If you are not really happy with that, then rather than counting thousands of cells from people, producing lots of problems for yourself, you might be better off doing more antenatal diagnoses.

The biology of trophoblastic disease: compete and partial hydatidiform moles

A. E. Szulman

INTRODUCTION

Trophoblastic diseases encompass the complete and partial hydatidiform moles as well as choriocarcinoma and the very rare placental site tumour. Of these, the hydatidiform moles are of prime relevance at this symposium for they are among the commonest manifestations of abnormal trophoblast and are associated with a sizeable proportion of pregnancy wastage.

The modern view of the pathogenesis of hydatidiform moles links them causally to an abnormal and hyperactive trophoblast as responsible for excessive water-logging of the villous stroma and as vulnerable, because of its initial dyscrasia, to malignant change.[1] The trophoblast however, even in its normal pristine state must be regarded as a peculiar and unique entity. In embryologic terms it may be viewed as the first organ of the developing zygote capable of multiple functions.[2] Among the most important of these are the penetration of the uterine lining and anchorage of the conceptus, and the secretion of hCG as well as of several steroid hormones that maintain pregnancy. One measure of this early competence is the stoppage of menstruation some 5 days after implantation. Expressing another unique attribute is the freedom of the trophoblast from allele-specific HLA and ABO antigens at its cell surfaces;[3,4,5] this allows for its undisturbed penetration of the decidual bed and of the local arterioles,[6] as well as for the steady embolis-ation into the intervillous blood spaces and hence into the maternal pulmonary circulation.[7]

Its protean nature and invasive properties are reflected in the unusual morphology of the trophoblast that contributes significantly to the difficulty in distinguishing between its benign and malignant phases and largely frustrates attempts at prognosis in the case of complete moles.[1]

The secretion of hCG characterises the normal trophoblast from its earliest implantation stages and is retained in hydatidiform moles as well as in chorio-carcinoma. hCG maternal blood levels thus provide a reliable means of ascertainment of its presence in the maternal organism irrespective of anatomical location. The clinical convenience of measurement of the beta-hCG levels in maternal blood is only marred by their lack of specificity with respect to the trophoblast's benign or malignant status. The non-committal nature of the concept of postmolar residual trophoblastic disease is born out of this latter circumstance.[8]

Molar pregnancies never lead to a viable infant as the embryo/fetus perishes *in utero* both in the complete and the partial mole for reasons (and at times) peculiar to each syndrome. This is to be expected since the two kinds of mole are the result of two different compound chromosomal errors. Enacted at fertilisation they lead to distinctive genomic constitutions that commit either conceptus to its own spectrum of morphology and biological behaviour.[9] Thus, the complete mole is the familiar, albeit rare, well-authenticated syndrome associated with 46 chromosomes of totally paternal origin (androgenetic diploidy).[10] It can lead occasionally to chorionic cancer. The partial mole by contrast—a much commoner condition—has a karyotype of 69 chromosomes with an extra haploid set of paternal origin (diandric triploidy)[11] and is innocent of cancerous sequelae. The two karyotypes correlate well with the two distinctive clinico-pathological entities respectively, as described below. As there is no transition between diploidy and triploidy, no transition between the two kinds of mole is possible and the term "transitional mole" has no validity.[12]

THE COMPLETE HYDATIDIFORM MOLE

This is the well-established syndrome characterised by a large "bunch of grapes" placenta without an ascertainable embryo/fetus.[8,9,12,13] The diagnosis is usually apparent macroscopically, and microscopic confirmation raises little difficulty. It hinges on the diagnostic triad of: 1) trophoblastic hyperplasia, usually marked in degree and random in distribution, that involves both the cyto-trophoblast and the syncytial layers; 2) rapidly accumulating villous oedema that creates multiple "cisterns", i.e., well-demarcated central fluid collections rimmed by maturing mesenchyme of decreasing vascularity and cellularity; 3) early embryonic demise so that no erythrocytes ever appear in such vessels as remain extant in the more recent "younger" villi.[13,14]

The trophoblastic hyperplasia and dysplasia vary in degree from case to case but their assessment is of no prognostic value in individual cases and should not influence decisions as to follow-up and therapy.[15]

The cisternal fluid resembles interstitial fluid elsewhere in the body with an addition of hCG and other hormones;[16,17] procoagulant substances have been found recently. It is of low osmotic and oncotic pressure and appears to be the product of the trophoblast.

The trophoblast and villi of the complete mole are capable of penetration beyond the usual implantation site so that both the myometrium and its veins may be involved.[18] Only occasionally does this process lead to uterine perforation and catastrophic haemorrhage. More frequently, the degree of invasiveness is slight and may be clinically inapparent. The venous involvement may show up clinically as vulvo-vaginal metastases or as pulmonary vascular embolisation, the latter only rarely massive or acute enough to require treatement.[19] Minor, subclinical pulmonary embolisation is more common than generally appreciated since a significant number of patients with clinically non-embolic residual disease was found recently to have pulmonary lesions by CAT-scan tomography.[20] In fact, minor degrees of "invasive mole" are probably quite common; they may resolve spontaneously within a period of time or may require chemotherapy applied according to the prevailing protocol.

The total frequency of invasive mole is difficult to estimate, but it is fair to guess that it is the pathological substrate of the majority of cases of residual tropho-blastic disease, a clinical entity mainly based on an evaluation of the post-molar hCG recession curve. Choriocarcinoma accounts for a small residue of cases of 2-5%. It is rarely clinically distinguishable from invasive mole, because the modern treatment remains similar for both diseases and biopsies are seldom, if ever, taken.[8]

In spite of the invasiveness and the vascular embolic phenomena[21,22] the invasive mole is not a biologically malignant condition nor is it a half-way house to choriocarcinoma; the incidence of the latter in patients with an invasive mole is not greater than in patients with non-invasive moles.[15] The behaviour of the invasive mole, it can be argued, is accountable in terms of the above peculiar attributes of non-cancerous trophoblast. Experimentally the idea of biological benignity is well-illustrated in studies employing "nude", (immunologically incompetent) mice which survived transplantation of both complete and invasive moles, to succumb only to transplants of choriocarcinoma.[23]

The Embryo in the Complete Mole

No embryo is ever found in the usually massive molar specimen, but strong evidence for its early and short existence is provided by the now-agreed-upon derivation of the placental, extraembryonic mesoderm from the margin of the primitive streak of the 12-14 days presomite embryo proper. Thus derived, the mesoderm evaginates the trophoblast to form the villi and generates *in situ* capillaries that are to be subsequently connected to the developing cardiovascular system. Since the villous vessels normally display embryonic erythrocytes at the stage of circa 30 days post-fertilisation, and since none ever appears in the vessels of the complete mole, it follows that embryonic demise takes place during a very early period contained between these two datable events when the gestational sac is smaller than the hydatidiform villi characterising the (developed) mole.[8] The reasons for the early loss of the embryo proper will be referred to again in the section on genetics.

THE PARTIAL HYDATIDIFORM MOLE

The partial mole has only recently been delimited from what was held to be a wide-spectrum syndrome of "hydatidiform moles". It is a separate entity definable by morphological, cytogenetic and clinical criteria. Its description can conveniently use the terms of reference provided by the complete mole since the former can be viewed as an attenuated, bland version of the latter, as described below.

Pathological Anatomy of the Partial Mole

This is a conceptus consisting of placenta and fetus, both of which evince a characteristic constellation of morphological anomalies that provide a basis for diagnosis.[8,9] The placenta presents focal trophoblastic hyperplasia, usually moderate in degree and confined to the syncytial layer, and focal hydatidiform villous swelling with cistern formation. The fluid accumulation here is slow, and focal oedema may be more in evidence than the end-stage villous cisterns. In addition to these two features, which the partial mole shares with the complete mole, there are several other characteristics, the most important being scalloping of villous outlines and trophoblastic "inclusions" (in reality fjord-like incursions of surface trophoblast into the villous stroma). Since the fetus tends to die early (see below), evidence of sometime fetal existence is only rarely provided by the fetal remnants and usually relies on the presence, and surprisingly long post-mortem persistence, of erythrocytes in the placental vessels. As all these changes (except the last) tend to be focal, with areas of intervening normal or near-normal placenta, sampling for pathological examination should be extensive and include minimally 5 tissue blocks.[24]

Regarding macroscopic villous swellings, it is worth emphasising that it is a secondary, non-specific phenomenon often encountered in the absence of trophoblastic hyperplasia, and it must not be taken as a sufficient diagnostic criterion. Abortuses with swollen villi, accordingly, must be examined microscopically, focussing on the status of the trophoblast and on the other histological features given above. In practice, the macroscopic swelling of the villi in partial moles varies in degree and may be inconspicuous, especially in early voluntary abortions. In general, the diagnosis of partial mole is more difficult than that of the complete mole, as it depends on an assembly of several somewhat variable morphological features. In any event, it belongs to the pathologist who must ascertain the presence of several diagnostic microscopic features, with trophoblastic hyperplasia as a necessary condition.[14]

As stated, whereas no choriocarcinoma has been found in association with the partial mole, rare cases of invasive partial mole have been well authenticated.[25,26,27] These form the pathological substrate of postmolar residual trophoblastic disease, amenable to surgery and/or chemotherapy. None of the invasive moles has so far been accompanied by embolic phenomena.

The Incidence and Clinical Presentation of the Partial Mole

As stated above, this kind of mole remains much underdiagnosed.[28] It tends to be inconspicuous clinically, since bleeding may be both late and slight, and the uterus is almost invariably "small for dates". As the hydatidiform change of the villi may be sparse and slight, the partial mole is easily missed on sonography and many cases stay below the threshold to remain undistinguishable from "missed abortion". Apart from presenting in the guise of "missed abortion," an equally large number of partial moles present as spontaneous abortions with a long-retained dead fetus. A most interesting subset, accounting for just a few percent of patients, are women admitted at mid-pregnancy with large uteri containing live fetuses, some presenting with pre-eclampsia. These can hardly be missed, and diagnosis is usually made preoperatively.[25,26]

The high incidence of partial mole can be gleaned from a prospective investigation wherein meticulous morphology combined with detailed cytogenetic study resulted in an ascertainment several-fold greater than that obtained in retrospective research.[8] Cases from among early elective abortions and late "missed abortions" are especially liable to be missed because hydatidiform change in the villi is apt to be slight.

The Fetus in the Partial Mole

Unlike the complete molar syndrome, the fetus here survives much better even though it never establishes independent extrauterine existence. Fetal deaths cluster at 8-9 weeks menstrual age, and only rare individuals survive into the second trimester.[24] Survival until term is exceptional, and death takes place soon after delivery. In the usual cases of early fetal death post-mortem retention tends to be long, and fetuses dead at 8-9 weeks gestation are macerated and poorly preserved at spontaneous or surgical delivery many weeks later. Where available for examination, especially if born alive at about mid-pregnancy, the fetuses are inevitably growth-retarded and present an array of congenital anomalies characteristic of triploidy. Although these anomalies are not immediately life-threatening, death takes place within a short time, presumably owing to the biochemical imbalances of triploidy.

The breadth of the anatomical anomalies ranges from near-normality to multi-system involvement. The gross anomalies involve mainly the head (including the brain, face and eyes) and the extremities, where syndactyly of the 2nd and 3rd digits is highly characteristic. Cleft lip and palate are common, while abdominal wall and neural tube defects seem infrequent. Among the internal anomalies, cardiac septal defects and renal malformations head the list, together with hypoplasia of lung, adrenals, thymus and ovaries. In 69,XXY cases the external male genitals are ambiguous, while the testes show Leydig cell hyperplasia that is in response to increased hCG levels of the partial mole. The total picture, however, is independent of the existence of a partially molar placenta; in fact, a normal placenta (as seen in digynic triploidy; see under genetics) seems to favour fetal survival.[29]

No triploid infant can be saved for post-natal life except the rarest individuals with 69/46 mosaicism.[30] The importance of a correct diagnosis, however, lies in the fact that triploidy is a random event not linked to maternal age or to prejudicing future reproductive performance.

THE GENETICS OF THE HYDATIDIFORM MOLE

The genesis of a hydatidiform mole is determined at fertilisation. Depending upon the nature of the chromosomal error, there results a diploid complete mole or a somewhat related triploid zygote of partial mole.

The compound error leading to the complete mole consists of loss by the ovum of the maternal chromosomal haploid set of 23,X ("empty egg") and duplication of the paternal X-bearing haploid set without concomitant cytokinesis to provide the requisite number of 46 chromosomes.[10] The predominantly frequent female, XX, sex-chromosome complement is due to the fact that a Y-chromosome bearing a paternal haploid chromosomal set would result in 46,YY zygote that is non-viable. The occasional (circa 5%) complete moles with an XY sex-chromosome compement are the product of a fertilisation of an "empty egg" by two spermatozoa, bearing the X and Y chromosomes respectively.[31] There will be some XX moles resulting if both sperm bear the X-chromosome.

Implied by the foregoing is the totally paternal origin of the complete mole, its homozygous character in cases of monospermic fertilisation and its heterozygous (within the limits of the paternal genome) character in cases of dispermic origin. In either case, however, the mole is a total allograft on the maternal organism, instead of being a semi-allograft as in normal pregnancy. The immunological consequences of these situations remain obscure.

The difference between the homozygous (46,XX) and the heterozygous (46,XY and some XX) moles may be of biological importance as the heterozygotes are regarded by some observers as probably more prone to residual disease or to chorionic cancer.[32] The matter is as yet unresolved, and further studies are no doubt being conducted.

The partial mole resembles in its origin the heterozygous dispermic complete mole—with the important difference that the maternal haploid set of 23,X persists in the ovum. Two spermatazoa fertilise a seemingly normal egg, the resulting chromosomal number being 69, with all 3 possible sex-chromosomes combinations of XXX, XXY and XYY.[11,33] It must be observed that triploidy can also result from a normal, unispermic fertilisation of a diploid egg (digynic triploidy), in which case the placenta is non-molar even though the fetus bears the stigmata of a triploid.[11]

The finding of a partial mole with three paternal contributions to one maternal one[34] (triandric tetraploidy) confirmed the idea that the molar phenotype is associated with the dominance of the zygote by paternal chromosomes.[11,33] Thus, in a complete mole the ratio of male to female contributions is 2:0, while in partial moles it is 2:1 or 3:1. A reversal of the ratio to 1:2 makes for a non-molar triploid.

The explanation of the above observations came, surprisingly, from experiments on transplantation of pronuclei among murine eggs.[35,36] Freshly fertilised and enucleated eggs can be subjected to transplantation with various combinations of male and female pronuclei from other fertilised eggs. A combination of male and female exogenous pronuclei in an "emptied egg" gives a normal term fetus. Two female pronuclei allow for the development of the embryo past the implantation stage, but the trophoblast develops poorly and the conceptus perishes by the 8th day of pregnancy. The most telling type of experiment reproduces the situations seen in the complete mole, as it consists of placing two male pronuclei in an emptied egg. This combination leads to an overgrowth of trophoblast, while the embryo proper dies very early. The implication of these experiments is that there must be a differential chromosomal imprinting during gametogenesis: it activates genes in the paternal haploid set that promote the growth of the trophoblast and activates genes in the maternal set to "take care of" the embryo proper. The early demise of the embryo in the complete mole is thus explicable as being due to the absence of the maternal set of chromosomes, while the trophoblastic hyperplasia is accountable in terms of the dominance of the zygote by the paternal set of chromosomes. The better survival of the embryo/ fetus in the partial mole is ascribed to the presence of the maternal chromosomes. In sum, the complete mole is totally dominated by paternal chromosomes that have genes activated to promote trophoblastic growth in the absence of a maternal set that "takes care of" the embryo. The partial mole is only partially dominated by the 2 paternal sets of chromosomes that bring forth the phenotypic molar features. The persistence of the maternal haploid complement of chromosomes allows for the development of the embryo, sometimes up to term, but "dilutes" the total syndrome, and apparently protects against the development of chorionic cancer. Digynic triploidy, consonant with the above hypothesis, gives a non-molar conceptus with a relatively better embryo-fetus survival.

REFERENCES
1. Park WW, Lees JC. Choriocarcinoma (A General review with an analysis of 516 cases). *Arch Pathol* 1950; **49:** 73 and 205.
2. Hertig AT. *Human Trophoblast.* Springfield: C. Thomas, 1968.
3. Bulmer JW, Johnson PM. Antigen expression by trophoblast populations in human placenta and their possible immunobiological relevance. *Placenta* 1985; **6:** 127.
4. Sunderland CA, Redman CW, Stirrat GM. Characterization and localization of HLA antigens on hydatidiform mole. *Am J Obstet Gynecol* 1985; **151:** 130.
5. Szulman AE. The A, B, and H blood-group antigens in human placenta. *N Engl J Med* 1972; **286:** 1028.
6. Pijnenborg R, Bland JM, Robertson WB, Dixon G, Brosens I. The pattern of interstitial trophoblastic invasion of the myometrium in early human pregnancy. *Placenta* 1981; **4:** 303.
7. Covone AE, Mutton D, Johnson PM, Adinolfi M. Trophoblast cells in peripheral blood from pregnant women. *Lancet* 1984; **2:** 841.
8. Szulman AE. Complete hydatidiform mole and partial hydatidiform mole. In: *Gestational Trophoblastic Disease.* Eds. AE Szulman, HJ Buchsbaum. New York: Springer, 1987; pp.27 and 37.
9. Szulman AE, Surti U. The syndromes of hydatidiform mole. I. Cytogenetic and morphological correlations. *Am J Obstet Gynaecol* 1978; **13:** 665.
10. Kajii T, Ohama K. Androgenetic origin of hydatidiform mole. *Nature* 1977; **268:** 633.
11. Jacobs PA, Szulman AE, Funkhouser J, Matsuura JS, Wilson CC. Human triploidy: relationship between parental origin of the additional haploid complement and development of partial hydatidiform mole. *Ann Hum Genet* 1982; **46:** 223.
12. World Health Organisation. *Gestational trophoblastic diseases.* Report of a WHO Scientific Group. Technical Report Series 692. Geneva, 1983.
13. Szulman AE, Surtu U. The syndromes of hydatidiform mole. II. Morphologic evolution of the complete and partial mole. *Am J Obstet Gynecol* 1978; **132:** 20.
14. Szulman AE. Trophoblastic disease: complete and partial hydatidiform moles. In: *Pathology of the placenta.* Ed. EDVK Perrin. New York: Churchill Livingstone, 1984; pp.183-197.
15. Elston RC. The histopathology of trophoblastic tumours. *J Clin Pathol* 1976; **10:** 111.
16. Chew PC, Ratnam SS, Goh HH. Testosterone in major vesicle fluid and theca-lutein cyst fluid. *Br J Obstet Gynaecol* 1978; **85:** 218.
17. Kaplan SS, Szulman AE. Effect of hydatidiform molar vesicular fluid on blood coagulation. *Am J Obstet Gynecol* 1985; **153:** 703.
18. Lurain J, Brewer JI. Invasive mole. *Semin Oncol* 1982; **9:** 174.
19. Kohorn EI. Clinical management and neoplastic sequelae of trophoblastic embolization associated with hydatidiform mole. *Obstet Gynecol Survey* 1987; **42:** 484.

20. Mutch DG, Soper JT, Baker ME, Bandy LC, Cox EB, Clarke-Pearson DL, Hammond CB. Role computed axial tomography of the chest in staging patients with nonmetastatic gestational trophoblastic disease. *Obstet Gynecol* 1986; **68:** 348.
21. Jackson TJ, Enzer N. Hydatidiform mole with benign metastasis to the lung. Histological evidence of regressing lesions in the lung. *Am J Obstet Gynecol* 1959; **78:** 868.
22. Ring AM, The concept of benign metastasizing hydatidiform moles. *Am J Clin Pathol* 1972; **58:** 111.
23. Kato M, Tanaka K, Takeuchi S. The nature of trophoblastic disease initiated by transplantation into immunosuppressed animals. *Am J Obstet Gynecol* 1982; **142:** 497.
24. Szulman AE, Phillipe E, Boué JG, Boué A. Human triploidy: association with partial hydatidiform moles and non-molar conceptuses. *Hum Pathol* 1981; **12:** 1016.
25. Szulman AE, Surtu U. The clinicopathological profile of the partial hydatidiform mole. *Obstet Gynecol* 1982; **59:** 597..
26. Berkowitz RS, Goldstein DP, Bernstein MR. Natural history of partial molar pregnancy. *Obstet Gynecol* 1985; **66:** 677.
27. Gaber LW, Redline RW, Mostoufi-Zadeh M, Driscoll SG. Invasive partial mole. *Am J Clin Pathol* 1986; **85:** 722.
28. Matsuura J, Chiu D, Jacobs PA, Szulman AE. Complete hydatidiform mole in Hawaii: an epidemiological study. *Genet Epidemiol* 1984; **1:** 271.
29. Doshi N, Surtu U, Szulman AE. Morphologic anomalies in triploid liveborn fetuses. *Hum Pathol* 1983; **14:** 716.
30. Blackburn WR, Miller WP, Superneau DW, Cooley NR Jr, Zellweger H, Wertelecki W. Comparative studies of infants with mosaic and complete triploidy: an analysis of 55 cases. *Birth Defects* 1982; **18:** 251.
31. Surtu U, Szulman AE, O'Brien S. Dispermic origin and clinical outcome of three complete hydatidiform moles with 46,XY karyotype. *Am J Obstet Gynecol* 1982; **144:** 84.
32. Fisher RA, Lawler SD. Heterozygous complete with hydatidiform moles; do they have a worse prognosis than homozygous complete moles? *Lancet* 1984; **2:** 51.
33. Lawler SD, Fisher RA, Pickthall VJ, Povey S, Evans MW. Genetic studies on hydatidiform moles. 1. The origin of partial moles. *Cancer Genet Cytogenet* 1982; **5:** 309.
34. Surti U, Szulman AE, Wagner K, Leppert M, O'Brien SJ. Tetraploid partial hydatidiform moles: two cases with a triple paternal contribution and a 92,XXXY karyotype. *Hum Genet* 1986; **72:** 15.
35. Surani MAH, Barton SC, Norris ML. Experimental reconstruction of mouse eggs and embryos; an analysis of mammalian development. *Biol Repro* 1987; **36:** 1.
36. McGrath J, Solter D. Completion of mouse embryogenesis requires both the maternal and paternal genomes. *Cell* 1984; **37:** 179.

Discussion

Chairman: Professor T.J. Gill

Professor SCOTT: Could I ask Dr Szulman what information there is about the karyotypic situation in choriocarcinomas?

Professor SZULMAN: The situation is bad because we haven't got the raw materials for one thing, and the good investigation is being done on cell lines, some of which have been in culture for 15 to 20 years. I personally don't trust them. There has been so much change, so many comings and goings, that nobody can make much sense of it. People even find it difficult to determine what the sex component of these cell lines is. If you were to get some material from autopsy, it would have been treated very heavily with all sorts of chemotherapy, and that too could change the karyotype.

Professor JOHNSON: Some choriocarcinomas will be derived from normal pregnancy, and will have 50/50 maternal/paternal components. Other choriocarcinomas will follow from complete mole and will be androgenetic. Biologically there is no difference between the two in the natural situation.

Professor SZULMAN: Biologically there is some difference because those that follow a normal pregnancy are said to be much worse and much more vicious. But the argument here is weakened by the fact that these women would not have been followed as the patients with the hydatidiform moles are. Therefore, they usually come for medical attention late in the game. And one of the essential requirements for chemotherapy is to get these patients early.

Dr LOKE: I read a paper that claimed that XY heterozygotic moles appeared to have a greater predilection to become choriocarcinoma, as compared to XX moles.

Professor SZULMAN: Yes, there was a letter in the Lancet where they said that there was insufficient data, so it is not confirmed. But you see, the problem is that some people, especially in Japan, are very quick on the trigger. What they call trophoblastic disease is something in a patient whose hCG doesn't decrease substantially within six weeks. By contrast, others are prepared to wait for 100 to 120 days. In such circumstances there is no pathologic diagnosis, and whether it is choriocarcinoma or an invasive mole remains a mystery to the very end of the patient's days. We are very much handicapped there. Clinically it is very

317

comfortable and convenient to have the clinical entity of residual trophoblastic disease. As a pathologist, I am absolutely devastated.

Dr RHODES: A mole arising in choriocarcinoma is not a clinical entity in any domestic animal that I am aware of. Do you know of any animal models?

Professor SZULMAN: I can see that I am going to be devastated twice in one evening. There is no animal model, alas.

Professor STIRRAT: I am grateful to Dr Szulman for clarifying the mis-apprehension I had in my mind. I think that it is important for us to consider this bombshell a little bit further; the importance of the paternal set of chromosomes for the development of the trophoblast versus the importance of the maternal set for the development of the embryo. I really don't think that the significance of this has sunk in, and we would do well to reflect on it and see how it might affect our thinking, even in relation to the issue we were discussing earlier.

Professor SZULMAN: The mother takes care of the baby?

Professor STIRRAT: Yes.

Dr ANTCZAK: There is one natural example of this kind of differential use of maternal and paternal genomes that has been described, to my knowledge. In 1969 Dr Allen showed that the levels of gestational hormones in horse/donkey crosses were determined by the way you did the cross, that is, by the paternal genome. Horses have high levels of hormones, and donkeys have low levels of hormones; when you make a cross with the horse as a father you get high levels, and with the donkey as a father you get low levels. These observations have been confirmed by experimental embryo manipulations.

Dr LOKE: I wonder if Dr Szulman will make some comments about the condition which I have always considered to be the converse of the mole. That is the ovarian teratomata which is parthogenetic and entirely maternal, but yet it produces a tumour which has 3 germ layers, rather than just trophoblast.

Professor SZULMAN: I have very sad memories, because at one time I thought that moles were due to maternal replication. I took my cue from the fact that the incidence of carcinoma in moles is about 1-4%, and it is the same in the teratoma. So, we thought we had something in hand, but it turned out that it really was just another example of parthenogenesis.

Dr HEAP: Could I ask you, Professor Szulman, whether it is possible that there may be a model in the androgenetic preparation that Dr Azim Surani has described? Have you had an opportunity to look at the pathology of that placenta in terms of trophoblast hypertrophy?

Professor SZULMAN: I have some slides on the way, so I cannot comment at the moment.

Professor GILL: After summing up I am going to ask Professor Mowbray to show his pedigrees from several families in the Gulf and continue the discussion on that basis. First, we have discussed the primary genetic mechanisms involved in the development of normal pregnancies, abnormal pregnancies and moles. These genetic mechanisms involve genes linked to the major histocompatibility complex or chromosomal abnormalities. They are the two best studied areas, but they need not be exclusive. Second, genetic modulation of cell surface antigens is important in tissue interactions and in development. Thus, we have put the focus very heavily on genetic mechanisms. But having said that, we are only at the beginning of where we want to go. What are these genetic mechanisms? What do the genes do? How is this regulation carried out? It is relatively easy to look at structural genes and to deduce the variations in the structural proteins that they control. It is very difficult to study regulation and quantitative expression of genes. It seems to me that in the field of developmental biology, when we move into the realm of molecular biology, gene control and the effects of gene ambalance are the critical areas to examine. In doing the experimental work in animals we are interested in seeing whether the same kinds of mechanisms pertain to humans, particularly if the genetic bases for repeated abortions can be documented in humans.

Professor MOWBRAY: Anyone familiar with the work done by Professor Johnson and me would know that there is a split from Professor Gill's views that probably the majority of abortions are genetically caused and that if you interfere with the immunological component of implantation you would possibly produce a large number of genetically abnormal children. That has been the worry he has raised in the past. Others have said: "It is all very well talking about the mice and the rats, but is there a human angle to it?" I would say that, yes, there is a human angle to it—the lethal recessive genes. They are uncommon, but you find them when you get inbreeding. Where do you get inbreeding? You get it in the Islamic world particularly. I have three families from the Gulf—two from Kuwait and one from Dubai—where there is a considerable degree of inbreeding and a pattern of family history which is quite unlike that which we see in other countries. For example, in one family there are seventy-one members. The proband had had five abortions and two live pregnancies; when I tested her immunity, it was absolutely normal. I said, as is usual with Gulf people, "Are you married to a first cousin?", and she said, "No, I am married to a second cousin." Her husband is one generation younger in the family than she is. If you look back into this family you will see that there are many males and few females. The products of three matings are five successful and five aborted pregnancies; five abortions and two live births; and five abortions and two live births. So it would seem to me that here we have a very good example of lethal recessive genes producing abortions. In this one family, unlike some of the others, all the children born are quite normal, except for three men who have oligospermia. In addition, one man married a woman not within the family, and they have seven live children and two abortions. The only thing against this pattern's fitting a simple lethal recessive, mendelian inheritance is that the fequency of abortion in these populations should be 25%; instead it is 50%, or somewhat higher. This pattern seems to recur in at least four generations. Nonetheless, this family is one example that I think is like Professor Gill's rats or mice. We are in the process of HLA-typing this family.

Professor GILL: We are obviously interested in these kinds of studies because they give us a way of looking at the relationship between animal immunogenetics and human immunogenetics. These extended Gulf families provide a very good system to examine, and this study does them some good as well as providing a model for us.

SECTION 6

TECHNIQUES, TREATMENT CRITERIA AND OUTCOME OF IMMUNOTHERAPY IN RECURRENT ABORTION

Chairman's introductory remarks

Chairman: Professor J. Mowbray

This morning we are talking about treatment, and what happens to treatment. Treatment being effective does not prove an immunological cause. The interpretation of the results of treatment may prove an immunological, psychological or any other sort of cause. What we are trying to do this morning is to demonstrate whether or not we modify the patient and whom.

The development of an immunological attack requires, in the immunological terminology of this time, sensitisation, which means the development of a cellular immune response which is aggressive and may damage trophoblast as being the exterior of the conceptus. Coincident with that, sometimes, is the development of protective antibodies, and in particular, antibodies against target cells epitopes which may block cellular attack, and antibodies which may block the immunising antigens. I do not think that it is appropriate, at the moment, to consider what is the immunising cell, but to leave it open. The only thing we know about cells which can immunise in the natural state is that they are fetal. They are fetal cells, and they are not necessarily trophoblast; they may be other fetal cells with this function. The only situation which would be bad would be to induce sensitised immunity without inducing the protective response. If you were to try and do this in the allograft situation where an enormous amount of work has been, and is being done on sensitisation, there is a route of sensitisation which is very much more efficient than any other, and that is to give the sensitising cells interdermally. If you do that you generate almost purely sensitisation without antibody. If you give it intravenously you tend to produce antibody without sensitisation. That has been well established with many species in terms of the allograft situation. We must establish what antibodies we are trying to generate to produce protection rather than sensitisation. If we get it wrong, we might sensitise people, and no matter what the cause of their previous abortions, they might have this as a new cause of abortion. If unbalanced by protective immunity, they would abort. I believe we have seen a small group of women of that kind. They are the women who have had two or more live children, did not have antibodies detectable, were immunised, and then all of them aborted their next pregnancy, although their previous pregnancy expectation was about 50%. These are not women I would like to treat. So the message that I personally would like to try and get over is if you immunise everybody, you may upset the balances. You have got to know what you are doing; we are only beginning to know what we are doing.

Success and failures of immunisation for recurrent spontaneous abortion

J. F. Mowbray

INTRODUCTION

In this paper I will discuss the causes of success and failure of immunisation with lymphocytes of paternal origin in the treatment of recurrent spontaneous abortion of apparently immunological origin. It is now clear that a large number of women have been, and will continue to be treated by immunisation with paternal lymphocytes, third party buffy coat or trophoblast microvesicle preparations. It is thus relevant to look first at what may be achieved. Initially we must consider, in the light of Lesley Regan's findings (this book), that the abortion rate of pregnancies is uninfluenced by their ordinal position, and is about 6% in each pregnancy in her study. The success rate of any treatment for recurrent abortion is unlikely to exceed this, unless it affects the causes of random loss as well as the recurrent ones. It is not impossible that this may be the case, and is a factor which we must discuss later. It is usually assumed, from somewhat suspect data, that single 'one off' abortions are predominantly due to genetic causes, mostly disjunctional failures. The resultant aneuploid pregnancies are unlikely to be affected by immunological manipulation.

Overall, the success following treatment is about 80% for the next pregnancy, whatever treatment is used.[1,2,3] This represents about 15% more than the sporadic loss rate by abortion. It should however be remembered that the maternal age of the recurrent abortion population attending for treatment is quite high (in our patients the mean age from 1980 to 1985 was 37). The rate of trisomy will be quite a lot higher in the older group, so that the true loss rate may be somewhat lower than 15%. This may mostly represent, and probably does, the inclusion in the treatment groups of couples with recurrent abortion for other causes than those which may be modified by immunological manipulation. Obviously we are now less likely to include the second trimester abortions associated with anti-phospholipid antibodies in such treatment groups, but there are others which may inadvertently be included. What then are we to use for selection criteria, and how may these be optimised to attempt the exclusion of the untreatable groups?

SELECTION OF RECIPIENTS

It is clear that the best results will be obtained by selecting as nearly as possible only those patients who will benefit from treatment. We have excluded patients with evidence of genetic cause, or who have evidence of a normal active immune response to paternal antigens.[4] Unander has chosen to exclude women with normal MLR blocking anti-idiotypic antibodies[5] and has shown that they do badly if they are immunised, and that is the finding in our group.[4] The rationale of the latter is that having multiple live births and abortions makes it more likely that an autosomal recessive lethal gene may be responsible for the condition (or on occasion possibly an X-linked lethal). Thus, at least two groups have excluded from immunisation couples who appear not to have the common antipaternal immunity problem. Without the use of exclusion criteria there is some evidence that overall success figures would be lower; as for example if we were to include patients with normal APCA or MLR blocking antibodies, and those who, not having those, have had more than one live child. The same would also be true when Unander's results are considered without the exclusion of the antibody positive women.

DOSE

We have tried using a smaller dose than our standard, in order to simplify treatment. Although the yield from 400 ml of blood is variable the range is between 250 and 480 million lymphocytes. When we tried using lymphocytes from 110 ml of blood we had yields which were obviously much lower, but overlapping with those from the larger amount of blood. Figure I shows that with a single immunising dose given before pregnancy, the success rate fell when doses of cells below about 110 million cells were given. It is of interest to note that the paper of Beer[6] which showed a worse than average survival rate was produced at a time when he was using doses of cells considerably below this limit. Although his route of administration was also different from the usual, as noted by Reznikoff[7] his success subsequently rose, possibly in part due to the use of larger cell numbers.

Obviously the results shown in Figure 1 cannot be extrapolated to the use of multiple doses, where the minimum effective dose would have to be determined for each treatment protocol. On theoretical grounds of one immunogen dose one would expect that although priming may require a large dose, further boost doses could probably be much smaller. We have chosen to give boosts when necessary, *vide infra*, of cells from 55 ml, with apparent effect.

FREQUENCY OF DOSAGE

Multiple doses have been used by several groups, and was always the routine for Taylor and Faulk,[8] although each dose is of course from a different donor. Reznikoff[7] has shown a benefit from repeated injection in three of her patients. She has repeated injections until cytotoxic antipaternal antibody was detectable, up to a maximum of three doses. Her published data do not, however, allow one to assume that seroconversion was the necessary effect correlated with success. The process of repeating doses alone could explain her finding.

Figure I

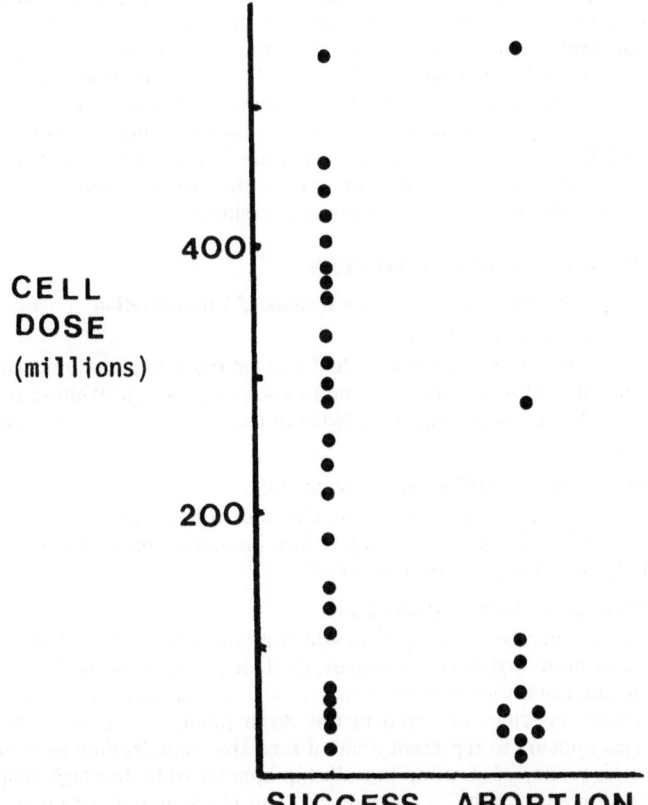

Effect of increasing dose of paternal cells on success of immunisation.

Sophie Alexander has used repeated doses of cells with a good result, and obviously feels that it is beneficial.[3] For reasons initially of economy, and to prevent exsanguination of the husband, we have in general used one dose, as described above. When however we had found a specific failure group, we decided to use a boost dose in them. This group was of women who did not show APCA seroconversion after immunisation, and who took more than three months to become pregnant. The results in this group were not better than the control women in our original controlled trial. We have been running a study of giving this group of patients 50 million paternal cells at the start of the next pregnancy. To date, the success rate of the next pregnancy in this group has risen from 30%[4] to about 80%. The success or failure of the next pregnancy is the same whether or not the boost dose has resulted in seroconversion of the APCA. It should be noted however, that an initial 400 million cell dose only produces a 25% conversion rate when given in pregnancy, compared with 65% when given outside. It may thus be difficult to see yet any correlation with seroconversion produced by the boost and protection, as conversion is relatively uncommon. I have stated before my view that if I were to start again I would probably use two doses, but if I had done so from the start we would not have treated nearly as many couples, as the labour and costs per patient would be about double. There is no reason to think that APCA conversion would be a marker of success. We have only found it to be a marker for prolonged protection, rather than the shortlived one found with our dose regime in those without seroconversion.[4]

RESULTS IN OUR SERIES AND OTHERS

Groups of Recurrent Abortion with Poor Results of Immunisation

a) Those with more than one live child.

We have immunised 13 women who had two or more live children with the current partner in addition to three or more abortions. Seven of these became pregnant and 6 aborted that pregnancy. None of these women had APCA before immunisation.[4]

b) Those with detectable APCA before treatment.

Albeit using third party immunisation, Unander has found that immunising women who have MLR blocking activity before immunisation is associated with abortion of all the subsequent pregnancies.[5]

c) Those with a family history of abortion

We have seen a number of couples in which a family history of abortion was present. One or more first degree relatives, or their partners has had more than one abortion, and usually some live children as well. In one family tree it was seen that when cousin marriage occurred in this Arab family, there were frequent abortions. This appears to represent a lethal recessive gene leading to abortion, although the frequency of abortion in a sibship appears to be too high (approximating to 50% rather than the 25% expected). This phenomenon, of a higher loss rate than expected, has been seen in two other families, where approximately half of the pregnancies in an affected partnership abort.

In these families, it appears that one or both partners are carrying an abnormality into the marriage, and we have considered them as different from the common partner specific effect, which is amenable to immunisation. We have not treated such couples, and although the number of subsequent pregnancies is small, the fractional success appears to be about 50%.

d) Women aborting with more than one husband, and husbands with more than one wife that abort repeatedly.

We have assumed that these are also carrying an inherited factor into the marriage and have not treated them. There are too few pregnancies after seeing them to make any conclusions about this group. It is obviously one of considerable interest, as it might contain women who were unable to respond appropriately to any paternal antigens, or those with a genetic fault leading to recurrent abortion. As the group is not large it will probably require a collaborative study between centres to gain enough material for useful conclusions to be drawn.

e) Women with 6 or more consecutive abortions

Susan Cowchock in Philadelphia (personal communication) has found that women with a large number of abortions fared poorly with immunisation. Table 1 shows that a similar phenomenon is found in our series, where the high success rate with 3 to 6 abortions before treatment falls with higher numbers. It is important to note that this may be a consequence of the abortions themselves, since the women we have treated successfully with lower numbers of abortions would enter the high abortion number group, if they had had time for more pregnancies before we saw them. It looks almost as though the condition of abortion becomes 'grooved in' with multiple abortions. Until we have more satisfactory ways of subdividing the whole group (by more specific immunological testing) it is difficult to study this group, and to see if their immune response to fetal/paternal antigens alters with increasing numbers of abortions.

Table 1

Effect of number of abortions before immunisation on success of next pregnancy. Although numbers are small it appears that success is low with more than 6 abortions.

No. of Abortions	Fractional Success	%
3	87/108	81%
4	49/64	77%
5	24/37	65%
6	15/16	94%
7	4/8	50%
>7	2/11	18%

WHO ARE THE FAILURES

Within the group of couples who do not have any of the reasons for exclusion described above we still do not have perfect success rate. As already stated, women immunised with a single dose of paternal cells in the start of pregnancy do very well. When immunisation is delayed to six weeks or beyond, the success rate falls (Figure II). It is likely that delaying this far means that irreversible damage has occurred before this time. For this reason we try to check a recent blood hCG value before treating late to ensure that, at least monitored that way, maternal attack on the conceptus is not apparent. Nevertheless something in development appears to occur abruptly at about the six week period which makes the conceptus particularly liable to maternal attack. A good candidate for this would be the dependence of the embryo for its survival on villous placenta, rather than diffusion from the decidua which is the early form of nourishment of the embryo.

Figure II

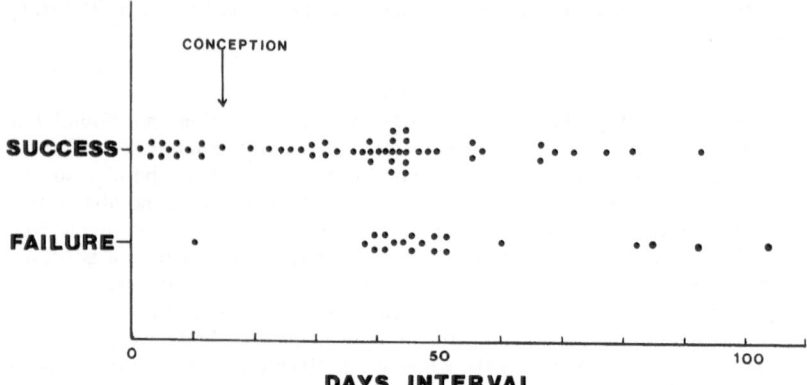

DAYS INTERVAL

Outcome in women immunised in pregnancy. The high success rate in early pregnancy declines rapidly about 25 days after conception.

THE NEED FOR FOLLOW UP OF THE CHILDREN

To date I have only considered success or failure as the birth of a viable child, or abortion. One must take the longer view, and in the light of comments by Gill *et al*[9] and others we must continue to follow the development of all children born after any intervention in couples with recurrent abortion. As the oldest children are not yet adult, it is an appropriate time to consider again the development of a Registry, perhaps under the auspices of the Royal College of Obstetricians and Gynaecologists, to record, collate and examine the children born to recurrent aborting couples. I would consider this study group very worthwhile if that were to be an outcome.

REFERENCES

1. Mowbray JF, Gibbings C, Liddell H, Reginald PW, Underwood JL, Beard RW. Controlled trial of treatment of recurrent spontaneous abortion by immunisation with paternal cells. *Lancet* 1985; 1: 941-943.
2. Reznikoff-Etievant MF, Durieux I, Huchet J, Salmon C, Netter A. Recurrent spontaneous abortions, HLA antigen sharing and anti-paternal immunity. Immunotherapic assay. In: *Immunologie de la reproduction: relation materno-foetale.* G Chaouat Ed. Colloque INSERM 1987; 154: 187-202.
3. Alexander S. Success and failure of immunisation in the treatment of recurrent spontaneous abortion. In: *Early pregnancy loss—mechanisms and treatment.* Eds. F Sharp, RW Beard. London: RCOG, 1988; pp.355-363.
4. Mowbray JF, Underwood JL, Michel M, Forbes PW, Beard RW. Immunisation with paternal lymphocytes in women with recurrent miscarriage. *Lancet* 1987; 2: 679-680.
5. Unander AM, Lindholm A. Transfusions of leukocyte-rich erythrocyte concentrates: a successful treatment in selected cases of habitual abortion. *Am J Obstet Gynecol* 1986; 154: 516-520.
6. Beer AE, Quebbeman JF, Ayers JW, Haines RF. Major histocompatibility complex antigens, maternal and paternal immune responses and chronic habitual abortion in humans. *Am J Obst Gynecol* 1981; 141: 987-999.

7. Reznikoff MF. Human MHC antigens and paternal leucocyte injections in recurrent spontaneous abortions. In: *Early pregnancy loss—mechanisms and failure.* Eds. F Sharp, RW Beard. London: RCOG, 1988; pp.375-384.
8. Taylor C, Faulk WP. Prevention of recurrent abortion with leucocyte transfusions. *Lancet* 1981; **2:** 68-70.
9. Gill TJ, MacPherson TA, Ho HN, Kunz HW, Hassett AC, Stranick KS, Locker J. Immunological and genetic factors affecting implantation and development in rat and human. *Proc Second Banff Conference on Reproductive Immunology.* Eds TJ Gill, TE Wegmann. Oxford: Oxford Universtiy Press, 1986. pp. 137-155.

Discussion

Chairman: Professor A. Beer

Dr REDMAN: I would just like to make a general comment. Yesterday David Clark said that the correct model that we should be using for a mammalian pregnancy was not that of graft/host relationship, but of tumour/host relationship. What you said at the beginning of your talk demonstrates how right he is. The reason being that human trophoblast lacks conventional MHC. Therefore, as far as we know it is not susceptible to T cell directed immune responses, not only in terms of stimulation and proliferation, but in terms of CTL. This means that your model of CTL attacking trophoblast just as far as we know today can't be true. Now it might be true if TLX were a new antigen that had the ability to direct T cell responses. TLX is an antigen that we have heard about for many years. It is still undefined, although yesterday Tom Gill coupled it as an MHC antigen, it can't even be said to be that. Everybody agrees that trophoblast and lymphocytes share antigens, but the functional significance of that sharing is totally undefined. So I think it very highly speculative to think of TLX as providing an explanation for invoking T cell responses. This means that we have to look at other sorts of immune responses, and of course the ones that are pertinent are the ones involving non-T non-B cells. What you are doing with your immunisations in terms of possibly modifying those responses, I think involves an completely different pattern of thinking and speculation. That is the first point. The second point involves side effects—you mention runting as a side effect.

Professor MOWBRAY: A possible side effect.

Dr REDMAN: Well, as a possible side effect . . .

Professor MOWBRAY: No. It isn't a possible side effect in immunisation.

Dr REDMAN: As a possible side effect that worries people who might be treating these patients. But you have discounted it because of the evidence that you see in front of your eyes. I would just like to remind this group that GVH may not be overt; it can be very mild at the beginning and may not present in this way. But in terms of experiments it can cause long term problems like lymphomas and leukaemias. This might be a long term danger that these children run. And it is as pertinent in that respect that in the past people have documented increased HLA-sharing in couples or families where the children have suffered that particular problem. So we do have to be careful about the long term implications of this kind of treatment.

Professor MOWBRAY: I am sure you are right, and this is one of the reasons why I am particularly anxious that a registry be set up in the world to follow children born after, not only immunisation, but any other active treatment of recurrent abortion, to establish whether such a problem arose. I would say that there has been a fairly large survey of the effect of blood transfusion in women on the long term follow-up of their children to see if there was an increased incidence of leukaemias or lymphomas, because of the possibility of the transmission of oncogenic viruses in blood transfusion, and in that study, which extends to a little over 15 years follow up, there isn't anything. That doesn't mean that it won't occur at 20 or 30 years. As was said by the man who initially showed that glycerol could be used for cryopreserving cells, "The study of longevity is of necessity a long term project". That is also true of the follow-up of these cases. Can I just say one thing about the CTL. It is partly tautology to say that trophoblast has no Class 1/Class 2. Cells may generate CTL against antigens which are recognised as being on the Class 1 background of the fetal cell which is immunised. In other words, that could be a cross-reacting cell. I did not actually say TLX, I said cross-reacting. I wasn't specifying anything except that if the antigen were present on the lymphocyte, and were present on the trophoblast, and you generate cells, you could potentially damage them.

Dr REDMAN: You can't do it because there is no MHC restriction. The MHC restriction of CTL is in the context of HLA A and B which is absent from trophoblast. So those CTL cannot use trophoblast as their targets, whatever the route of immunisation.

Professor MOWBRAY: Yes. But, cytotoxic cells can be generated against allogeneic cells, and will kill C1 targets.

Dr REDMAN: Yes, but only if those F1 targets carry HLA A and B. The trophoblast does not.

Professor MOWBRAY: As far as I know they only carry one specificity.

Dr ANTCZAK: Either one . . .

Dr REDMAN: A and B will do, but the trophoblast has neither.

Professor MOWBRAY: Yesterday Tom produced a little evidence that maybe sometimes there is expression of an AA antigen on the trophoblast surface, and indeed, as I understood it, he suggested maybe there could be a mechanism which might allow expression in the F1.

Dr REDMAN: Not a lot is known about the human. And although the human trophoblast does express an MHC-like antigen, it is known that that is not A or B.

Professor MOWBRAY: I accept that.

Dr CHAOUAT: I agree with you that the decrease of MHC or the lack of MHC expression on the trophoblast can make it weakly susceptible. There are many other simplifications which have been made about the immune system. One of those simplifications is that an IA negative target is not recognised, which is simply not true.

And there are a lot of examples *in vitro* and *in vivo* where you can have the function of other antigen-presenting cells which would, as an alternative, present antigen. There have been descriptions of classical cells with alpha/beta receptors, or gamma/delta receptors which can kill in a *T* cell-like MHC-restricted fashion. The best example is EBV infected target which George Klein has perfectly demonstrated to be killed in a perfectly MHC restricted fashion by non-MHC restricted CTL's of a perfect CTL target. Last, we don't know quite what they are, but they apparently have *T* cell receptors, and they kill a variety of targets in a perfectly MHC-restricted fashion. If we prove that trophoblast is not a target for such a cell, you cannot say that a minor surface antigen of the cell which in some tumour situations, or in some allograft situations has been demonstrated to be able, in some cases, to do enormous damage. It cannot be held responsible for the damage. So, I want, because of our simplification, the rigorous definition of classical *T* cells because this minor subset has been shown to be involved in some cases, and caused changes in some organs or in tumour rejection. There are some NK cells, which we believe to be NK, which are of perfect *T* cell lineage. I discussed that again with Jan Klein yesterday afternoon, and he admitted they were *T* cells in fact, and they kill in an MHC non-restricted fashion.

Professor BEER: I think that we are continuing to fool ourselves. There is a lot of evidence out there; a lot of trophoblast has been studied. And I know of no really convincing case of trophoblast being killed by a cytotoxic immune response. It may be totally unnecessary for the trophoblast to suffer cytotoxic immune damage. We have looked now at 21 placentas of women who have failed paternal leucocyte immunisation, in whom the pregnancy was electively terminated at the time of fetal death so that the tissue was fresh. Kurt Banashka has helped me in this study. The only abnormality we see in any of these placentas are abnormalities around the anchoring cells deep in the decidua which he calls the *x* cells. Now I don't know a lot about the *x* cells, but I do know that they have monoclonal antibodies, the major basic protein of the eosinophil, and something in my patients who are failing paternal leucocyte immunisation, are showing abnormalities around these *x* cells. If immune responses are necessary it may be that something is restraining these cells from releasing their parasitic-type factor that could stimulate the uterus to get rid of the placenta. And it may not be nearly as complicated as we are trying to make it with blocking antibodies and change in lymphocyte subsets. I think we have to be novel in our rethinking the whole business of reproductive immunology. I think I know the literature, and I don't see any new tests that are being applied to the trophoblast making it more interesting to me as a tissue susceptible to cytotoxic attack. That is not to say that I am not interested in the role that immunity plays in a successful pregnancy. I certainly am.

Mr CHAPMAN: You started out saying that we should talk about "why", or justify why you are doing immunisation. So let's go back to your discussion. One thing was that you suggested that 75% of recurrent abortions were due to an immunological problem. And you base that on the evidence that 75% of your patients get pregnant when you modify the immunity.

Professor MOWBRAY: No, it isn't. It is 75% of the total population, not of the ones that are immunised, because there is a group that was not immunised. That is not my only reason. This group of women cannot demonstrate the normal immune responses, that normal women make. That doesn't prove that the lack of this response has caused them to abort, but it is in that group. Then take the fraction that is in this group and multiply them up.

Mr CHAPMAN: The other point that I was concerned about was the slide about immunising during pregnancy. You showed a number of patients being immunised during the cycle in which they got pregnant. If a woman got pregnant and had a longish cycle, how did you show that?

Professor MOWBRAY: If they have gone a day over on their cycle we have done hCG's.

Mr CHAPMAN: You are underestimating; you are excluding the group of patients who may have been in what was a successful conception, but we didn't detect that they were pregnant.

Professor MOWBRAY: Because they became very early losses.

Dr ANTCZAK: I disagree with almost all of your theory, but I agree with all of your results. But the most astounding piece of evidence is this 44 days to achieve conception. If your data is correct, then us vets ought to be immunising every cow, sheep, pig or horse in the world en bloc. It would save farmers millions or billions of dollars worldwide.

Pregnancy outcome in couples with recurrent abortions following immunological evaluation and therapy

A. E. Beer

SUMMARY

Three hundred and sixty five couples with 3 or more spontaneous primary abortions were immunologically evaluated after their clinical workup and revealed no aetiology for their recurrent losses. One hundred and seventy three women in this group qualified for paternal leucocyte immunisation. The remainder received no therapy. Reproductive performance following workup and therapy revealed: 100/121 women immunised with paternal leucocytes established a pregnancy and delivered live infants; 21/121 aborted an additional time following immunisation. Subsequently these women were immunised twice with HLA incompatible leucocytes from the same non-paternal female donor and were retested immunologically. Of these 15/21 have delivered live infants. Six women aborted their pregnancy following non-paternal leucocyte immunisation. Thirteen/51 women qualifying for and awaiting treatment established a pregnancy and delivered, the remainder aborted an additional time. Twelve couples established a second pregnancy one year or longer following leucocyte immunisation. Six of the women not reimmunised aborted this pregnancy, the six reimmunised with paternal leucocytes delivered a second live infant. We conclude: 1) The incidence of a live born infants in couples with 3 or more spontaneous abortions is very low; 2) Paternal leucocyte immunisation results in an 83% live birth incidence; 3) Reproductive outcome following paternal leucocyte therapy correlates with *in vitro* immune response profiles; 4) Non-paternal leucocyte therapy is highly successful in women previously failing paternal leucocyte therapy and in women who experienced severe intrauterine growth retardation following paternal leucocyte immunisation. We suggest that this subgroup of 21 couples aborting an additional time post paternal leucocyte therapy may share the same trophoblast lymphocyte crossreactive (TLX) antigens. As a result the female is incapable of initiating the pregnancy associated responses necessary for the immunoprotection and growth stimulation of the trophoblast. Leucocytes from the non-paternal donor initiated measurable immune responses in most and this response was associated with improved reproductive outcome. The immunological significance of these findings is discussed.

INTRODUCTION

In the past, the placenta was regarded as an inert or immunosuppressive barrier between the maternal and fetal circulations.[1] More recently it has become clear that a specific maternal immune reactivity against the fetus can be measured, and this response seems to facilitate fetal survival. Other exciting data relevant to this thesis suggests that spontaneous abortion in mice, horses, and humans[2] can be prevented by immunisation of the female with lymphocytes of the appropriate genotype. It is beyond the purpose of this contribution to do more than summarise what I consider to be the immunological features of successful and unsuccessful pregnancies that can be supported by data in the literature. Without these position statements the subsequent data, discussions and conclusions regarding immunotherapy may be less clear. These features are:[3]

1. Complex immunoregulation during pregnancy leads to the production of a protective rather than a destructive maternal immune response and factors that interfere with the function of immune cytotoxic effector cells capable of destroying or damaging target tissue.

2. The trophoblast, the fetal tissue at the maternal interface that completely surrounds the fetus, expresses in a modified form, the major and minor histocompatibility and developmental (oncofetal) antigens that are essential for recognition by the local maternal immune system and the subsequent elicitation and expression of a local and systematic non-cytotoxic immune response.

3. Once maternal immunological recognition has occurred, a phenomenon of immunotrophism is initiated. T lymphocytes activated in the mother by placental antigens produce lymphokines and other cells produce antibodies that augment trophoblast cellular proliferation and feto-placental growth.

4. If these processes are not initiated, the critical features for the immuno-protection of the trophoblast are not achieved and it fails to proliferate in a manner necessary to support the fetus or it is rejected by allo- or autoimmune reactivity initiated in the mother; however, this latter process has never been convincingly demonstrated.

Post-fertilisation reproductive wastage in humans is very high. Most pregnancies terminate within the first 28 days and are never recognised clinically. Of those that are, 15-25% terminate in spontaneous abortions. These statistics are supported further by the observed 80% implantation failure rate following embryo transfer in *in vitro* fertilisation candidates. Although specific conditions, thought to be related to pregnancy losses, can be documented in one half of the couples, the remainder demonstrate no genetic, structural, endocrinological or microbiological aetiologies. [4-8]

A healthy couple has a 60% chance of establishing a pregnancy in any ovulatory cycle.[9] Of these couples, 25% will have a clinical pregnancy. It is thought that over 90% of pregnancy losses occur without the knowledge of the woman. Of pregnancies that are clinically recognised the incidence of spontaneous abortions is between 15-25%.[10] There are many aetiologies for this early embryonic mortality that must be considered by the clinician. A large number of couples who lose their pregnancies repeatedly have measurable abnormalities of immunity when compared to normal couples having their pregnancies electively terminated or to those couples who sustain a normal pregnancy to term.[7]

With the incidence of pregnancy loss so high and the aetiologies so numerous, it is understandable that the clinician is confused and frustrated as he attempts to unravel the aetiology for the disappointed, and often grieving couple. Recent studies have led to the increased awareness of the role of immunological factors in the establishment of a successful pregnancy. It is presently thought that these measurable immunological factors are associated with pregnancy losses in over 50% of normal couples who have experienced three spontaneous losses; however, the precise nature of these abnormalities is still open to debate, as is the type of immunotherapy currently being advocated. Much of the controversy that exists regarding the success of immunotherapy arises because the spontaneous cure rates in patients with documented reproductive failures is not precisely known. What follows is an assessment of the literature as it exists.

The chance that a next pregnancy will be successful in a normal couple that have no living children and who have experienced 3 consecutive spontaneous abortions is variously reported. All studies to date can be faulted, but suggest the following.[11] If a woman has experienced 3 or more consecutive abortions it is almost certain that the losses are caused by a recurrent factor; however, claiming that the aetiology is immunological because no other aetiology can be established is not fully justified. Many workers in the field of immunotherapy for reproductive problems have jumped to this conclusion without much supportive immunological data. The conclusion is further reinforced by the reported successes of immunotherapy that are very high at present.

The risk of a 4th abortion after a 3rd is estimated to be 73% and increases to a 94% risk for a fifth spontaneous abortion after a 4th. These statistics were based on data available in 1938 before there were any accepted therapies for recurrent spontaneous abortions.[12] Even more pessimistic estimates of a 16% spontaneous cure rate after 3 consecutive spontaneous abortions or an 84% recurrence rate were reported by Eastman.[13] In a Kinsey Study based on pregnancy histories obtained from a large group of women interviewed, 60% reported losing a third pregnancy after experiencing 2 consecutive spontaneous abortions, and 79% reported aborting a 4th pregnancy after experiencing 3 spontaneous abortions. James[14,15] reported only 26% of control patients who had experienced 3 or more abortions delivered live infants without therapy. This was compared to an 84% success rate in couples undergoing the therapy in vogue during that period. He concluded from his own data and the data of others that the risk of a fourth pregnancy loss following a third in a couple with no children was 58% or greater.[16]

Although genetic abnormalities are common causes of abortions, they are observed infrequently in couples that have experienced 3 spontaneous abortions. This greatly lower incidence of chromosomal abnormalities in fetuses of recurrent aborting couples (5-6% compared to the 50% incidence in sporadic aborting couples) is further evidence for a specific aetiology (possibly immune) in couples with recurrent losses.[17]

In later studies, when specific aetiologies for recurrent spontaneous abortion were suspected and therapy regimens advocated, it was found that almost any type of therapy resulted in successful pregnancies in 80% of couples treated. Warburton and Fraser summarised the situation in 1961 and suggested that the subsequent pregnancy success rates claimed from the varied therapies could be accounted for by the spontaneous cure rate typical of this disorder.[18] They concluded that the probability of a subsequent abortion after three consecutive abortions was only 20% or an 80% cure rate. These figures are similar to those of recent studies of the Stray-Pedersons claiming that "tender loving care" was as effective a therapy in achieving a subsequent live birth for the couple as any reported in the literature.[19]

As a clinical scientist involved in a large immunotherapy program for recurrent spontaneous abortion, this debate and these widely varying statistics are of major interest. There are now reproductive performance statistics of control recurrently aborting couples appearing in the literature. These are cited in Table 1. These suggest that the risk of a fourth spontaneous abortion in an untreated woman who has experienced three consecutive abortions is between 65% and 90%. There are double-blind and blinded cross over studies currently in progress that should soon provide the clinician with more reliable data regarding spontaneous cure rates in these couples as well as the effectiveness of immunotherapy.

Table 1

Results of immunotherapy on subsequent reproduction in women with recurrent spontaneous abortions

Study	Cytotoxic Antibodies	No. of Abortions	Source of Lymphocytes	Live Births	%	Offspring Status
Faulk	not done	3-10	Husband	4/4	(100)	Normal
Mowbray	0/49	3-8	Wife (control)	10/27	(37)	Normal
			Husband	17/22	(77)	Normal
Beer	19/121	3 or >	Husband	100/121	(83)	15% IUGR
		3 or >	None	13/51	(25)	Normal
Beer	21/21	4 or >	3rd Party	15/21	(72)	Normal
Johnson	0/18	3 or >	Trophoblast Vesicles	14/18	(78)	Normal
Carp	0/0	3 or >	Husband	19/27	(70)	Normal
		3 or >	none	1/10	(10)	
Reginald	not done	3 or >	none	97/334	(29)	28% IUGR
Unander	not done	3 or >	3rd Party	22/38	(58)	Not Rep.
Stray-Pedersen	not done	3 or >	Psyc. Support	32/27	(86)	Normal
			Non Psyc. Support	8/24	(33)	Normal

The immunological parameters of interest to us in these couples included sharing of Class I and Class II HLA antigens, mixed-lymphocyte culture (MLR) reactivity of maternal cells to paternal and third-party antigens, the presence of MLR-blocking activity in maternal serum, the presence or absence of leucocytotoxic antibodies and the responses of maternal decidual and peripheral blood lymphocyctes to mitogens.

In the present study we identified a group of women who were presumed to have had immunologically mediated abortions. They were immunised with lymphocytes from their partners, a procedure that has previously been claimed to exert an anti-abortion effect in clinical and experimental studies. We report on the relationship between maternal immune responses and reproductive outcome in 4 study groups: 1) 20 couples having their pregnancy electively terminated; 2) 121 normal couples with 3 or more abortions in which the woman was immunised with paternal lymphocytes and established a pregnancy; 3) 21 women from this latter group who were subsequently reimmunised with non-paternal donor lymphocytes after failing to respond to paternal lymphocyte immunisation and experiencing another pregnancy loss; and 4) 51 women immunologically evaluated and who qualified for treatment but established another pregnancy before immunisation could be accomplished.

MATERIALS AND METHODS

Patient Selection

A total of 365 couples with 3 or more abortions were drawn from the United States, South America, Great Britain, Europe, and the Middle East. The workup of these patients has been described elsewhere.[8,5] Control couples were selected from among patients having their pregnancies terminated electively at the Planned Parenthood Clinic of mid-Michigan. Ten were primigravidas and 10 were multigravidas. They were chosen after they were screened for evidence of previous spontaneous abortions, infertility or strong risk factor status for infertility. Blood samples were drawn from each partner and sharp decidual uterine curettage was performed on each woman after the pregnancy termination procedure to obtain decidual tissue for recovering decidual lymphocytes.

Couples were presumed to have possible immunological mediated abortion if they met any of the following criteria and did not have an identifiable medical cause for recurrent spontaneous abortion: 1) sharing of three or more HLA Class I and Class II antigens, 2) a 30% or greater decrease in response of the woman's lymphocytes in MLR to her partner's stimulator cells, as compared to third-party controls, and 3) the absence of specific blocking activity for MLR responses to paternal antigens.

Women meeting these criteria were offered immunisation with their partner's leucocytes as described previously.[30] Four weeks following their second immunisation they were restudied immunologically. Couples were advised to attempt another pregnancy after the second immunisation regardless of the post immunisation results. One hundred and seventy five women have been immunised in all.

Tissue Typing

Tissue typing of both members was performed for Class I (A,B,C locus) antigens and Class II (DR) antigens according to the NIH modification of the Terasaki technique.[20]

Mixed Lymphocyte Culture Assays

One-way mixed lymphocyte cultures were performed as we have reported previously.[8,5] The following cell cultures were included: female stimulator/

female responder; female stimulator/female responder + PHA; male stimulator/ female responder; 3rd party stimulator/female responder; non-paternal-donor stimulator/female responder; male stimulator/male responder; male stimulator/ male responder + PHA; 3rd party stimulator/male responder; female stimulator/ male responder; 3rd party stimulator/3rd party responder; 3rd party stimulator/ 3rd party responder + PHA; male stimulator/3rd party responder; female stimulator/3rd party responder; non-paternal-donor stimulator/3rd party responder. Harvested decidual lymphocytes were also included in certain of the combinations above and were stimulated with PHA.

Mixed Lymphocyte Culture Blocking Assays

Some of the cell cultures were repeated using serum from the female participants at the same concentrations as for the pooled AB serum. Additional female serum was heat-inactivated in a water bath at 56°C for 30 minutes and then used in the corresponding cell cultures including decidual lymphocytes as stimulators and responders.

Leucocyte Immunisation

One hundred and twenty one women meeting our criteria were immunised with 50×10^6 paternal leucocytes intradermally on two occasions separated by 6 weeks. Repeat immunological analyses were performed 4 weeks following the last immunisation and women failing to demonstrate a serum MLR blocking response of greater than 30% were re-immunised with paternal leucocytes and re-studied. Couples were counselled to establish another pregnancy regardless of the results. Twenty-one women who failed to respond to paternal leucocyte immunisation and who aborted an additional time post paternal leucocyte immunisation were reimmunised with 50×10^6 leucocytes from the same non-paternal donor on two occasions and every 6 weeks through the 24th week of pregnancy. The HLA type of the non-paternal donor was: A 2,3/ B51,51/ C $-/-/$, Dr 1,1. Immunological studies were repeated post-immunisation, during pregnancy and at delivery or at a repeat abortion.

RESULTS

The reproductive outcome as of October 1, 1987 experienced by women who were immunised with paternal leucocytes is outlined in Table 2.

Table 2

Subsequent reproductive outcome of couples with
recurrent spontaneous abortions
(No treatment, paternal and non-paternal leucocyte immunisation)

	Paternal	Non-Paternal	None
Pregnancies	121	21	51
Delivered	100 (83%)	15 (72%)	13 (25%)
Repeat Abortion	21 (17%)	6 (28%)	38 (75%)

Elective Pregnancy Termination

In 20 women electing pregnancy terminations and in 21 women with a repeat abortion post paternal leucocyte immunisation decidual lymphocytes were harvested and assayed as responders in MLR in normal serum and in heat inactivated serum. The lack of serum suppression is evident in Table 3 in women failing paternal leucocyte immunisation at the time of a repeat abortion when compared with those having their pregnancies terminated.

Table 3

Decidual lymphocytes in MLR from women electing pregnancy termination
and at a repeat abortion post immunisation with paternal leucocytes

Stimulator/Responder

	Unheated Maternal Serum	Heat Inactivated Maternal Serum
Elective (20)	52.8%	46.9%
Recurrent (21)	21.0%*	0.0%*

*P less than 0.001

We next analysed alterations in one-way MLR reactivity by heat inactivated female serum in three groups of women. Those electing pregnancy terminations, those immunised with paternal leucocytes and delivered, and those experiencing a repeat abortion post paternal leucocyte immunisation. The results are graphed in Figure I. All women electing pregnancy termination in the first trimester had significantly higher blocking activity than women in the other two groups. Women who delivered post leucocyte immunisation developed blocking activity in MLR that was the same as those electing pregnancy termination. The levels increased significantly by the time of delivery. Women who aborted an additional time demonstrated blocking in MLR that was one half that measured in women who went on to the successful completion of their pregnancies.

Figure I

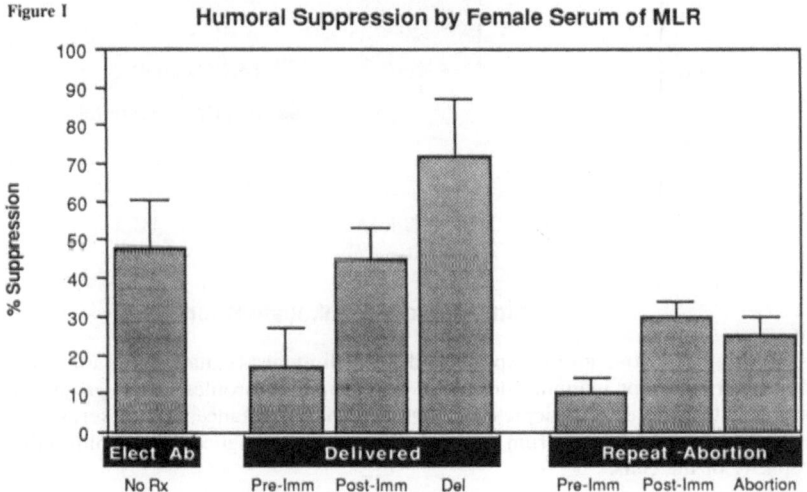

Humoral Suppression by Female Serum of MLR

At present, women who fail to develop significant MLR blocking in both normal serum and heat inactivated serum following paternal leucocyte immunisation are offered non-paternal donor leucocyte immunisation before attempting another pregnancy.

The 21 women who failed paternal leucocyte immunisation were immunised with non-paternal leucocytes from the same donor and were retested. The data is shown in Figure II for those 15 who have delivered a live born child. In this group no MLR blocking activity was demonstrated pre-immunisation with paternal leucocytes. Post immunisation, female serum potentiated the MLR and enhancement of the responses were seen. Following non-paternal donor immunisation strong MLR blocking activity was demonstrated to both the husband and the 3rd party stimulator.

Figure II

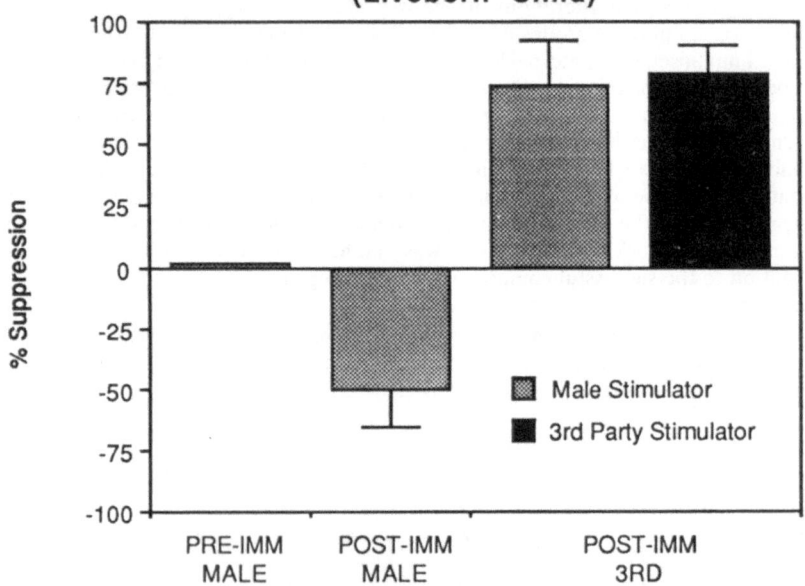

Suppression of MLR by Female Serum Pre- and Post-Immunization (Liveborn Child)

Six couples in this group experienced an additional pregnancy loss following non-paternal donor immunisation. The MLR immune profiles in this group are significantly different and depicted in Figure III. In all instances female serum and heat inactivated female serum did not suppress but enhanced the proliferative capacity of the cells.

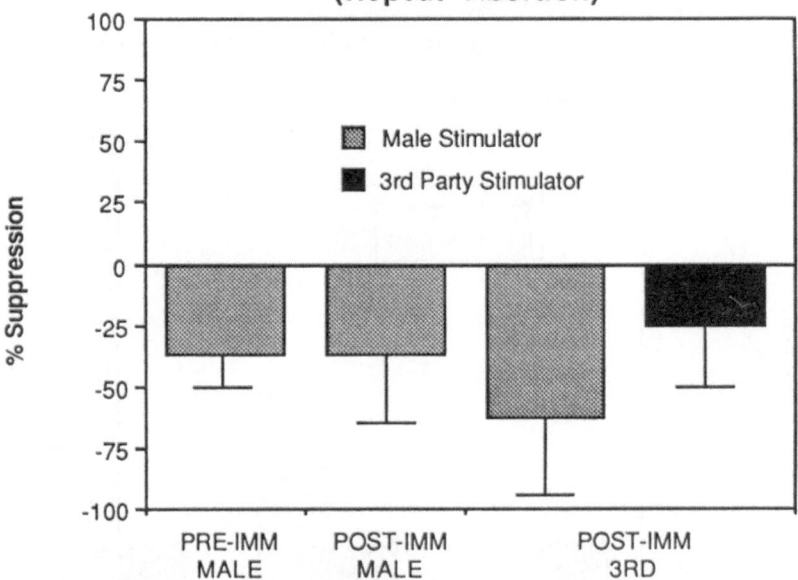

Figure III

Suppression of MLR by Female Serum
Pre- and Post-Immunization
(Repeat Abortion)

Immunization (Leukocyte Source)

We tested the paternal antigen specificity of the female serum MLR blocking activity in cultures involving 3 individuals of differing HLA types in all possible stimulator/responder combinations in MLR. The serum of all women who delivered following non-paternal donor leucocyte immunisation significantly blocked MLR reactivity of all stimulator/responder cell populations tested. Serum from the 6 women similarly treated who aborted an additional time post-non-paternal donor leucocyte immunisation demonstrated no blocking activity in any MLR stimulator/responder cell populations tested. PHA induced mitogenesis was not inhibited by female serum.

Antileucocytotoxic Antibody Production

Figure IV shows the incidence of antipaternal leucocytotoxic antibodies in the serum of women in the three groups. The incidence of antileucocytotoxic antibody was increased to 40% in women immunised with paternal leucocytes who subsequently delivered a child. This incidence was not increased further in those women who received a third immunisation. Of major interest was the finding of 100% incidence of leucocytotoxic antibodies post immunisation in the group of women who aborted an additional time. The presence of antipaternal leucocytotoxic antibody and the absence of MLR blocking factors was predictive of a subsequent pregnancy loss following paternal leucocyte immunisation and appears to correlate with the absence of anti-idiotypic antibodies to maternal T cell receptors (work in progress).

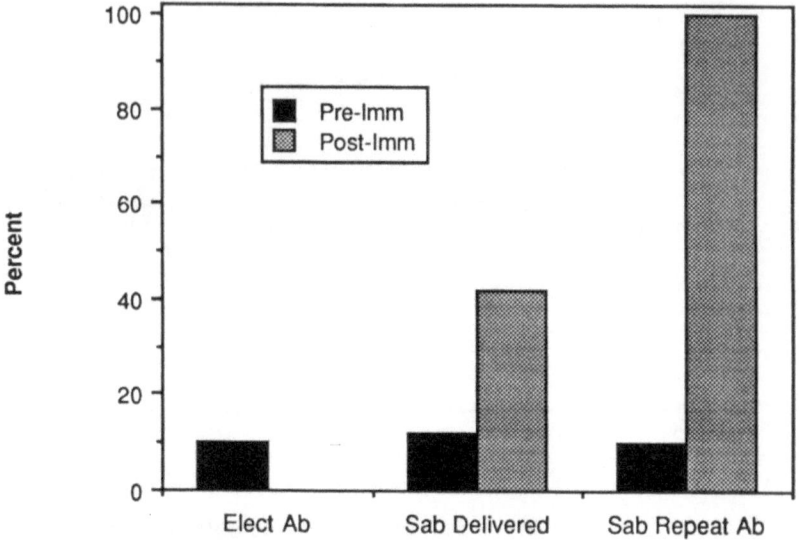

Figure IV **Incidence of Leukocytotoxic Antibodies**

DISCUSSION

Factors in pregnancy serum that are immunoregulatory may be: 1) Serum factors that induce the generation of cell mediated suppressor cells or products in *in vitro* cultures;[21] 2) IgG blocking antibodies to trophoblast/lymphocyte crossreactive antigens;[22] 3) Antibodies to paternal HLA antigens that block paternal stimulator cells;[23] 3) Factors that inhibit T helper cells from releasing IL-2 following allogeneic stimulation;[24] 4) Anti-idiotypic antibodies that block HLA receptors on maternal immunoblasts stimulated by paternal DR antigens; [25] and 5) Non specific suppressors of lymphocyte mitogenesis.[26] The results of the present study confirm the presence of a potent factor in early pregnancy serum and in the serum of recurrently aborting women who carry a successful pregnancy post immunisation with leucocytes that suppress MLR of decidual and peripheral blood lymphocytes. Studies of the HLA antigen profiles of the couples and third party controls make it unlikely that HLA polymorphic antigens as defined by typing sera are targets for the serum factors suppressing the MLR. These findings support the hypothesis that the immunoregulatory factor in pregnancy serum is an antibody to an allotypic TLX antigen or to a broadly shared Class I determinant.[22] It has been shown that sera from multiparous women contain antibodies reactive only with activated, PHA stimulated T cells and have no reactivity with resting T or B cells.[27] Here also the reactivity of these sera bore no relationship with HLA Class I or Class II MHC antigens. It was concluded that the antibody seen consistently in the sera of all pregnant women defined developmental antigen(s) presented to the immune system of the mother during pregnancy. These studies have been confirmed by Konoeda *et al* (1986) who analysed public epitopes from serum isolated from 50,000 placentas.[28] These epitopes were as immunogenetic as the private HLA Class I epitopes by the frequency with which antibodies were produced against them. Again their specificity bore no relationship with Class I MHC polymorphic determinants.

Other types of antibody and systems of antibody mediated suppression of the immune response have been described. Idiotypic control of the immune response was first suggested by Jerne (1974).[29] Anti-idiotypic antibodies stimulate as well as suppress immune responses to a variety of antigens under differing conditions, and their presence during pregnancy has been documented.[30] Maternal T lymphocytes primed *in vitro* to allogeneic paternal HLA-DR antigens express idiotypic receptors for these antigens. Sera collected from parous women contain autoantibodies that react specifically with maternal T lymphoblasts alloactivated against the HLA-DR antigens of the father or a third party of the same DR type as the father. Such anti-idiotypic antibodies to HLA-DR receptors were found both in women who developed anti-HLA antibodies and in women who did not. They can be identified very early in a first pregnancy. These antibodies inhibit the lymphocytotoxic activity of the corresponding anti-HLA-DR antibodies from both autologous and homologous sera. Studies to date suggest that the development of anti-idiotypic antibodies to HLA during pregnancy is a general phenomenon seen in all women tested.[31,32] We are currently investigating whether the MLR blocking factor is an anti-idiotypic antibody that can be demonstrated when maternal T-immunoblasts are generated to paternal DR locus antigens. Studies in progress indicate that recurrently aborting women who sustain pregnancy to term following leucocyte immunisation do develop anti-idiotypic antibodies reactive with maternal T-immunoblasts. We are currently testing to determine if the high incidence of antileucocytotoxic antibodies in women who abort consistently following paternal leucocyte immunisation correlates with their lack of the corresponding anti-idiotypic antibody. It has also been shown that anti-idiotypic antibodies induced by blood transfusions prior to organ allografting blocked the antigen specific receptor on T cells and caused suppression of the recipients response against the donor's alloantigens *in vitro* as demonstrated by graft survival and *in vitro*, as determined in mixed lymphocyte culture reactions.[33]

Tissue extracted from the decidua of uterine subsystems has been shown to suppress antibody production *in vitro* and block MLR reactions.[34] Suppressor cells isolated from the decidua have also been shown to down-regulate immune responses against paternal antigens. Although decidual lymphocytes harvested at the time of pregnancy termination were suppressed *in vitro* by pregnancy serum, they were as responsive in all assays as peripheral blood leucocytes. Future studies of local immunoregulation in early gestation in humans must address the types and the activities of lymphocytes in the decidua of an early first pregnancy. Based on these findings, we do not recommend that a couple attempt another pregnancy post immunisation with paternal leucocytes unless female serum MLR blocking activity of 40% or greater is seen. Non-responding couples in this category who abort an additional time post immunisation are offered non-paternal donor leucocyte immunisation. When a single non-paternal donor was utilised 75% of the women responded and delivered a child. Whether the remaining individuals are genetic non-responders, or by chance shared the same determinants discussed above with both spouse and non-paternal donor is being explored.

ACKNOWLEDGEMENTS

This work was supported in part by grants HD 19908 and HD 16207.

REFERENCES
1. Chaouat G, Kolb JP, Wegmann TG. The murine placenta as an immunological barrier between the mother and the fetus. *Immunol Rev* 1983; **75**: 31-60.
2. Chaouat G, Kiger N, Wegmann TG: Vaccination against spontaneous abortion in mice. *J Reprod Immunol* 1983; **5**: 389-392.
3. Beer AE, Quebbeman JF, Hamazaki Y, Semprini AE: Pregnancy outcome in human couples with recurrent spontaneous abortions: The role(s) of HLA antigen sharing, ABO blood group antigen profiles, female serum MLR blocking factors, antisperm antibodies and immunotherapy. In: *Immunoregulation and Fetal Survival*. Eds. Gill TJ, Wegmann TG. New York and Oxford: Oxford University Press, 1987; pp 286.
4. Menge AC, Beer AE. The significance of human leucocyte antigen profiles in human infertility, recurrent abortion, and pregnancy disorders. *Fertil Steril* 1985; **43**: 693-695.
5. Beer AE, Quebbeman JF, Ayers JWT, Haines RF. Major histocompatibility complex antigens, maternal and paternal immune responses, and chronic habitual abortions in humans. *Am J Obstet Gynecol* 1981; **141**: 987-999.
6. Beer AE. Immunopathologic factors contributing to recurrent spontaneous abortion in humans (editorial). *Am J Reprod Immunol* 1983; **4**: 182-184.
7. Beer AE: How did your mother not reject you? *Ann Immunol* 1984; **135D**: 315-318.
8. Beer AE, Semprini AE, Zhu X, Quebbeman JF. Pregnancy outcome in human couples with recurrent spontaneous abortions: 1) HLA antigen profiles; 2) HLA antigen sharing; 3) Female serum MLR blocking factors and 4) Paternal leukocyte immunization. *Exp Clin Immunogenet* 1985; **2**: 137.
9. Edmonds DK, Lindsay KS, Miller JF, Williamson E, Wood PJ. Early embryonic mortality in women. *Fertil Steril* 1982; **38**: 447-453.
10. Warburton D, Fraser F. Spontaneous abortion risks in man: data from reproductive histories collected in a medical genetics unit. *Hum Genet* 1964; **16**: 1.
11. Graves WL. Psychological aspects of spontaneous abortion. In: *Spontaneous and Recurrent Abortion*. Eds. MJ Bennett, DK Edmonds. Oxford: Blackwell Scientific Publications, 1987; pp 214.
12. Malpas P. A study of abortion sequences. *J Obstet Gynaecol Br Empire*. 1938; **45**: 932-949.
13. Eastman NJ. Habitual abortion. In: *Progress in Gynecology*. (Eds.) JV Meigs, SH Sturgis. New York: Grune and Stratton, pp 262.
14. James WH. Control data for evaluating the efficacy of psychotherapy in habitual spontaneous abortion. *Br J Psychiatry* 1963; **109**: 81.

15. James WH. Notes toward an epidemiology of spontaneous abortion. *Am J Hum Genet* 1963; **15:** 223.
16. MacNaughton MC. The probability of recurrent abortion. *J Obstet Gynaecol Br Commonw* 1964; **71:** 784.
17. Elias S, Simpson JL. Evaluation and clinical management of patients at apparent increased risk for spontaneous abortions. In: *Human Embryonic and Human Death.* Eds. I Porter, EB Hook. New York: Academic Press 1980; pp 331.
18. Warburton D, Fraser FC. On the probability that a woman who has had a spontaneous abortion will abort in subsequent pregnancies. *J Obstet Gynaecol Br Commonw* 1961; **68:** 784-788.
19. Stray-Pederson B, Stray-Pederson S. Etiologic factors and subsequent reproductive performance in 195 couples with a prior history of habitual abortion. *Am J Obstet Gynecol* 1984; **148:** 140-146.
20. Terasaki PI, Bernoco D, Park MS, Ozturk G, Iwaki Y. Microdroplet testing for HLA-A,-B,-C and-D antigens. *Am J Clin Pathol* 1978; **69:** 103-120.
21. Chaouat G, Voisin GA. Regulatory T cell subpopulations in pregnancy. I. Evidence for suppressive activity of the early phase of MLR. *J Immunol* 1979; **122:** 1383-1388.
22. McIntyre JA, Faulk WP. Allotypic trophoblast-lymphocyte cross-reactive (TLX) cell surface antigens. *Human Immunol* 1982; **4:** 27-35.
23. Nicholas NS, Panayi GS, Nouri AM. Human pregnancy serum inhibits inter-leukin-2 production. *Clin Exp Immunol* 1984; **58:** 587-595.
24. Domingo-Garcia CG, Domenech N, Aparicio P, Palomino P. Human pregnancy serum inhibits proliferation of T8-depleted cells and their interleukin-2 synthesis in mixed lymphocyte cultures. *J Reprod Immunol* 1985; **8:** 97-110.
25. Suciu-Foca N, Reed E, Rohowsky C, Kung P, King DW. Anti-idiotypic antibodies to anti-HLA receptors induced by pregnancy. *Proc Natl Acad Sci USA* 1983; **80:** 830-834.
26. Figueredo MA, Palomino P and Ortiz F. Lymphocyte response to phytohemagglutinin in the presence of serum from pregnant women: correlation with serum levels of alpha-fetoprotein. *Clin Exp Immunol* 1979; **37:** 140-144.
27. Kim SJ, Christiansen FT, Gosar I, Silver DM, Pollack MS, Dupont B. Frequency of alloantibodies reacting with PHA activated T lymphocytes, unexplainable by known HLA activities. *Human Immunol* 1980; **4:** 347-355.
28. Konoeda Y, Terasaki PI, Wakisaka A, Park MS, Mickey MR. Public determinants of HLA indicated by pregnancy antibodies. *Transplantation* 1986; **41:** 253-259.
29. Jerne NK. Towards a network theory of the immune system. *Ann Immunol* 1974; **125c:** 373-379.
30. Reed E, Bonagura V, Kung P, King DW, Suciu-Foca N. Anti-idiotypic antibodies to HLA-DR4 and DR2. *J Immunol* 1983; **131:** 2890-2894.
31. Suciu-Foca N, Rohowsky C, Kung P, King DW. Idiotype-like determinants on human T lymphocytes alloactivated in mixed lymphocyte culture. *J Exp Med* 1982; **156:** 283-288.
32. Klatzmann D, Gluckman JC, Foucault C. Modification of mixed lymphocyte reactivity after blood transfusions in man. *Transplantation Proceedings* 1983; **15:** 1016-1018.
33. Clark DR. Local suppressor cells and the success or failure of the "foetal allograft". *Ann Immunol* 1984; **135D:** 21-24.

Discussion

Chairman: Professor J. Mowbray

Dr ANTCZAK: I would like to ask you if you have done absorption experiments with some of those sera? Can you absorb out the blocking acitivity with either the mother's cells or the donor cells?

Professor BEER: The sera can be appropriately absorbed. The leucocytotoxic antibody will be absorbed out with resting paternal cells. However, the MLR blocking activity is only absorbed out if we activate the cells, or if the cells are actually mitogen stimulated, suggesting that the blocking may be to an activation antigen. In studies with Nicole and Fisher Pocock it appears that this may actually be an anti-idiotypic antibody that is only recognised when we activate the maternal cells with paternal leucocytes, and then that will confirm the presence of binding of the antibody in maternal serum to these receptors.

Dr ANTCZAK: That is why I asked about absorbing with the mother's own cells.

Professor BEER: I am sorry. I thought you asked, "Can it be absorbed by the cells"? I have not absorbed this in any other way.

Professor BEARD: Could I just discuss with you briefly the growth retardation problem, because there is no doubt about it that when a subject is presented to a group of immunologists it fills them with great anxiety. But I really do think that before you perhaps start to imply as you do, that immunisation is producing growth retardation, then one really needs more data. Growth retardation basically can be divided into two groups—those babies that are cell-deficient and have not gone through the normal amount of cell divisions, and those, for example the rubella-type babies, who have the normal complement of cells, but the cells are small, due to intrauterine starvation. Now you can really only tell the difference those two groups of babies by follow-up studies. And one of the first things you look for is catch-up growth after delivery. Those babies are the ones that apparently do normally and do not suffer. Among the babies that remain permanently small, some turn out to be developmentally abnormal, but the great majority are simply small individuals. Without follow-up data of that sort it is impossible to imply anything about the growth-retarded babies. The second point to make is that we are not the only group that have essentially found that the weight distribution of babies after immunisation is normal. Margareta Unander has also found that pregnancies in her study are entirely normal.

351

Professor BEER: I totally agree, Professor Beard, and I hesitated to present the limited data, but at a meeting like this I feel that I must open my doors and give you what I have. You must also realise that our group is quite different from any other. We selected patients for sharing the three antigens, individuals who were already hyporesponders in MLR to other groups. So this may be a very unique selected group that is in no way comparable to yours. I am only making those statements based on the data that I have presented.

Professor ALBERMAN: I just wanted to ask how we can relate this to the findings that I reported, which is that you get growth retardation after a succession of abortions quite independently of immunisation. I wonder how that relates to your findings. Secondly, what I have missed very much is any examination of the genetic causes in any of the treated and untreated groups. Because there must be a group of women or their partners with chromosomal anomalies that gets lost, and I would like to know whether the ones that you have treated who lose their fetuses are chromosomally normal or abnormal. And finally, I am totally confused trying to synthesise anything I have heard with these prolongation principles, as has been found by so many people before an abortion. It might be explicable by the fact that there have been repeated early abortions which have not been picked up, but I wonder whether in the three groups that you were reporting from the beginning, is it possible that the untreated group are the ones that took much longer to become pregnant; otherwise they would have come into your treated group. Or would they have become pregnant earlier anyway?

Professor BEER: Those are beautiful questions; I wish that I had the same kind of beautiful answers. It is possible that the intrauterine growth retardation that you reported, and that I have seen, is background coincidence, having nothing to do with the immunisation. I am ready to accept that. I accept your data, and I think my data, independent of immunisation, may only be reconfirming that. The third question, regarding those that were waiting for me to return to establish a pregnancy, I think are really kind of a "cheap" control group for presentation of data I had available. I am sure they are individuals who were living their lives in a way so as to postpone their pregnancy until I returned, and really do not comprise à control group. This study group should resist the temptation to say that Beer has shown that 75% of all women with previous abortions abort again. And your middle question—I just can't answer; I do not have the data.

Professor GILL: I would just like to make a comment along the lines of the ones made by Professor Mowbray and Professor Beer to plead for the presentation of data in a clear and well-worked-out form. It seems to me a lot of the discussions over the past two and a half days, and prior to this time, are confusing experimental observations and mechanisms. People have been looking at organ graft rejection for forty years, and the mechanisms still are not well worked-out. It is still difficult to tell whether an organ is rejected because of a cellular or a humoral response or what the mechanisms are. Even in very well worked-out systems, the kinds of parameters that people talk about at Class 1 restriction, Class 2 restriction, etc. come from *in vitro* test tube phenomena. You need not see them to have an effect on an organ graft. The same I think is true in pregnancy. You know that if you expose transplantation antigens on the surface of any tissue, it is going to elicit a response. The distribution of transplantation antigens in the placenta is complex; either it is constitutively suppressed, or actively suppressed, and these can be changed. We are dealing with mechanisms that are very complicated, and may involve immunological phenomena or may not. But I think that it is very important to get clear cut data, well worked-out systematically, and developed by the registries or corroborative studies that pull these data together. I think we have had too much discussion of the types of mechanisms which in areas that would have been much better studied over a much longer period of time, are still unclear.

Professor CLARK: I was quite puzzled by the discrepancy in the predictability of leucocytotoxic antibodies, at least the antibodies detected in that test, between your results and those reported by James Mowbray. As I was thinking about this, I realised that, in fact, you are doing intradermal paternal leucocyte immunotherapy. Those of us who do basic immunology know that the intradermal route is one of the most effective ways of inducing immune responses, particularly those of a *T* cell.

Professor BEER: That is why I chose it.

Professor CLARK: . . . whereas, an intravenous route is more likely to induce a classic type of response. I wonder if maybe some of the problems that you have seen with growth retardation, if you think these are immunological, might be related to the induction of harmful kinds of immune responses that are being prevented when some cells are also being given by the intravenous route. I do not think this issue of routing of immunisation has come up, but I suspect that it may be quite an important one.

Professor BEER: I can only answer that the route of immunisation was chosen based on all knowledge available in the field of transplantation at that time. It is a very effective way of stimulating a cell-mediated immune response that related to graft rejection. I was looking at the fetus as an allograft, and therefore, I chose the most effective route to incite the immunity. If we look on it as tumour graft, you may be absolutely right; intravenous injection may be far superior to intradermal administration.

Professor CLARK: Wouldn't you like to produce immunological enhancement rather than immunological rejection?

Professor BEER: I don't know.

Professor JOHNSON: Just carrying on from that point, I think that there is severe concern about this question of IUGR which cannot be brushed under the carpet. There is quite a marked contrast in results. There is a recent paper from Mario Cauci that claims that 4 out of 7 patients following white cell immunisation have had pregnancies that were complicated by IUGR. And this may well be associated with routing of the immunisation or timing of the immunisation. What I would like to ask is whether you happen to know which protocol Mario Cauci used? Did he use yours or James Mowbray's protocol?

Professor BEER: I am not familiar with that data at all.

Ms UNDERWOOD: I discussed it with him in Toronto this time last year. As far as I remember, just to really confuse everybody, he gives a very much smaller dose, and he gives all his cells intravenously. He does give a very small number of cells.

Professor JOHNSON: There is a potential correlation between intradermal and intravenous immunisation, and also with prolonged immunisation going on into pregnancy.

Dr ANTCZAK: You pose very good questions about who, how and how often. You say that you are looking at very different groups of people. Both of you are immunising very different groups of people. The bottom line to me is that your results are essentially the same. You are both getting 75% success with different populations studied. You have minor differences, but the major effect of treatment gives essentially identical results. I would like to have you make one of those charts that you made at one of the other meetings.

Professor MOWBRAY: The chart in Paris. I think the thing it did show was that Professor Beer's selection of patients was different from most of us. We all had minor differences amongst us about who one would accept for treatment.

Dr ALLEN: Could you medics tell we non-medics the definition of growth retardation that you are talking about here? Is that any different from the growth retardation seen in babies of a heavy-smoking woman who drinks a lot?

Professor BEARD: The definition is a statistical one based on the birth weights relative to gestational age of a defined population of pregnant women. Most people define a growth retarded baby as one that is on or below the tenth centile. A more rigorous definition is babies whose weight for gestation is outside the limits of two standard deviations.

Belgian experience with repeat immunisation in recurrent spontaneous abortions

S. A. Alexander, D. Latinne, M. Debruyere, E. Dupont, W. Gottlieb, K. Thomas

INTRODUCTION

Recurrent spontaneous abortion, distressing to the mother and enigmatic to the obstetrician, has known successive phases of interest and neglect. These have ranged from denying the benefit of any therapeutic measure,[1] to various unvalidated therapeutic approaches, mainly hormones. In addition, there is no generally agreed definition of recurrent abortion,[2] so that simple comparisons of outcome from various groups is almost meaningless.

More recently interest has focused on immunological causes especially for the first trimester (early) recurrent abortion. Almost simultaneously, teams started sensitising women who recurrently aborted, in a manner not dissimilar from that which is done in presensitisation of transplant recipients by blood transfusions.

Because things have happened simultaneously, protocols vary quite markedly from one unit to the other. Immunising material includes paternal lymphocytes[3] or donor lymphocytes,[4] pooled donor lymphocytes[5], leucocyte-rich erythrocyte concentrates[6] syncytiotrophoblast membrane preparation[7] and possibly others.

Not only do the immunogens vary from one department to the other, but also, the dose, route and number of doses. The general rationale underlying the various protocols has been to combine effectiveness in terms of immunisation with avoidance of untoward side effects. Though protocols were largely empirical, basically derived from the experience that has been acquired in transplant patients. In these, minor immunisation accidents have been described, including pyrexia; such accidents seem less likely to occur with small doses and the intravenous route. Because of the potential hazards of hyperthermia, this approach was chosen in the Belgian immunising groups.

PATIENT SELECTION

One hundred patients were referred to either the Catholic University of Louvain or the Free University of Brussels for repeated pregnancy failures: each one had been pregnant on at least three occasions, but had failed to deliver a live child.

A. Personal obstetric history

Spontaneous abortions were classified as early (before the 12th week) or late (after the 13th week) and primary (all pregnancies ended in spontaneous abortions) or secondary (at least one live birth). This classification is often adopted in relation to recurrent spontaneous abortion, but it is somewhat ambiguous: to which group should women with a personal history of stillbirth, ectopic or molar pregnancies be allocated? Most women had rather dramatic histories, and quite a few seemed to have accumulated problems which were probably merely coincidental, like recurrent miscarriages, infertility or early neonatal death. No hasty conclusions should be drawn from this kind of information, because, as in other centres caring for recurrent pregnancy failure, the Belgian women belong to a highly selected population. Characteristics are nevertheless described in Table 1 and compared with characteristics in 100

Table 1

Personal and family history in 100 women with recurrent pregnancy failure (RPF) compared to 100 consecutive antenatal women (C)

	RPF	C
First Trimester Miscarriage—< 3	23%	NR
3-4	61%	NR
5-8	16%	
Prior Live Birth—With Other Man	4%	NR
—With Same Man	4%	NR
Second Trimester Abortions	8%	1%
Terminations	8%	8%
Cosanguinous parents	2%	0%
DES Exposure	1%	0%
Family History of Malformation or Handicap	9%	8%
Mother or Sister has/had RPF	7%	0%

NR = not relevant because RPF: self selected group

consecutive antenatal patients. One recurrent aborter has been exposed to DES. This has also been observed by Carp in the Israeli immunisation group. The most interesting point seems to be that nearly one in ten women described RSA to be a family problem. This has been observed by Johnson.[7] Though the true incidence of recurrent spontaneous abortion is not known, the highest reported rate[8] is 0.4% in 14000 reproductive histories. A positive family history in 8% of our patients is clearly higher than one would expect. If the familial trait in recurrent spontaneous abortion can be confirmed in other centres, it might point towards a genetic component determining a susceptibility to variable paternal challenge such as Sutherland *et al*, 1981,[9] have shown for pre-eclampsia. Family histories did not reveal much else. Two couples were blood related. These consanguineous couples are at increased risk of preterm birth, perinatal mortality and congenital anomalies[10] and it is questionable whether any intervention aimed at avoiding miscarriages is warranted in these couples.

B. Laboratory investigations

A very exhaustive testing of candidates was performed; this was aimed more at gaining insight into the problem than at direct clinical decision making. Investigations were made in accordance with guidelines given by Mowbray, Stray-Pederson, Harger, Poland and others.[3,11,12,13] Results can be seen in Tables 2 and 3, and were in keeping with what has been described by the aforementioned authors.

Table 2
General investigations in recurrent spontaneous abortion (N = 72)

Hysterosalpingogram
Normal in all early recurrent spontaneous abortions

Spermiogram
Teratospermia
Decreased count   7 cases
Decreased mobility

Parental karyotype
1 Turner Mosaic
2 Translocations

Infection (Serology + Swabs)
No Chlamydia; AIDS; Herpes.
Ureaplasma or Mycoplasma in 50% of women (= local prevalence)

Endocrinology
Increased Androgens (Testo, Free Testo, DHEAS, 17OHP, Androtestosterone, at end of Luteal phase) in 1/3 of women.
No Anomalous OGTT or Thyroid tests.
No Subclinical Pregnancies (HCG).

Table 3
Immunological investigations in
recurrent spontaneous abortion (N = 72)

Lymphocytotoxic Antibodies
(CMC-NIH standard reaction)
+ in 3 women before immunisation.

"Autoimmune" Anomalies
Minor coag. defects   7
Specific markers   1
    Anticardiolipin
    Lupus anticardiolipin
    Antinuclear antibody

Parental karyotype was normal in all but three cases: one Turner mosaic and two translocations. All these patients were accepted for immunisation and were offered amniocentesis for fetal karyotyping.

Hysterosalpingogram (HSG) was strictly normal in all women with early recurrent miscarriage. This is not in keeping with published data: in these anomalous HSGs are present in 15% of cases,[11,14] and even 27%.[12] To what extent recurrent spontaneous abortion can be ascribed to the malformations, and whether surgical correction of these is a first choice intervention is an open question.[15]

358 Study Group: Early Pregnancy Loss

Sperm analysis was abnormal in 7 cases. It is questionable whether these patients are good candidates for immunotherapy.

Bacteriological assessment included endocervical swabs but not endometrial biopsies were performed. There were no cases of herpes, listeria mono-cytogenes or chlamydia. Almost half the patients were positive for either Ureaplasma urealyticum or Mycoplasma hominis. This prevalence rate is the same as that found in the antenatal clinic.

Serological tests for HIV and Brucella abortus were performed; they were all negative. Though they have been recommended, their utility may be questioned.

Endocrinological assessment included oral glucose tolerance test (OGTT), thyroid tests, HCG at end of cycles to diagnose subclinical pregnancies and assays for LH, FSH, estradiol, progesterone, 17OH progesterone, DHEAS testosterone, free testosterone and androstenedione, these were repeated every 3 days starting at ovulation.

All GTTs were normal. This is in agreement with data from Crane and Wahl,[16] which showed that spontaneous—including repetitive—abortion was not more frequent in women with frank or gestational diabetes.

There were no subclinical pregnancies nor abnormal thyroid tests.

Almost one-third of tested patients showed an increase in one or more of the androgen assays on at least one occasion. This is difficult to interpret, because we have no normal controls. Yet if this were an effect of random variation one would expect to see values not only above the normal range, but also below. This observation is in keeping with that made by Beard to the effect that ultrasound scanning in recurrent abortion showed an excess of polycystic ovaries.

Patients were tested for anticardiolipin, lupus anticoagulant and antinuclear antibody. Only one patient was positive. This again is very variable from one unit to another. Though the test is well standardised, anticardiolipin is present in more than 10% of patients in Unander and Lindholm's series,[6] while results from Reznikoff-Etievant et al[17] are similar to ours.

Table 4

HLA sharing in recurrent spontaneous abortion			
	A	B	DR
—Our data (N = 72)			
(True couples)	50%	30%	42%
(Sham couples)	34%	18%	30%
—Review MF Reznikoff (N = 154)			
SRA	51%	38%	48%
Controls	44%	28%	29%
"Rare" antigen sharing			
—Our data (N = 72)			
True couples		13%	
Sham couples		2%	
Rare: Present in 10% of population			
Total HLA sharing			
	RSA	Controls	
—Our data (N = 72 + 72)	21%	5%	
—Reznikoff data (N = 109 + 47)	15%	4%	

There is much discussion as to what is an adequate marker of immunological recognition for antipaternal antibodies in normal pregnancy. The Belgian group followed Mowbray's protocol[3]: cytotoxic crossmatch of maternal serum against paternal lymphocytes was performed using the NIH crossmatch technique (complement mediated colouring). Three women were positive, two of them were nevertheless accepted for immunisation.

Like many authors[18] we had excess HLA sharing in our couples, this was true for group I and group II MHC complexes and remained true for rare antibody sharing (Table 4).

PROTOCOL

Fifty-nine patients were immunised with Lymphoprep gradient purified lymphocytes from the father. The Belgian protocol differs quite considerably from other protocols.

Route of administration

A purely intravenous route was selected. This approach was dictated by two considerations. Firstly, there have been descriptions, following subcutaneous immunisation, both of severe, if exceptional, anaphylactic reactions, and of pyrexia occurring not infrequently. Uncertainties persist concerning the possible teratogenic role of hyperthermia in early pregnancy.[19] This double risk was felt to be unacceptable. Secondly, a wide experience had already been gained by one of us (MD) with intravenous immunisation to generate antibodies for typing of renal transplants.

Dosage

All over the world, varying quantities have been used. The Belgian protocol used 50 million paternal lymphocytes, which is similar to the quantity injected by Beer *et al*,[4] but ten times less than the quantities used by Mowbray *et al*[3] or Reznikoff-Etievant's[20] team.

Repeat immunisation

Immunisation was repeated monthly or until cytotoxic antibodies appeared. The total number of immunisations received by a single patient ranged from one to twenty. A few patients were given donor lymphocytes when paternal ones failed to bring on cytotoxic antibodies.

RESULTS OF IMMUNISATION

Fifty-nine women were immunisd using this protocol. Antibodies appeared in 64% of cases. This is a lower conversion rate than those obtained by Mowbray or Reznikoff, who both achieved more than 80% conversion, using a multiple route (IV; SC; ID) and lymphocytes from one pint of blood. A cumulative graph of the rate of conversion with successive immunisations shows that up to the 5th immunisation the rate is linear (Figure I). After the 5th immunisation the rate slows down, and after 9 immunisations no more women developed cytotoxic antibodies. When non-converting women were treated with donor lymphocytes, a few more converted.

There was no relation between the appearance of cytotoxic antibodies and HLA sharing. Two-thirds of the women developed cytotoxic antibodies; this was true both of the 15 women who shared 3 or more HLA loci and of the 44 who had two or less than two common HLA sites.

Figure I

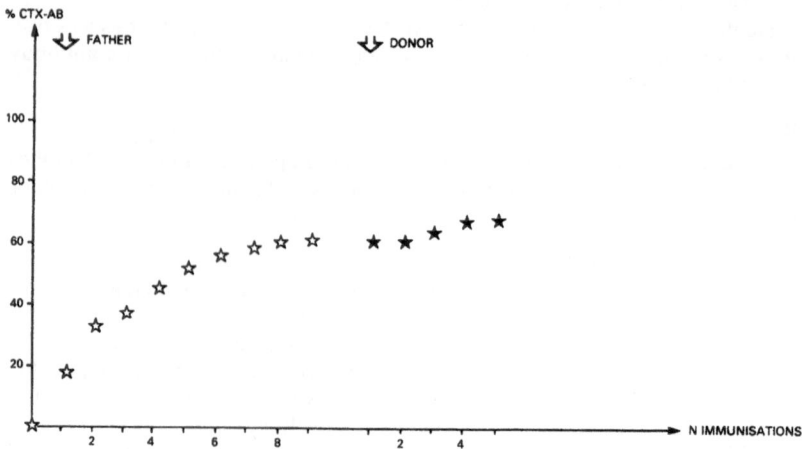

OUTCOME

Immunised women became pregnant, and in 24 of them pregnancy went beyond 16 weeks. The success rate of 80% is therefore similar to that reported by other groups.[6,21] For comparability's sake, we shall consider only women who had experienced 3 or more RSA; of these 26 became pregnant, and in 20 cases pregnancy continued beyond 16 weeks, which is still 80% success.

Again, a classification problem arises: one woman was immunised, had a repeat miscarriage, went on with immunisation and then had a successful pregnancy. A third category has to be established for women with mixed outcome.

A total of 27 pregnancies which did not end in recurrent early spontaneous abortion was recorded for 24 immunised women (three women were pregnant twice). There were four late fetal bad outcomes: one Turner's syndrome, one non-immune hydrops fetalis, one anencephalic and one abruptio placentae.

There were 23 live born babies, one severely growth retarded, the mother having developed preeclamptic toxaemia. Among the other babies there was no excess of preterm births or small for dates.

One father committed suicide just after delivery, while mother and child were still in hospital. Psychological stress in infertility treatment is a well known problem. Though this unfortunate case may well be unrelated to our management, we feel it worth reporting, in the hope that other centres involved in immunisation should recognise and treat emotional disruption related to treatment.

Table 5 shows pregnancy outcome in relation to HLA sharing and to CTX antibodies. Successful outcomes were not more likely when there was an excess of HLA sharing. If this remains true in a larger series, the validity of one of the selection criteria used by Beer 1987 (sharing three of more HLA Class I and Class II antigens) should be questioned.

Table 5

Pregnancy outcome in relation to HLA sharing and CTX antibodies

		Failures	Success	Total
HLA sharing < 3		4	18	22
≥ 3		2	6	8
	Total	6	24	30
CTX AB −		2	10	12
+		4	14	18
	Total	6	24	30

It was also surprising to us that there was no relation between developing CTX antibodies and successful outcome. In Reznikoff's 1987 group[17] successful outcome was significantly more likely when cytotoxic antibodies were developed.

CONCLUSION

In the Belgian group, immunisation of recurrent aborters was performed, using a repeated small quantity of immunogen by the intravenous route. Fewer women developed antibodies with this protocol than with more widely diffused protocols, yet results in terms of pregnancy outcome are similar to those of the best groups.

There are still many uncertainties regarding immunisation in human recurrent aborters: What is the true prevalence of recurrent abortion? How likely is a woman to have a successful pregnancy without treatment? What is the importance of the placebo effect?

A first answer to this comes from the St Mary's double-blind randomised trial,[22] in which women received either their own or their husband's lymphocytes. There was a dramatic difference between the groups, with 63% repeat miscarriages in the placebo group and 23% in the treated group! Because of small numbers in each group (respectively 27 and 22), the lower confidence limit (P = 95%) is 0.98, i.e. it is still possible that there was no benefit to the paternally immunised groups. There is scope for a multicentre randomised controlled trial. Some centres will find it difficult to participate. Their assumption is that, in 1987, immunisation is the best treatment we can offer women with early recurrent miscarriages. For these centres many more practical questions arise: should one test the immune status of the women with cytotoxic antibodies? Using which technique? With mixed lymphocyte reaction? Is there a case for reviewing punctuation? What quantity of immunogen should one give? By which route?

Should one repeat immunisation? Until antibodies appear? In pregnancy? What is the role of HLA sharing? Of CTX antibodies? For these units there is a need to mount an international register; similar registers have been established and allowed much more progress, in the field of renal transplantation and chorion villous sampling.

REFERENCES
1. Hawkins DF. Sex hormones in pregnancy. In: *Obstetric therapeutics. Clinical pharmacology and therapeutics in obstetric practice*. Ed. DF Hawkins. London: Baillere Tindall, 1974; pp.106-150.
2. Stirrat GM. Recurrent abortion—a review. *Brit J Obstet Gynaecol* 1983; **90:** 881-883.
3. Mowbray JF, Gibbings CR, Sidgwick AS, Ruszkiewicz M, Beard RW. Effects of transfusion in women with recurrent spontaneous abortion. *Transplant Pro* 1983; **XV:** 896-899.
4. Beer AE, Shekar SS, Quebbeman JF, Xhu X. Paternal and nonpaternal leukocyte immunization in women with recurrent spontaneous abortions: Immune responses and subsequent pregnancy outcome. In: *Immunologie de la réproduction: relation materno-foetale*. Ed. G Chaouat. Colloques INSERM, 1987; **154:** 161-178.
5. Taylor C, Faulk WP. Prevention of recurrent abortion with leucocyte transfusions. *Lancet* 1981; **2:** 68-69.
6. Unander AM, Lindholm A. Transfusions of leucocyte-rich erythrocyte concentrates: A successful treatment in selected cases of habitual abortion. *Amer J Obstet Gynecol* 1986; **154:** 516-520.
7. Johnson PM, Kirkpatrick DC. HLA sharing in pregnancy. *Lancet* 1984; **2:** 1122-1123.
8. Naylor AF, Warburton D. Sequential analysis of spontaneous abortion. II. Collaborative study data show that gravidity determines a very substantial rise in risk. *Fertil Steril* 1979; **31:** 282-286.
9. Sutherland A, Cooper DW, Howie PW, Liston WA, MacGillivray I. The incidence of severe pre-eclampsia amongst mothers and mothers-in-law of pre-eclamptics and controls. *Brit J Obstet Gynaecol* 1981; **88:** 785-791.
10. Naderi S. Congenital abnormalities in newborns of consanguinous and non-consanguinous parents. *Obstet Gynecol* 1979; **53:** 195-199.
11. Stray-Pedersen B, Stray-Pedersen S. Etiologic factors and subsequent reproductive performance in 195 couples with a prior history of habitual abortion. *Amer J Obstet Gynecol* 1984; **148:** 140-146.
12. Harger JH, Archer DF, Marchese SG, Muracca-Clemens M, Garver KL. Etiology of recurrent pregnancy losses and outcome of subsequent pregnancies. *Obstet Gynecol* 1983; **62:** 574-581.
13. Poland BJ. Recurrent spontaneous abortion. *Eur J Obstet Gynecol Reprod Biol* 1984; **16:** 369-375.
14. Tho TP, Byrd JR, McDonough PG. Etiology and subsequent reproductive performance of 100 couples with recurrent abortion. *Fertil Steril* 1979; **32:** 389-395.
15. Underwood JL, Mowbray JF. Treatment of recurrent spontaneous abortion. *Clin Immunol Aller* 1985; **5:** 33-42.
16. Crane JP, Wahl N. The role of maternal diabetes in repetitive spontaneous abortion. *Fertil Steril* 1981; **36:** 477-479.
17. Reznikoff-Etievant MF, Durieux I, Huchet J, Salmon Ch, Netter A. Recurrent spontaneous abortions, HLA antigen sharing and anti-paternal immunity. Immunotherapic assay. In: *Immunologie de la réproduction: relation materno-foetale*. Ed. G Chaouat. Colloques INSERM, 1987; **154:** pp.187-201.
18. Oksenberg JR, Persitz E, Amar A, Schenker J, Segal S, Nelken D, Brautbar C. Mixed lymphocyte reactivity nonresponsiveness in couples with multiple spontaneous abortions. *Fertil Steril* 1983; **39:** 525-529.

19. Smith DW, Sterling KC, Sedgwick Harvey MA. Hyperthermia as a possible teratogenic agent. *J Paediatr* 1978; **92:** 878-883.
20. Reznikoff-Etievant MF, Simmoney N, Janau A, Darbois Y, Netter A. Treatment of recurrent spontaneous abortions by immunisation with paternal leucocytes. *Lancet* 1985; **1:** 1398.
21. Mowbray JF, Underwood JL. Immunisation with paternal cells for recurrent spontaneous abortion. In: *Immunologie de la réproduction: relation materno-foetale.* Ed. G Chaouat. Colloques INSERM, 1987; **154:** pp.179-186.
22. Mowbray JF, Liddell H, Underwood JL, Gibbings C, Reginald PW, Beard RW. Controlled trial of treatment of recurrent spontaneous abortion by immunisation with paternal cells. *Lancet* 1985; **1:** 941-943.

Discussion

Chairman: Professor J Mowbray

Dr CARP: Can I just put it to you that you mention that it took a long time in some patients for them to develop cytotoxic antibody after repeated doses. That is probably a dose-related effect, because we found in our population when we used a 50 cc immunising dose with two immunisations, only 36% of patients converted; at 75 cc it went up to 65% of patients; and with 100 cc and two immunisations it went up to 78% of patients. So we put up the dose.

Dr ALEXANDER: I am sure that the route you select, and the quantity you give is going to have an effect on your conversion of cytotoxic antibodies. What I am not sure is if the appearance of cytotoxic antibodies has anything to do with the outcome.

Professor MOWBRAY: It doesn't in your series, or in our series, whereas in Professor Beer's series it shows an adverse effect.

Dr CARP: In our series it does help, quite significantly.

Professor BEER: How can you say that, Dr Carp, and how can we be so caught up with cytoxic antibodies? It is a very easy test to do, and I think we are making a big deal out of it in trying to say that its presence is associated with a good outcome or a bad outcome. I don't think any of us can say that.

Professor ALBERMAN: First of all, thank you enormously for a paper that I can understand. There were implications there that I think shouldn't be lost, and taken together with James Mowbray's comment that the binovular twinning rate may go up because the second set is lost. The fact that you have a Turner and an anencephalic in that small series makes me very worried that we may be stopping the normal protective mechanism.

Dr RHODES: Maybe I misunderstood your results, but you said that you started with 59 couples that you immunised, and 30 had a pregnancy. How does that work out to an 80% success rate?

Dr ALEXANDER: To arrive at the success rate—out of the women who become pregnant, you count how many deliver a live child. That is how you calculate the success rate.

Dr RHODES: You are not calculating from the total number that entered the trial?

Dr ALEXANDER: That would depend on your recruitment rate. If you suddenly started, and just immunised 100 women and none were pregnant 8-9 months after being immunised, you would have 0%.

Dr RHODES: Among the groups of challenge that you have been discussing is one that I find absent that is used in livestock production, which is putting the lymphocyte challenge right into the uterus. I wondered if that was feasible in the human?

Dr ALLEN: What route would they use?

Dr RHODES: Intrauterine.

Dr ALLEN: Yes, but just into the cavity, or injection into the myometrium?

Dr RHODES: By passing an AI rod loaded with lymphocytes right into the uterus.

Dr ALLEN: That is awkward!

Professor MOWBRAY: Each intrauterine artificial insemination must put 50,000 paternal lymphocytes into the cavity.

Dr RHODES: In the pig, which is the species that this is done in, they have used both porcine lymphocytes, or bovine lymphocytes, and they are reporting an increase of two offspring born per litter.

Mr EDMONDS: I would like to comment on that, because it may have nothing to do with the uterus because those lymphocytes will be in the peritoneal cavity. And if you just look a few hours later you will find them there, so you might as well just inject them intraperitoneally.

Dr RHODES: But is a mucosal challenge of the uterus not an appropriate way to deliver the lymphocyte challenge?

Professor MOWBRAY: Are you not extrapolating spermatazoa to lymphocytes.?

Dr ALLEN: Not at all. If you take latex particles and place them at the cervix, two hours later you will find them in the peritoneal cavity, so it doesn't really make much difference.

Professor BEER: I would like to defend Allen. I have done a lot of intrauterine immunisations, and essentially it is as effective with lymphocytes as injecting by other routes. So we place our application of leucocytes into a rat or mouse uterus and not into the peritoneal cavity as in the human.

Dr PAGE-FAULK: Can I simply say that the absence of cytotoxic antibody following what is a considerable dose of antigen has been viewed by some investigators as simply meaning the presence of autoanti-idiotype to the necessary toxic antibody. There have been groups that have looked into this rather more seriously, and have shown that you can remove the anti-idiotype from the cytotoxic antibody and show that the lymphocyte cytotoxic antibody is actually there. Now if we believe some of the existing or growing dogma in mammalian reproduction, the presence of autoanti-idiotype is rather more good than bad. So, I would not be surprised that you found a rather low incidence of lymphocyte cytotoxic antibodies. I would only be surprised if you found a high incidence.

Dr ALEXANDER: Sixty percent and 80% is of the same order of magnitude.

Professor BEARD: What is the view of the medical community about this as an on-going form of therapy?

Dr ALEXANDER: There is much demand. More demand than we can treat among a third of these 16 cases of patients who got immunisation after only two abortions. It is not the National Health System; you can't say "No".

Professor BEARD: Do you believe that you need to do all the investigations as a preliminary that you are doing now before doing the full immunisation? Or have you been able to weed out some?

Dr ALEXANDER: I would be scared of not doing them all.

Immunotherapy in recurrent spontaneous abortion: who, how, outcome

C. G. Taylor, J. G. Hill, N. A. Maclachlan, J. K. Wilson, P. R. Apps, M. F. Robards.

INTRODUCTION

The first report of successful pregnancies following immunotherapy in patients with recurrent spontaneous abortion (RSA) was published by the Pembury Unit.[1]

WHO

Couples were tested to exclude anatomical, hormonal, chromosomal and other recognised causes of RSA. They were then immunologically investigated. HLA typing of both partners was performed. The presence of antipaternal lymphocytotoxic antibody was determined, if found it was considered to be a contraindication to random donor white cell therapy. A group a couples was therefore identified and considered suitable for this treatment.

HOW

Immunotherapy for these couples suffering RSA involved administration of white cell concentrates from random donors as previously described by Taylor and Faulk.[1] Whole blood was taken into standard acid/citrate/dextrose donor packs and kept for at least three days to reduce the risk of cytomegalovirus infection. All blood was tested for HBsAg by the 'hepatest' technique and also, since testing has been available, for HIV infection. The buffy coats from each unit were removed but the lymphocyte population was not separated from the other white cells, since to do this would increase the chance of accidentally infecting the white cell concentrates. The patients were typed for ABC, Rhesus, Kell, Duffy, Lewis, Kidd and MNSs blood groups. The erythrocyte groups of the donor units were selected in order not to stimulate red cell antibodies in the mother, and all red cells were cross-matched against maternal sera. Prior to pregnancy, transfusions were given on two occasions three weeks apart. Once pregnancy was confirmed further transfusions were given at three week intervals until sixteen weeks gestation. Viability of the fetus was confirmed by ultrasound scan prior to each transfusion.

All complications of blood transfusion were discussed with the patients, including hepatitis and HIV infection. Fully informed consent for treatment was obtained from both partners.

OUTCOME

All the mothers in this series have remained well since therapy. The outcome of pregnancies occurring in mothers with a history of RSA prior to immunotherapy is associated with small-for-gestational age infants, prematurity, a high perinatal mortality rate and an increase in congenital abnormalities.[2-7] These parameters in our series are shown in Figures I-III.

Figure I

Histogram demonstrating distribution of gestational age at time of delivery

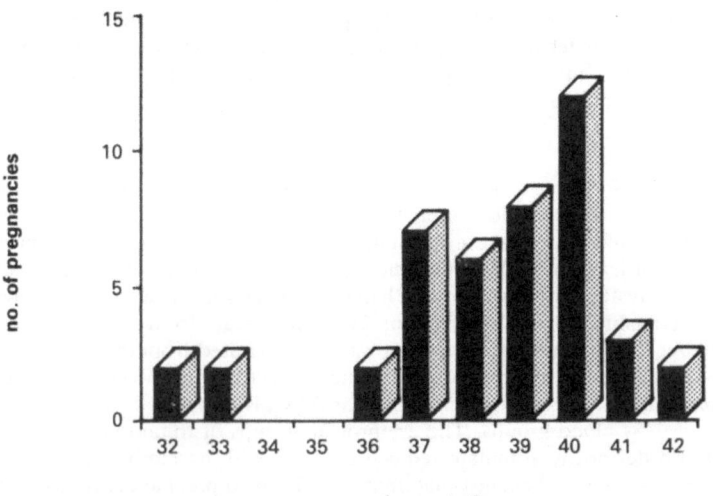

weeks gestation

Figure II

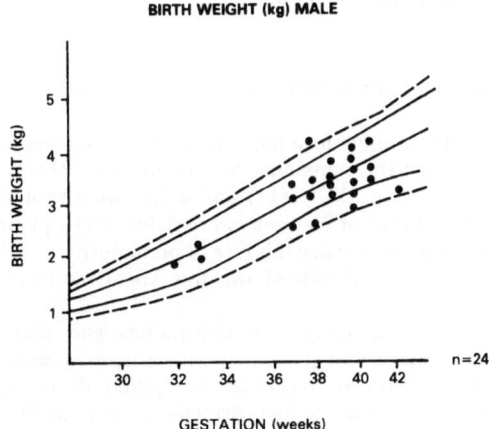

Figure III

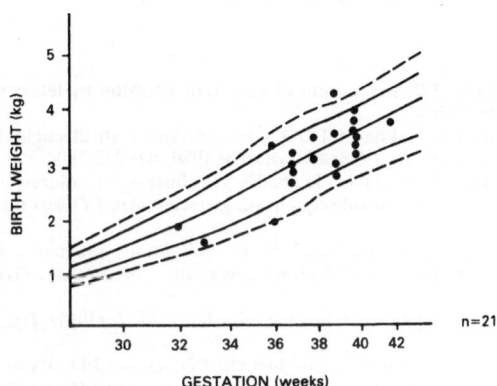

LOW APGAR SCORES

Mean score at 1 minute:- 7.9 (SEM ± 0.26)
Mean score at 5 minutes:- 9.3 (SEM ± 0.11)

CONGENITAL ABNORMALITIES

There were three infants with congenital abnormalities; these were hypospadias, cleft lip and palate and oesophageal atresia.

DISCUSSION

Following treatment with third party leucocytes the incidence of SGA infants is not increased.

Seven infants were delivered before the 37th week of pregnancy. Two of these were twins (32 weeks). Of the remaining 5, 1 infant was delivered following a suspected placental abruption (33 weeks) and 2 following spontaneous labour (33 weeks). Both infants borns at 36 weeks were delivered by planned caesarean section. Excluding the twin pregnancy this rate of prematurity is slightly above the normal population rate. As is clearly shown the Apgar scores of these infants were normal.

There were 3 babies with congenital deformities and also one with an inherited disorder. The mother of the infant with a tracheo-oesophageal fistula suffered ulcerative colitis, and she received selazopyrine during her pregnancy. The child with the cleft lip and palate had corrective surgery and he is developing normally. A mild case of hypospadias occurred in a baby whose uncle also had this condition. One child inherited osteogenesis imperfecta from his father. Despite genetic counselling the parents chose to proceed with treatment. It appears that there is an increased incidence of congenital abnormalities in this group of infants which may represent a higher rate than the standard population rate.

The data we have accumulated during this long term follow up enables us to state confidently that immunotherapy has had no significant adverse effects on either the development of the infants or on the mothers' health.

REFERENCES
1. Taylor CG, Faulk WP. Prevention of recurrent abortion by leucocyte transfusions. *Lancet* 1981; **2:** 68-70.
2. Alberman E, Roman E, Pharoh POD, Chamberlain G. Birthweights before and after spontaneous abortion. *Br J Obstet Gynaecol* 1980; **87:** 275-280.
3. Pontelakis S, Papadimitriou G, Doxiadis S. Influence of induced and spontaneous abortion on the outcome of subsequent pregnancies. *Am J Obstet Gynecol* 1973; **116:** 799-805.
4. Funderburk S J, Guthrie D, Meldrum D. Suboptimal pregnancy outcome among women with prior abortions and premature births. *Am J Obstet Gynecol* 1976; **126:** 55-60.
5. McNaughton M. Pregnancy following abortion. *Br J Obstet Gynaecol* 1961; **68:** 789-792.
6. Schoenbaum SC, Manson RR, Stubblefield PG, Domy PD, Ryan K. Outcome of delivery following induced and spontaneous delivery. *Am J Obstet Gynecol* 1980; **136:** 19-24.
7. Reginald PW, Beard RW, Chappel J, Forbes PB, Liddell HS, Mowbray JF, Underwood JL. Outcome of pregnancies progressing beyond 28 weeks gestation in women with a history of recurrent miscarriage. *Br J Obstet Gynaecol* 1987; **94:** 643-648.

Discussion

Chairman: Professor J Mowbray

Professor GILL: I didn't quite get the comparisons with the normal population that you used.

Dr TAYLOR: That is published data from several sources on what one might expect in a pregnancy which has occurred without treatment. Most people are treated, but when one is presented with a woman finally who has had a string of previous abortions, presumably she has not had immunotherapy. Several authors report those kind of abnormal findings. So it would seem to be part of the pathogenesis of spontaneous recurrent abortion. We did perhaps correct the birthweight problem. One would have to have 200 babies or more to really find a significant number.

Professor GILL: Is it high relative to what you would expect?

Dr TAYLOR: High relative to the normal population, yes.

Professor GILL: How about as compared to spontaneous aborters who are not treated?

Dr TAYLOR: Well, if one believes the information, probably not.

Professor GILL: It is about the same? Both of them are higher than normal?

Dr TAYLOR: I think that inference can be drawn, yes.

Professor BEARD: Can we just get the figures right? We are dealing with 45 babies, and there are one or two anomalies in what you have said. In my calculation, you had 14 babies that were less than 38 weeks, which is the definition of prematurity.

Dr TAYLOR: I am not quite sure of this definition of prematurity; I am not sure if it applies.

Professor BEARD: I think you have to take them out. As you can see in the less than 37 week group you have got something like 7, and you have got 6 more in the 37-38 week group, so that is 13 or 14. This gives a prematurity rate of 30% which is three times the normal rate.

Dr TAYLOR: I actually think that we still have problems with prematurity, and I wouldn't disagree with your remarks. The only thing that we appear to have corrected is the actual birthweights, which I think is significant. But as for prematurity, I think there is more than a hint of its continuing as a problem.

Professor BEARD: The only other point that I want to make is that all the published work on these series showing the outcome of pregnancies in women who have a tendency to miscarry, whether they have had one or more, show that there is no significant increase in the incidence of malformations. So that if we are starting to show malformations, (our group hasn't, but we have heard two presentations where this is the case) then that would be about three times above the normal background rate.

Dr BILLINGTON: I understand that you have some experience in treating patients with pre-existing cytotoxic antibody, and I wonder if you could tell us about this. I am asking because we have heard this morning evidence that the existence of these has no predictive value whether they appear before pregnancy or after immunisation. I wonder whether at the present moment there is any justification for excluding women from treatment who do have pre-existing antibody.

Dr TAYLOR: We have found very little correlation between success or failure. I personally don't think it has a predictive value. Some time ago I treated a small number of women with cytotoxic antibody, and we had no success at all. But that was a small number of cases, and I wouldn't want to comment on the success rate, which was literally zero, which is in contrast to immunotherapy now.

Human MHC antigens and paternal leucocyte injections in recurrent spontaneous abortions

M. F. Reznikoff-Etievant, I. Durieux, J. Huchet,
C. Salmon and A. Netter

INTRODUCTION

A large proportion of recurrent spontaneous abortions (RSAs) remain unexplained; but recently many observations during both normal and pathological pregnancies underline the possibility of an immunological aetiology.

Immune responses to foreign antigens do not differ very much in pregnant or non-pregnant women; so far, a variety of immunological mechanisms have been investigated to explain the paradoxical tolerance of the mother to the fetus. Among these, enhancing, anti-idiotype and blocking antibodies have been observed to protect the fetal placental unit in normal pregnancies and to be deficient in unexplained early fetal losses.[1,2,3] An alloantigenic system has been described which is perhaps linked to the major histocompatibility complex.[4] It corresponds to a trophoblast antigen cross-reacting with leucocytes (TLX) and is supposed to stimulate enhancing immune factors. This concept may explain the increased HLA compatibility reported within couples who suffer from idiopathic RSAs[5-12] although not in all studies.[13-20]

In the light of the immunological explanations of RSAs, and the enhancing effect of blood transfusions in organ transplantation, immunomodulating therapies have been tested in RSA women, by injecting either the husband's leucocytes[21,22,23] or unrelated ones.[24,25,26]

Within this context, we report the results of our HLA studies in RSAs combined with twenty other studies, and also our results of antipaternal immunisation with paternal leucocytes injections in these patients.

PATIENTS AND METHODS

a) HLA Study:

1) In our own work, 129 caucasian women with three or more confirmed RSAs of unknown aetiology were selected. All these abortions occurred with the same partner, in the first trimester of the pregnancies. There were 111 women with

primary abortions, having had no previous live birth and 18 women with secondary abortions, having had one living child and then three or more abortions.

Gynaecological, endocrinological, chromosomal or infectious reasons for habitual fetal loss, cosanguinity and arterial hypertension were excluded. Furthermore, none of these women had abnormal thyroid function tests, lupus anticoagulant, pathological anti-nuclear antibody nor clinical evidence of an auto-immune disease. Forty-seven normally fertile couples were specially selected for having had at least 2 or more normal children and no history of fetal loss. HLA-A, B and DR typing were performed as previously described.[5]

2) We gathered the results of 13 previously published results[7-19] and 7 personal communications, willingly sent to us in 1986 for this study (Blangero et al, 10 RSA couples; Bonneau et al, 12 RSA couples; Fizet et al, 26 RSA couples; Gerencer, 105 RSA couples; Gebuhrer et al, 35 RSA couples; Johnson et al, 104 RSA couples; Roche et al, 16 RSA couples).[27] That is to say 21 studies including our own were collated to make up a total of 1154 RSA couples. Full clinical investigations were carried out on 831 couples. One hundred and sixty-six couples were not investigated for lupus anticoagulant, anti-nuclear antibody and thyroid function tests. Finally, 157 couples were selected as having had RSAs without precise clinical selection criteria. There were 1071 control couples with 2 or more normal children and no history of abortion.

b) Antipaternal Immunisation:
We studied the anti-HLA and anti-paternal antibodies in 129 women with RSAs; 111 of them had primary RSAs and 18 had secondary RSAs in the first trimester of the pregnancy. Anti-HLA and anti-paternal immunisation was performed as previously described.[5,23] Husband's T and B lymphocytes as well as T and B autologous lymphocytes were used through the lymphocytotoxicity test to detect the anti-paternal antibodies in the wives' sera.

c) Paternal Leucocyte Injections:
Seventy-two among the anti-paternal negative women were immunised with their husbands' leucocytes. Two hundred million cells were prepared by Ficoll/Triosil separation and 150 million were injected intravenously. Fifty million were injected by ID and SC routes.[23] One to three injections were given after an interval of one month, until anti-paternal antibodies were produced. These antibodies were sought 3 weeks after each injection. No more than three injections were given even if the women did not produce any evidence of antipaternal antibodies.

RESULTS
a) HLA Study
1) Figure I shows a significantly increased HLA-DR homology in RSA couples. This result is similar in both primary and secondary abortion groups.

Figure I

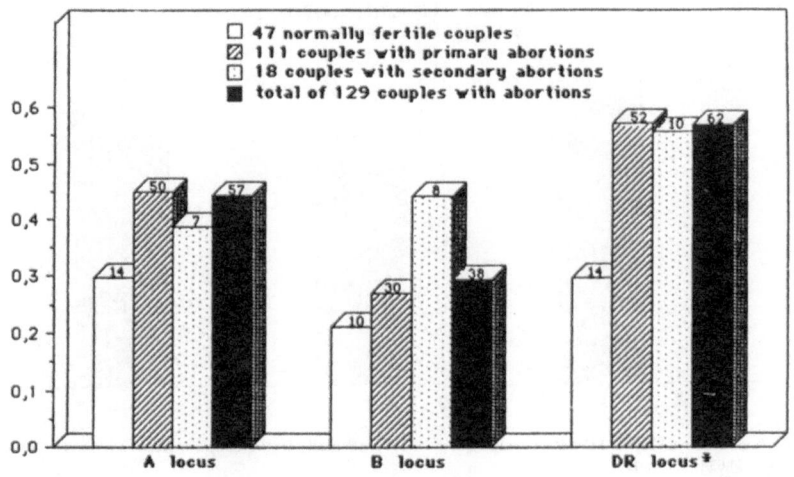

HLA antigen sharing in 129 couples with recurrent abortions
*only 91 out of the primary abortions were tested for the DR locus $-\chi = 9.29$ (p < 0.01)

We do not confirm our previous findings of a significantly increased HLA-Dr5 in both partners of RSA couples.[5] We observe an increased number of HLA antigen shared in this RSA group compared with the control couples, but the result is not statistically significant (Table 1).

Table 1
Number of HLA antigen sharings in RSA couples and normally fertile couples.
*X = 3.50

	number of antigen sharings	
	0 to 2	3 to 6*
RSA couples	93 (85.7%)	16 (14.6%)
47 control couples	45 (95.7%)	2 (4.3%)

2) The results of the 21 studies are the following:

There is no unanimity about the possible association between a particular HLA antigen and RSA: statistically increased Dr5 in both partners and slightly increased HLA-A9 in the wives are reported by Gerencer[6] and confirmed in a larger study by the same authors (personal communication); elevated HLA-B35,[9] HLA-B58[18] and HLA-A10.[15]

Figure II

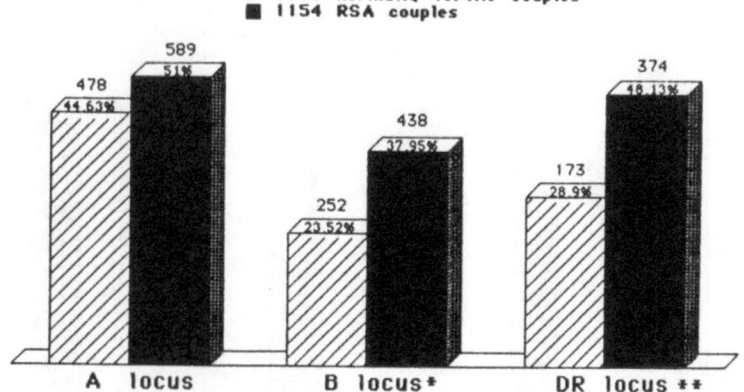

☑ 1071 normally fertile couples
■ 1154 RSA couples

HLA antigen sharing in 1154 RSA couples and in 1071 normally fertile couples. Results from 21 studies.
* X = 54.03 (p < 0.001)
**777 RSA couples and 598 control couples were tested for the DR locus
('78 RSA couples and 62 control couples were tested for Dw)
X^2 = 79.17 (p < 0.001)

There is a higher increase of HLA DR and B antigen sharing in RSA couples compared with the controls (Figure II).

By gathering studies with the appropriate information:

a) References 12, 18, 26, 2 personal communications (Blangero and Roche) and ours, we observe an increased number of HLA antigens shared among the RSA couples (Table 2).

Table 2

Number of HLA antigen sharings in RSA couples and normally fertile couples, results of 5 studies.

| | number of antigen sharings | |
	0 to 2	3 to 6*
302 RSA couples	265 (86.6%)	41 (13.4%)
182 control couples	180 (99%)	2 (1%)

*X^2 = 21.49 (p < 0.001)

b) Johnson's personal communication and ours, show that the results are similar in both primary and secondary RSAs (Table 3).

b) Anti-Paternal Immunisation:

Anti-paternal antibodies were present in 36 out of the 129 RSA women (27.9%). Indeed, only 24 primary aborting women had antipaternal antibodies (21.6%), compared with 12 out of 18 secondary aborting women were (66.6%).

Table 3
HLA antigen sharing in couples with secondary abortions.
Results of 2 studies.

	HLA antigen sharing at locus		
	A	B*	DR**
58 RSA couples	25	22	28
	43.83%	37.9%	48.27%
98 control couples	41	24	27
	41.83%	24.5%	27.55%

* NS
** $X^2 = 6.66$ (P < 0.01)

These antipaternal antibodies are reactive specifically with the husband's B lymphocytes; they are always active at 37C; in a few cases (4%) they are also active at 22C and 4C. Seventy-two percent of them are absorbed on pooled platelets. We did not find any known HLA specificity for 30 of the 36 anti-paternal positive sera.

Figure III

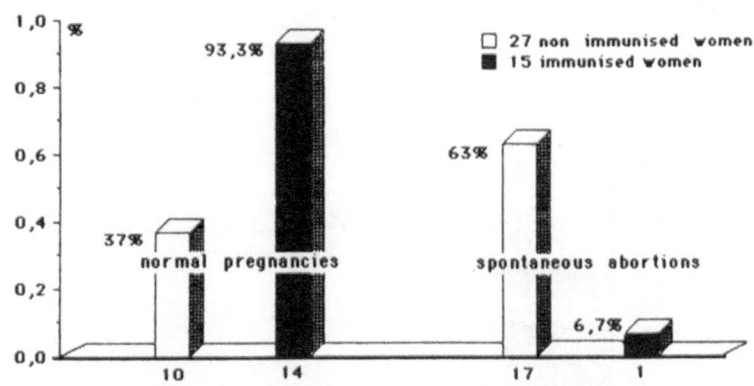

Outcome of 42 new pregnancies and anti-paternal immunisation
129 women have been tested after 3 or more RSAs
27.9% had antibodies against the husband's lymphocytes

Figure III shows that:

1) Anti-paternal immunisation, in women with RSAs, may be a good indicator for a normal outcome of the next pregnancy, since 14 of the 15 women (93.3%) with anti-paternal antibodies who became pregnant, gave birth to healthy babies.

2) On the other hand, in anti-paternal antibody negative women, 63% suffered from a further abortion.

c) **Injection of Husband's Leucocytes:**
After full treatment, the antibody response was as shown in Table 4; the women with secondary abortions seemed to respond more easily to the paternal antigens than the primary aborted women, since 71.5% of the secondary aborting women respond to the first injection compared to only 21.6% in primary aborting women.

Table 4

Number of paternal leucocyte injections necessary to have detectable antibodies.

	Primary abortions n = 65	Secondary abortions n = 7
Immunised women		
after 1 injection	14 (21.6%)	5 (71.5%)
2	19 (29.2%)	0
3	25 (36.9%)	2 (28.5%)
Non immunised women		
after 3 injections	7 (12%)	0

Thirty-five of the 72 treated women became pregnant and 33 delivered normal babies or were beyond the critical period for habitual abortions. The results are shown in Figure IV; the success rate is 84.6%.

Figure IV

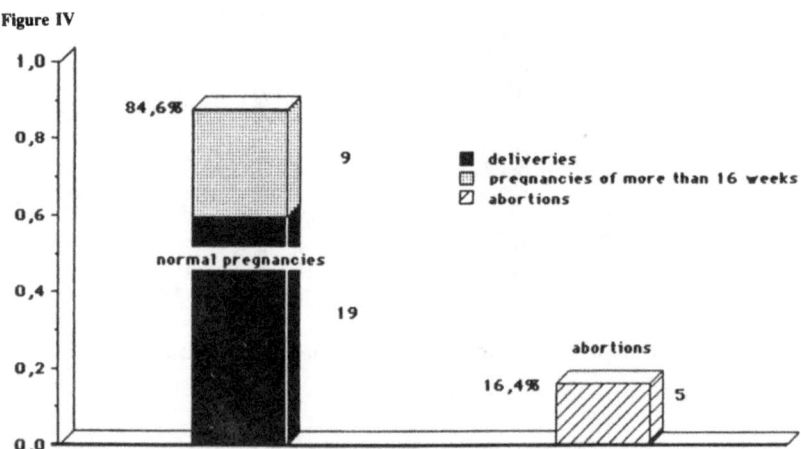

Husband's leucocyte injections. Evolution of 32 new pregnancies.

If we consider the anti-paternal response of the treated women (Figure V), it appears that women with detectable anti-paternal antibodies have a 92.8% chance of having a subsequent normal pregnancy, which is 40% in treated women without antibody, and 37% in unimmunised and untreated women (Figure III).

Figure V

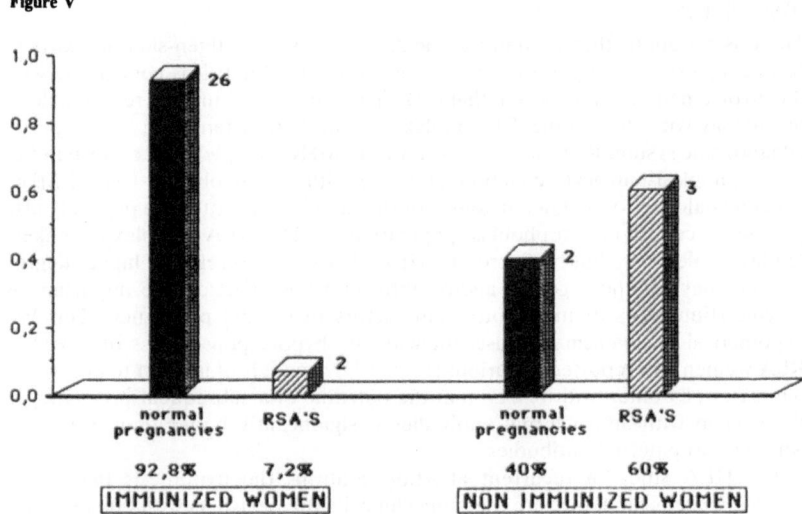

Husband's leucocyte injections. Outcome of a new pregnancy according to the anti-paternal immunisation.

All the babies were normal and had a normal birth weight, although toxaemia occurred in one case (Table 5).

Table 5

Pregnancies and neonates after paternal leucocyte injections
to 72 women.

---

35 pregnancies

19 deliveries: 1 toxaemia, birth at 36 weeks of a boy weighing 2500g.
in good health at 3 years.
18 normal pregnancies:
deliveries between 38 to 41 weeks
11 boys and 7 girls
birth weight: 3330 ± 250g
in good health at 3 months to 3 years
5 RSAs
11 pregnancies evolve normally, 9 are between the 5th and the 8th month

---

The importance of anti-paternal immunisation is underlined in 3 treated women who became pregnant before the end of treatment. These 3 women became pregnant after the first injection despite our recommendation, did not develop anti-paternal antibodies, and all 3 aborted again. Then they received 2 more injections, and developed anti-paternal antibodies; 2 became pregnant and delivered normal babies.

DISCUSSION

There is no doubt that an unusual incidence of HLA antigen-sharing exists in RSA couples; this is open to several interpretations. First, it is compatible with the involvement of a recessive lethal MHC gene or genes[28] in recurrent fetal loss, by analogy with the murine T/t complex. It is also consistent with the proposed alloantigenic system that may be linked to the MHC complex and correspond to the trophoblast-leucocyte common TLX[4] or with a trophoblastic Class I MHC antigen analogue to the Qa antigens[29] of the mouse. The latter are probably also present on certain cytotrophoblast populations.[30] The HLA complex is unlikely to play a role *per se* but the increased HLA sharing could reflect a higher degree of homology for those genes, and/or antigens whose part can be important as specific stimulators of immunotolerant factors in normal pregnancy. This last hypothetical mechanism is consistent with the hyporesponsiveness observed in RSA women and reported in various studies;[1,3,12] and it is of interest to observe in our series of women with RSAs, that the outcome of a subsequent pregnancy in the women with anti-paternal antibodies is significantly better than in women without anti-paternal antibodies.

The HLA study in recurrent abortion confirms the hypothesis that RSAs without a live birth before are the same clinical entity as RSAs with one live birth before, though the latter seem to develop anti-paternal protecting immunisation more easily. More extensive HLA studies in secondary abortions are necessary however to corroborate this point of view.

HLA homology is not a good selective criterion for immunotherapy, as it may also reflect genetic causes of RSAs. The best criterion at the moment, seems to be the lack of paternal immunisation, as has been already used;[22,23] moreover, immunisation of women with pre-existent anti-paternal antibodies seems to hinder the normal outcome of the next pregnancy.[25]

With this immunological selection in our series, only 37% of the RSA women would probably have had normal pregnancies without injections (Figure III), versus 84.6% after repeated paternal leucocyte injections (Figure IV).

This immunotherapy is harmless during pregnancy, at birth or for the child's health; although intra-uterine growth retardation or neonatal immunodeficiency after paternal leucocyte injections have been reported by another group,[8] none of these complications were observed in our experimentation nor in the extensive Mowbray therapeutic study. The reason for this disparity in the therapeutic results is perhaps the consequence of the use of different routes for the injections and the different number of cells injected by Beer: the subcutaneous route only and 10 times fewer paternal cells injected.[8]

REFERENCES
1. Rocklin RE, Kitzmiller JL, Garavoy MR. Materno-fetal relation. II Further characterization of an immunologic blocking factor that develops during pregnancy. *Clin Immunol Immunopathol* 1982; **23:** 303-315.
2. Suciu-Foca N, Reed E, Rohowsky C, Kung, P, King DW. Anti-idiotypic antibodies to anti-HLA receptors induced by pregnancy. *Proc Natl Acad Sci USA* 1983; **80:** 830-834.

3. Power DA, Mason RJ, Stewart KN, Noble ND, MacLeod A, Shewan G, Gatto GRD. B lymphocyte antibodies associated with successful pregnancy: evidence for MHC linkage. *Transplant Proc* 1983; **15:** 890-892.
4. Faulk WP, McIntyre JA. Immunological studies of human trophoblast: Markers, subsets and functions. *Immunol Rev* 1983; **75:** 139-175.
5. Reznikoff-Etievant MF, Edelman P, Müller JY, Pinon F, Sureau C. HLA-DR locus and maternal-foetal relation. *Tissue Antigens* 1984; **24:** 30-34.
6. Gerencer M, Kastelan A. The role of HLA D region in feto-maternal interactions. *Transplant Proc* 1983; **15:** 893-895.
7. Aoki K. HLA-DR compatibility in couples with recurrent spontaneous abortions. *Acta Obstet Gynaecol Jpn* 1982; **34:** 1773-1778.
8. Beer AE, Semprini AE, Xiaoyu Z. Quebbeman JF. Pregnancy outcome in human couples with recurrent spontaneous abortions: HLA antigen profiles; HLA antigen sharing; female serum MLR blocking factors; and paternal leukocyte immunization. *Expl Clin Immunogenet* 1985; **2:** 137-153.
9. Komlos L, Zamir R, Joshua H, Halbrecht I. Common HLA antigens in couples with repeated abortions. *Clin Immunol Immunopathol* 1977; **7:** 330-335.
10. McIntyre JA, McConnachie PR, Taylor CG, Faulk WP. Clinical, immunologic, and genetic definitions of primary and secondary recurrent spontaneous abortions. *Fertil Steril* 1984; **42:** 849-855.
11. Thomas ML, Harger JH, Wagenner DK, Rabin BS, Gill TJ III. HLA sharing and spontaneous abortion in humans. *Am J Obstet Gynecol* 1985; **151:** 1053-1058.
12. Unander AM, Olding LB. Habitual abortion: parental sharing of HLA antigens, absence of maternal blocking antibody, and suppression of maternal lymphocytes. *Am J Reprod Immunol* 1983; **4:** 171-178.
13. Caudle MR, Rote NS, Scott JR, Dewitt C, Barney MF. Histocompatibility in couples with recurrent spontaneous abortion and normal fertility. *Fertil Steril* 1983; **39:** 793-798.
14. Casciani CU, Pasetto N, Forleo R, Adorno D, Valeri M, Piazza A. HLA sharing in couples with recurrent abortion. *Expl Clin Immunogenet* 1985; **2:** 65-69.
15. Jeannet M, Bischof P, Bourrit B, Vuagnat P. Sharing of HLA antigens in fertile, subfertile and infertile couples. *Transpl Proceed* 1985; **17:** 903-904.
16. Lauritsen JG, Kristensen T, Grunnet N. Depressed mixed lymphocyte culture reactivity in mothers with recurrent spontaneous abortion. *Am J Obstet Gynecol* 1976; **125:** 35-39.
17. Oksenberg JR, Persitz E, Amar A, Brauther C. Maternal-paternal histocompatibility: lack of association with habitual abortions. *Fertil Steril* 1984; **42:** 389-395.
18. Vanoli M, Fabio G, Bonara P, Eisera N, Pardi G, Acaia B, Smeraldi RS. Histocompatibility in Italian couples with recurrent abortions of unknown origin and with normal fertility. *Tissue Antigens* 1985; **26:** 227-233.
19. Weitkamp LR, Schacter BZ. Transferrin and HLA: spontaneous abortion, neural tube defects, and natural selection. *N Engl J Med* 1985; **313:** 925-932.
20. Johnson PM, Barnes RMR, Risk JM, Molloy CM, Woodrow JC. Immunogenetic studies of recurrent spontaneous abortions in humans. *Expl Clin Immunogenet* 1985; **2:** 77-83.
21. Beer AE, Quebbeman JF, Ayers JWT, Haines RF. Major histocompatibility complex antigens, maternal and paternal immune responses and chronic habitual abortions in humans. *Am J Obstet Gynecol* 1981; **141:** 987-999.
22. Mowbray JF, Reginald PW, Gibbings C, Liddell H, Underwood JL, Beard RW. Controlled trial of treatment of recurrent spontaneous abortion by immunisation with paternal cells. *Lancet* 1985; **1:** 941-943.
23. Reznikoff-Etievant MF, Simmoney N, Janaud A, Darbois Y, Netter A. Treatment of recurrent spontaneous abortions by immunisation with paternal leucocytes. *Lancet* 1985; **1:** 1398.

24.   Taylor CG, Faulk WP, McIntyre JA. Prevention of recurrent spontaneous abortions by leukocyte transfusions. *J Roy Soc Med* 1985; **78:** 623-627.
25.   Unander AM, Lindholm A. Transfusions of leukocyte-rich erythrocyte concentrates: A successful treatment in selected cases of habitual abortion. *Am J Obstet Gynecol* 1986; **154:** 516-520.
26.   McIntyre JA, Faulk WP, Nichols-Johnson VR, Taylor CG. Immunologic testing and immunotherapy in recurrent spontaneous abortion. *Obstet Gynecol* 1986; **67:** 169-175.
27.   Reznikoff-Etievant MF, Durieux I, Huchet J, Salmon C, Netter A. Recurrent spontaneous abortions, HLA antigen sharing and anti-paternal immunity. Immunotherapic assay. In: *Immunologie de la réproduction: relation materno-foetale.* Ed: G Chaouat. Colloque INSERM, 1987; pp.187-202.
28.   Awdeh ZL, Raum D, Yunis EJ, Alper CA. Extended HLA/complement allele haplotypes: evidence for T/t-like complex in man. *Proc Natl Acad Sci USA* 1983; **80:** 259-263.
29.   Gazit E, Gothelf Y, Gil R, Orgad S, Pitman TB, Watson ALM, Yang SY, Yunis EJ. Alloantibodies to PHA-activated lymphocytes detect human Qa-like antigens. *J Immunol* 1984; **132:** 165-169.
30.   Redman CW, McMichael AJ, Stirrat GM, Sunderland CA, Ting A. Class I major histocompatibility complex antigens on human extra-villous trophoblast. *Immunology* 1984; **52:** 457-468.

Discussion

Chairman: Professor J. Mowbray

Professor GILL: I would reiterate a couple of points that I made before on the HLA-sharing data. The first—the fact that it shares at all in our hands a three-love side and in your hands at two-love side. The fact that it shares a different love-side and that there is no association with any particular antigen makes it highly unlikely to be antigen-sharing by itself is as important, but rather as a marker for sharing that segment of the chromosome. I think the most reasonable hypothesis is that there are silent lethals in the MHC. This has been shown in the mouse and in the rat. The fact that there is no t complex in the human is irrelevant, because the t has to do with segregation distortion, and suppression of recombination. It has nothing to do with the lethals. What we are interested in, in spontaneous abortion, is the lethals. And thirdly, there is no firm evidence for Qa-Qla system in the humans. There are a few very fine suggestions in the order of softness as there are for t complex. So I think that the most reasonable interpretation is that the sharing of that segment of the chromosome in couples with spontaneous abortions is sharing of excessive lethals.

Professor HARRIS: Talking of HLA associations makes one think of all the disease associations, and some striking analogies in a way. One of the most powerful tools in looking for associations has been sib sharing of HLA antigens. So that in diabetes mellitus, for example, there is a great excess of affected sibs, both of whom have diabetes, who share the same parental haplotypes. In Hodgkin's disease, even more striking, the association in the general population is very weak. Yet the association when you do get that rare entity—affected sibs—they almost always share the two haplotypes. So the logical experiment, if it were possible, would be to do HLA typing of pairs of abortuses (and one realises how difficult it would be to get the material), but pairs of abortuses ought to have a great excess of sharing, of both haplotypes of the parents. It might be easier in a way to go to some of your families, in the Gulf and elsewhere, and look at the sibs that actually survive from high abortion parents. If this idea is correct then they ought to differ more than one would expect statistically.

Professor MOWBRAY: That is one of the things we wanted to look at. We have, however, looked a little bit at something else, which is—is there an excess of a

385

particular HLA haplotype in the children born after immunisation compared with the one child born previously? But of course, we only had one to look at there, so that it really becomes rather difficult. We need two or three more.

Dr REZNIKOFF: We do that.

Professor JOHNSON: Just two points. I cannot let the statement that there is no evidence for Qa-Qla antigens in man go unchallenged. Recently Moore and Demaris have mapped that area of chromosome 6, and have shown that there are at least fifteen different gene loci there. Many of them, admittedly, are pseudo genes or gene fragments, but at least two are fully transcribable genes. And there are now monoclonal antibodies becoming available that appear to detect the serological product of those genes—as Class 1-like molecules that are not regular HLA A, B, C molecules. So I think that there is now becoming firm compulsive, both genetic and serological, evidence for Qa analogues which are in the same genetic region. The second point is to the immunogenetics in spontaneous abortion. It is really a plea—we are hindered by the fact that we are doing serology and looking at HLA A, B, C, Dr antigens that have been defined in the classical transplantation rejection scenario. Now there are molecular biological reagents we can do RFLPs through that area to cover comprehensively many of the gene loci. And if the concept, whichever way it is stated, is a recessive gene that is present within MHC, or some kind of deletion that may have an effect on viviparity, then the way of conclusively showing that is to go through the gene loci doing RFLP analysis, which is not a great deal of effort. And I would just make a plea that that work is done.

Professor HARRIS: And concentrate on the Class 2 routine because that is what we share.

Dr REZNIKOFF: It may also be that it reflects something else.

Professor MOWBRAY: May I also make another plea, which is that if there is an antigenic determinant which is important, the husband must become homozygous for it. So that looking at homozygosity in the husband is at least as important as looking at HLA sharing in primary aborters.

Professor GILL: That would correspond with Peter's comment.

Professor HARRIS: Why does he have to be homozygous?

Professor MOWBRAY: Because they are primary aborters.

Professor HARRISON: I find it strange that we have had three clinical papers this morning, and no one has commented on the clinical data or challenged the results. This afternoon I am going to challenge the positive results, but I would like to make one comment. Two speakers have said that they have groups of people who got pregnant while they were away, etc, etc, and they drew some conclusions from that data. If you want to use placebo groups or groups in that way, the conditions should at least be the same as those you are treating. To me there is a very significant thing missing in those untreated, and that was the two speakers themselves. And I would like to think that this illustrates that they both have a very powerful placebo effect on their patients.

Dr REZNIKOFF: I must say that in France we will begin again a controlled trial.

Dr BILLINGTON: For the record, can I refute the opening statement of this speaker, which has also been stated by the other people in the last two and a half days? The statement that an intact immune system is essential for a successful pregnancy. We have plenty of data from experimental animals which have been *B* cell depleted or suppressor cell depleted, scid mice—a whole range of animals which have very severely depleted immune systems that have successful pregnancies.

Dr REZNIKOFF: Yes, I know that, but it is just because many years before they said that pregnancy occurs because a woman is not able to reject it. But I agree with you, of course.

Professor GILL: In the Qa/tla business, I am not saying that they don't occur. The demand system I believe was an *in vitro* system and it hasn't been shown to be expressed *in vivo*. There are a lot of pseudo genes out there, RFLP mapping can be a terrible quagmire. RFLP mapping in organ matching for transplantation has almost been as good as serological mapping. Where RFLP mapping has been very good is in the diabetes mellitus story where it is focussed down on a particular range of the genome so that one can study in detail this small area of the genome. But to undertake RFLP mapping of the whole MHC would be a tremendous task.

Professor JOHNSON: RFLP mapping with limited cutting by restriction endonuclease is not an great task.

Trophoblast membrane infusion (TMI) in the treatment of recurrent spontaneous abortion

P. M. Johnson, G. H. Ramsden, K. V. Chia

INTRODUCTION

Before discussing trophoblast membrane infusion (TMI), it is necessary to identify the groups of patients studied. Much information has been published recently about treatment in recurrent spontaneous abortion (RSA) but, unfortunately, the clinical definition has sometimes varied between centres and this has made comparisons difficult. We have investigated women with three or more (mean 4.7) confirmed consecutive first-trimester spontaneous abortions with the same partner. Known cytogenetic, endocrine, gynaecological, infectious or other medical causes that may contribute to recurring early fetal loss have been excluded by both clinical and laboratory investigation; this has included hystero-salpingogram, thyroid function tests, cervical cultures and karyotypic analyses. No woman was included who was known to have a history of aneuploidic pregnancy loss, detectable serum anti-nuclear autoantibody, lupus anticoagulant autoantibody,[1] clinical evidence of autoimmunity or an abnormal full blood count. Thus, they fall into an, as yet, unexplained group of RSA patients.

These women have been further divided into two main groups: so-called primary (1°) RSA patients are those with no viable pregnancy beyond 28 weeks and no previous elective abortions, and so-called secondary (2°) RSA patients are those with one live birth preceding the unbroken series of spontaneous pregnancy losses. It must be stressed that their identification is essentially one of exclusion of other known causes that could lead to the common end-product of early fetal loss, and it is unjustified to assume a single common cause in the remaining unexplained RSA women. Furthermore, patient selection has often varied between centres. Thus, McIntyre et al.[2] characterised 2° RSA women as posses-sing serum anti-paternal lymphocytotoxins and polyspecific lymphocytotoxins, which could have resulted in the inclusion of some patients with subclinical auto-immune disease. The immunotherapy trial of Mowbray et al.[3] also made no men-tion of the study of lupus anticoagulant-type autoantibodies with phospholipid-related specificities.

We have investigated nearly 200 couples each with between 3 and 17 spontaneous abortions, of which 95 were classified as 1° RSA and 35 as 2° RSA. The remainder were omitted from this classification because the further clinical or laboratory investigation brought to light an exclusion, such as thyroid disease, collagen disorders or cyanotic heart disease. Two women had marked thrombocythaemia that could have contributed to an adverse decidual vasculopathy and three women had lupus anticoagulant activity which could have contributed to previous pregnancy pathology (two of whom showed no clinical evidence of SLE).

A considerable amount of basic immunological data for pregnancy in man and experimental animals has now accumulated.[4-7] These studies have been widely interpreted as indicating that, in addition to other (often passive) mechanisms for survival of the fetal allograft, trophoblast cell surface antigens expressed at the feto-maternal interface may actively induce cellular and humoral immunoregulatory mechanisms in the mother that contribute to the paradoxical immunological success of viviparity. In addition, this immunological recognition could be impaired in a few women who suffer RSA because of restricted protection from transplantation rejection afforded to the early embryo.[2,7-10] In immunological terms, this could result either from intrinsic maternal hypo-responsiveness to appropriate fetal antigens (which would be partner-nonspecific) or from absent maternal recognition due to materno-fetal allelic identity for a relevant fetal antigen expressing genetic polymorphism (which would be partner-specific). We will discuss briefly the immunological and immunogenetic data derived from 1° and 2° unexplained RSA patients at this centre before discussing in more detail our clinical studies of trophoblast membrane infusion.

LABORATORY INVESTIGATIONS

Parental HLA sharing

This has been reported from some centres as being increased in couples with unexplained RSA, whereas other centres (including Liverpool) have not statistically observed this effect.[2,10-13] In practice, results from all centres have tended to fall just on either side of a line of significance at the 1% level, and the variation is well within limits that might be expected because of differences in the selection of control couples, study group numbers and tissue typing methodology (particularly the number of HLA-DR antigens assessed within the tissue typing antiserum panel). We have been unable to distinguish any features of clinical behaviour in unexplained RSA couples that correlate with the degree of parental HLA matching.

HLA homozygosity

We have observed a significant increase in apparent HLA-B antigen homozygosity for 1° RSA women.[11] This has been confirmed at the same level of statistical significance in a further cohort of patients, as well as an increased frequency of apparent homozygosity of the A3B1 phenotype of the fourth component of complement (C4) for both the male and female partners in unexplained RSA (Johnson *et al*, unpublished observations). Both HLA-B and

C4 are located quite closely within the major histocompatibility complex (MHC) region on the short arm of chromosome 6, and hence this data could reflect an action of recessive genes in this region. Whilst this may await confirmation, however, we have been unable to distinguish any features of clinical behaviour in unexplained RSA couples that correlate with HLA-B or C4 locus homozygosity.

Immunological hyporesponsiveness

There have been earlier reports that 1° RSA may be characterised by a decreased prevalence of serum lymphocytotoxic antibodies (LCA) than may be expected. Thus, an incidence of approximately 10% was considered low by comparison with multigravid women having term pregnancies. However, a recent study[14] has shown an even lower prevalence of LCA in a matched group of recurrent elective aborters compared with recurrent spontaneous aborters. Data for 2° RSA is contradictory,[2,12] probably because of different local patient selection; the prevalence of serum LCA in 2° RSA at this centre is closely comparable with that for 1° RSA (Johnson *et al*, unpublished observations).

An intriguing observation of apparent selective immunological hypo-responsiveness has been the significantly lower prevalence of serum antibodies to cytomegalovirus (CMV) in unexplained RSA women compared with their male partners or age-matched female controls.[15] This was not the case for serum antibodies to *Herpes simplex* virus. In addition, there was also a markedly impaired lymphocyte proliferative response to CMV in CMV-seropositive RSA women compared with CMV-seropositive female controls.[15]

Lymphocyte subsets

Because of the above data, it was also logical to investigate different peripheral blood T-lymphocytes in unexplained RSA. Again, there have been conflicting reports in the literature on small numbers of patients. We have found no evidence for any significant difference in either absolute numbers or relative percentages of CD4-positive or CD8-positive T cell subsets in either 1° or 2° RSA compared with controls.[16] Assessment of T-lymphocyte subpopulations would appear not to be useful in monitoring RSA patients, and could be too insensitive to reflect any local tissue alterations relevant to immunoregulatory control at materno-fetal interfaces.

TROPHOBLAST MEMBRANE INFUSION (TMI)

Background

Recent studies have suggested that repeated intravenous and/or intradermal immunisation with large amounts of intact viable allogeneic peripheral blood leucocytes may favour subsequent successful reproductive outcome in unexplained RSA patients.[2,3,9,10] Only one controlled trial has been performed to date[3] and the strength of 'placebo effect' remains to be fully assessed. In addition, the cell source (paternal or third-party leucocytes), dose and route of administration, as well as selection criteria for inclusion, has varied between centres. Although convenient, this approach in healthy immunologically competent women may have clinical limitations. For example, concomitant platelet antigen sensitisation might compromise subsequent pregnancies. In addition, sensitisation to fetal HLA or other antigens may be associated with increased risk of intrauterine growth retardation (IUGR) or, theoretically, neonatal immunodeficiency following maternal isoimmunisation.[7,17] Severe IUGR in pregnancy has been reported following leucocyte immunisation.[10,12] Finally, this approach includes transfusion-related risks of viral transmission by viable leucocytes, namely for CMV and human immunodeficiency virus (HIV).[15] Congenital CMV is the commonest infective cause of fetal malformation, reflecting its ready transplacental passage, and hence the CMV-immune status of RSA women is of considerable interest when considering leucocyte immunisation during the peri-conception period.[15] Congenital abnormalities have also been associated with parental HLA sharing,[18] and it may also be relevant that leucocyte immunisation may increase apparent fertility and twinning rates (Mowbray, personal communication).

We have introduced an alternative approach for active immunisation to negate fetal allograft rejection which is based on a single intravenous infusion with an isolated placental syncytiotrophoblast microvillous membrane (StMPM) preparation.[19] The clinical disadvantages of leucocyte immunisation may outweigh the inconvenience of isolation of StMPM preparations. This approach of trophoblast membrane infusion (TMI) has the advantages of (i) being a mimic of natural events of fetal cellular contact with the maternal immune system in normal pregnancy, (ii) using an HLA-negative cell source lacking blood group antigen expression, and (iii) using a highly purified non-nucleated cell fraction.[19] Both LCA-negative 1° and 2° RSA parents have been included in this study of TMI.

Trophoblast membrane vesicle preparation

The full methodology for the sterile StMPM preparation from term placentae of uncomplicated healthy pregnancies is described in detail elsewhere.[19] Donor retroplacental blood was always tested for HBsAg and antibodies to HIV or syphilis. Throughout the StMPM isolation procedure, meticulous detail was paid to maintaining sterility using aseptic conditions, pyrogen-free solutions, antibiotics and UV-irradiation.[19] The final preparations were assessed for microbial activity under both aerobic and anaerobic conditions, and could be stored lyophilised prior to reconstitution for use. Standard coagulation techniques were used to assess any thromboplastin activity.

Patient selection

Initial interview consisted of a full clinical history, including previous blood transfusions, allergic hypersensitivity and familial history of reproductive disorders. Laboratory investigations included HLA tissue typing, blood grouping, lymphocytotoxic, anti-erythrocyte, anti-sperm, anti-cardiolipin and anti-viral antibodies, autoantibodies and blood coagulation studies (prothrombin time— PT, and activated partial thromboplastin time—APTT). When necessary, chromosome analysis, thyroid function tests, random blood sugar, endocervical swabs, hysterosalpingogram and endocrine (serum progesterone or prolactin) were also performed to obtain complete investigation.

Table 1

Selection Criteria for Trophoblast Membrane Infusion

Three or more consecutive confirmed spontaneous abortions with the same partner

No live birth, or a single live birth in the first pregnancy

Chromosomal, anatomic, microbiological, hormonal or other medical reasons (e.g. diabetes, thyroid disease etc.) for recurring spontaneous abortion having been excluded as far as possible

Absence of serum lymphocytotoxic antibodies (LCA) and acquired anti-red cell antibodies

Absence of serum anti-nuclear autoantibody and lupus anticoagulant-type autoantibody (the latter assessed by both anti-cardiolipin ELISA and by activated partial thromboplastin [APTT])

Total serum IgE level of less than 1000 iu/ml

Normal full blood count

Not currently pregnant

The complete criteria for admission to the TMI study are given in Table 1. HLA was not taken into account for patient selection. Any RSA patient with a total serum IgE level of 100-1,000 iu/ml was skin prick-tested on separate arms with a 1:10 dilution in pyrogen-free saline of the final StMPM preparation compared with pyrogen-free saline alone immediately prior to TMI.

Initially, consenting patients were only entered onto an open study but, since June 1985, all 1° RSA patients aged under 40 have now been included in a double-blind trial of trophoblast membrane infusion compared with a dilute lyophilised Intralipid preparation of identical appearance. The pregnancy outcome results given below necessarily refer only to those patients accumulated in the open study.

Infusion

This was performed as a day case procedure. An intravenous infusion with 1g wet weight sterile StMPM preparation pooled from two or more donors blood group matched with the recipient was given by slow infusion from a 250ml saline drip-pack over a period of greater than 1 hour. Pulse, temperature and blood pressure were recorded every ten minutes during the infusion, and hourly for the next three hours. All patients were assessed for full blood count and differential, as well as PT and APTT blood coagulation times before, during and two hours after treatment. These parameters remained within normal limits for all patients. Patients were advised to wait 1-3 months following infusion before considering conception, depending on whether or not they were positive for anti-CMV antibody. Patients were not advised of any requirement for attempting conception rapidly.

Treatment results

This approach to treatment has been applied without adverse reaction to 58 RSA patients in the open study, as well as those patients selected for the double-blind study. We have reported in full on the first 21 pregnant women, of whom 16 (76%) have achieved a live birth.[19] There has now been one further pregnancy loss and six further patients are currently in the second or third trimester of pregnancy (interestingly, including one LCA-negative patient given TMI and who previously had suffered two further first-trimester spontaneous abortions following leucocyte immunisation). Two patients have now had second children without further treatment or obstetric complication. The subsequent pregnancy outcome appears very comparable with that obtained following leucocyte immunisation.[2,3,9,10]

Figure I

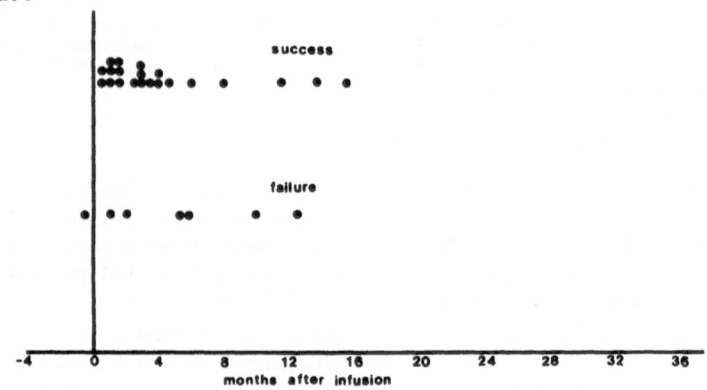

Term pregnancy (success) or repeated spontaneous abortion (failure) compared with time in months following TMI to conception.

Figure II

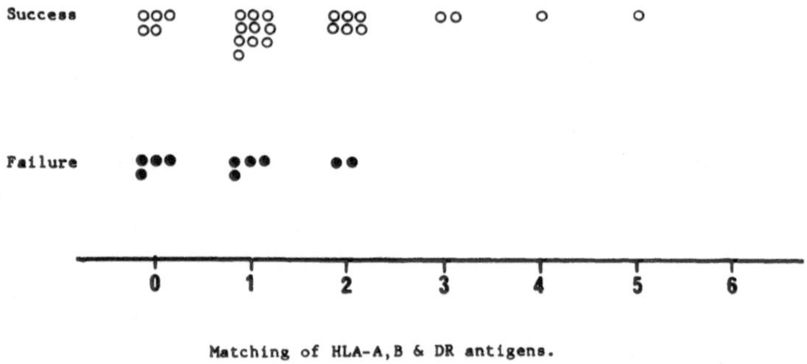

Term pregnancy (success) or repeated spontaneous abortion (failure) compared with the number of HLA-A, B & DR antigens shared between mother and father.

It has been of note that 2° RSA patients appear to respond as well as 1° patients.[19] The results to date have shown no correlation of pregnancy outcome either with the time span between infusion and conception. (Figure I) or with the degree of parental HLA sharing (Figure II). There have been no cases of ectopic pregnancy, IUGR, stillbirths, twins, congenital abnormalities or developmental problems in this open study of TMI. On investigation four to six weeks after TMI, no patient had developed serum LCA, anti-cardiolipin or anti-erythrocyte antibodies, anti-nuclear autoantibodies or markedly elevated total serum IgE levels.

Future perspectives

Central questions focus on what may be the most rational and safe approach to immunotherapy in RSA, as well as how to identify those patients who may benefit from within the undoubted clinical heterogeneity of the unexplained RSA patients pool. Further placebo-controlled or comparative studies need to be undertaken to determine efficacy, particularly in respect of the claims in favour of supportive psychotherapy in repeated spontaneous abortion at some centres.[20,21] Of equal importance is that attention should be paid to the need for better laboratory identification of suitable patients, their response to immunotherapy and monitoring through a subsequent pregnancy. At present, the immunotherapy approach presupposes the development of a relevant immunoregulatory response—which has been unfortunately elusive to identification by consistent and direct laboratory assays (as indeed, has been the identity of any immunological laboratory serological parameter characteristic of normal trophoblast survival in healthy pregnancy).[22] This is urgently required in order to improve selection of patients, and to avoid unnecessarily offering false hope to those unexplained RSA women who will not benefit from active immunotherapy.

ACKNOWLEDGEMENTS

This work was supported by Birthright and Mersey Regional Health Authority research project awards. We would like to thank Mrs. W. J. A. Francis and Mr. R. G. Farquharson, Consultant Gynaecologists, as well as the staff at Liverpool Maternity Hospital and Women's Hospital for their help and encouragement in this work.

REFERENCES

1. Lubbe WF, Liggins CG. Lupus anticoagulant and pregnancy.*Amer J Obstet Gynecol* 1985; **153**: 322-332.
2. McIntyre JA, Faulk WP, Nichols-Johnson VR, Taylor CG. Immunologic testing and immunotherapy in recurrent spontaneous abortion. *Obstet Gyecol* 1986; **67**: 169-175.
3. Mowbray JF, Gibbings C, Liddell H, Reginald PW, Underwood JL, Beard RW. Controlled trial of treatment of recurrent spontaneous abortion by immunisation with paternal cells. *Lancet* 1985; **1**: 941-943.
4. Bulmer JN, Johnson PM. Antigen expression by trophoblast populations in the human placenta and their possible immunobiological relevance. *Placenta* 1985; **6**: 127-140.
5. Stern PL, Beresford N, Thompson S, Johnson PM, Webb PD, Hole N. Characterization of the human trophoblast-leukocyte antigenic molecules defined by a monoclonal antibody. *J Immunol* 1986; **137**: 1064-1069.
6. Johnson PM, Stern PL. Antigen expression at human materno-fetal interfaces. In: *Progress in Immunology VI.* Eds. B Cinader and RG Miller. Orlando: Academic Press, 1987; pp.1056-1069.
7. Lancet editorial. Maternal blocking antibodies, the fetal allograft and recurrent abortion. *Lancet* 1983; **2**:1175-1176.
8. Johnson PM, Chia KV, Risk JM. Immunological question marks in recurrent spontaneous abortion. In: *Reproductive Immunology* 1986. Eds. DA Clark, BA Croy. Amsterdam: Elsevier Biomedical Press, 1986; pp 239-245.
9. Takakuwa K, Kanazawa K, Takeuchi S. Production of blocking antibodies by vaccination with husband's lymphocytes in unexplained recurrent aborters: the role in successful pregnancy. *Amer J Reprod Immunol Microbiol* 1986; **10**: 1-9.

10. Beer AE, Semprini AE, Xiaoyn Z, Quebbeman JF. Pregnancy outcome in human couples with recurrent spontaneous abortion: HLA antigen profiles, HLA antigen sharing, female serum MLR blocking factors and paternal leukocyte immunization. *Exp Clin Immunogenet* 1985; **2**: 137-153.
11. Johnson PM, Barnes RMR, Risk JM, Molloy CM, Woodrow JC. Immunogenetic studies of recurrent spontaneous abortions in humans. *Exp Clin Immunogenet* 1985; **2**: 77-83.
12. Cauchi MN, Koh SH, Tait B, Mraz G, Kloss M, Pepperell RJ. Immunogenetic studies in habitual abortion. *Aust NZ J Obstet Gynaec* 1987; **27**: 52-54.
13. Oskenberg JR, Persitz E, Amar A, Brautbar C. Maternal-paternal histocompatibility: lack of association with habitual abortions. *Fertil Steril* 1984; **42**: 389-395.
14. Biddle P, Friedman CI, Johnson PM. Lymphocyte-reactive antibodies and recurrent early pregnancy failure. *Amer J Obstet Gynec* 1987; **157**: 785-786.
15. Radcliffe JJ, Hart CA, Francis WJ, Johnson PM. Immunity to cytomegalovirus in women with unexplained recurrent spontaneous abortion. *Amer J Reprod Immunol Microbiol* 1986; **12**: 103-105.
16. Chia KV, Johnson PM. T-lymphocyte subsets in unexplained recurrent spontaneous abortion. *Fertil Steril* 1987; **48**: 685-687.
17. Bastian JF, Williams RA, Ornelas W, Tani P, Thompson LF. Maternal isoimmunisation resulting in combined immunodeficiency and fetal graft-versus-host disease in an infant. *Lancet* 1984; **1**: 1435-1437.
18. Aymé S, Mercier P, Dallest R, Mattei JF. HLA and trisomy 21. Confirmation of a trend of restricted HLA heterogeneity in parents of Down syndrome children. *Amer J Hum Genet* 1984; **36**: 405-412.
19. Johnson PM, Chia KV, Hart CA, Griffith HB, Francis WJA. Trophoblast membrane infusion for unexplained recurrent miscarriage. *Brit J Obstet Gynaec* 1988; In press.
20. Stray-Pedersen B, Stray-Pedersen S. Etiological factors and subsequent reproductive performance in 195 couples with a prior history of habitual abortion. *Amer J Obstet Gynec* 1984; **148**: 140-146.
21. Vlaanderen W, Treffers PE. Prognosis of subsequent pregnancies after recurrent spontaneous abortion in first trimester. *Brit Med J* 1987; **295**: 92-93.
22. Hole N, Cheng HM, Johnson PM. Antibody reactivity against human trophoblast membrane antigens in the context of normal pregnancy and unexplained recurrent miscarriage. *Colloque INSERM* 1987 **154**: 213-224.

Discussion

Chairman: Professor J Mowbray

Professor JENKINS: One simple thing . . . why doesn't pregnancy itself, Peter, improve the chance of success subsequently if what you are doing is giving the microvillous suspensions that have come from a previous pregnancy?

Professor JOHNSON: When we designed the double blind-study, we restricted it only to the primary aborters. We thought that it would be worthwhile having a look at the secondary aborters, and I am as surprised as anyone else that the secondary aborters are doing well. So it does worry me what the placebo rate in that group is. Is this actually active treatment?

Dr PAGE FAULK: Peter, you are immunising with live reconstituted microvilli, and then you are putting on your ELISA plate detergent solubilised microvilli, and you don't find any antibody in the recipients. Now, we find several trophoblast antigens against which we have pretty good monoclonals, which are lost subsequent to solubilisation. What if you just put the live microvilli back on the plate? Do you see antibodies?

Professor JOHNSON: We have yet to do that because of the poor reproducibility in our hands if you use the intact membrane fragment rather than a solubilised protein. But while I am talking to you I am gaining a few hints about the way you are doing it.

Dr PAGE FAULK: Because it is not dissimilar—this whole question of maternal antibodies.

Professor JOHNSON: And equally a negative doesn't mean that it is not there.

Dr SEMPRINI: Could I ask you why you exclude patients who are anti-HLA-antibody-positive, since you are using a system that by definition has nothing to do with the HLA system?

Professor JOHNSON: We exclude patients who are lymphocytic toxic antibody positive, and the reason for doing that has nothing to do with the debate that we heard earlier this morning whether the lymphocytic toxic antibodies are a good or a bad prognostic indication. It is purely that this is a new form of treatment, and when we developed that we were keen ourselves (and our ethical committee was keen) to ensure that we didn't put any patient at an unnecessary risk. Now I think that any kind of intravenous immunisation in the presence of an established antibody activity such as that, would in the initial development be putting the patient at an unnecessary risk. We did not know; and it is just the same reason that we exclude atopic individuals. I think that if you can prove that there really is a statistically significant effect of this treatment in as safe a population group as you can possibly define, then you may readdress that question, and say to the other groups—may they gain any benefit?

Professor STIRRAT: Could you address the question of the purity of your reagent? Is it highly purified? In the Smith, Brush and Luckett method, which I presume you are using, it is extremely difficult to get it purified. But of course it would bear on David Jenkins' question, because maybe it is not trophoblast membrane at all; but it is the membrane of other cells which are accompanying that which are tending to produce the relevant response, but not in any concerted way.

Professor JOHNSON: We assess the preparation by the usual kind of biochemical criteria, and as you know, in the past we have been happy that the degree of contamination of non-trophoblastic cell membrane has been minimal indeed. And also, that is why I put that slide up with the animal data. By deliberate directed immunisation into another species we do not develop anti-HLA antibodies. We are happy that the level of contamination with other cell surface membranes is undetectable within our laboratories.

Professor GILL: Did you say that the only criterion that you use for infusing was matching for the ABO blood groups?

Professor JOHNSON: The criterion for the actual trophoblast membrane preparation is ABO rhesus matches in the recipient.

Professor GILL: What kind of control do you use for these studies? Have you tried membranes from some other organs?

Professor JOHNSON: No. The initial study was a study of trophoblast membrane *in vitro*. The control now in the placebo, in the double-blind study, is an Intralipid preparation. These are vesicles that morphologically are indistinguishable from trophoblast membranes.

Dr BILLINGTON: Peter, you should also make the point that it is almost impossible to obtain comparable preparations from any other known tissue that it is possible to use.

Professor JOHNSON: Which would be comparable and ethical to use.

Professor HOWIE: Can I just say how pleased I was as a practising obstetrician to hear that you are doing double-blind, randomised trials of immunotherapy. I am not an expert in this field, but I have listened for two and a half days now, and I have enjoyed it because I like insoluble logic problems, and this has been an excellent exercise. For the clinicians, the bottom line is not what mechanism might operate, but whether immunotherapy really is an effective form of treatment for women who present with recurrent abortion. My understanding is that so far there has only been one randomised, one controlled trial, of immunotherapy which has been reported to date. And it is a well known experience of clinicians who have worked in any field that the first trial is not always the definitive trial. That is not offered as a criticism; it is just common experience that the first enthusiastic trial for whatever reason is not always replicated. And I still think that the major question is whether or not this treatment really works. Perhaps you would like to give your view of what you see as the future strategy for the correct mounting of trials to really tell clinicians whether this treatment is effective or not.

Professor MOWBRAY: There are trials, Peter Johnson's trial, Marie-Francoise Reznikoff's trial; Chris Redman is running a trial; Dr Daya has got one too. So there are quite a lot of excellent ones going along at the moment. They are not all on the same protocol.

Professor JOHNSON: One of the important things is that the message has to be given exactly as you just said it, because there is pressure from other groups— patients and referring obstetricians—that another trial is not necessary, and we, in terms of trying to persuade people into a double-blind study, have had patient resistance. I think that there have been some centres where they have been putting up proposals for double-blind studies that have had resistance from ethical committees. Perhaps it is important that we, as an assembly of experts, actually make some agreement that there is a need for further double-blind studies.

Professor MOWBRAY: The only person who could not do another double-blind study is me. I couldn't sit down to do another one ethically having shown that one treatment is better than the others. But everybody else should do one.

Dr HOWIE: Yes, I think that that is a very important point. If what this group showed is correct then it should be reproduceable by other groups replicating your study. And I think it is absolutely essential that that is done.

Dr B STRAY-PEDERSON: That is a comment that I very much agree with, but as to the statement that earlier trials which have been performed have been double-blind studies, that is not quite correct. Most of them have been performed with randomisation, preconceptionally, without paying any attention to control during the pregnancy.

Professor BEARD: Could I just reply to that, because you are commenting on our trial. It is true that we randomised before pregnancy, but the way in which such pregnancy was subsequently managed was a perfect randomisation method. The patients were all sent back to their individual obstetricians who looked after them in multiple different ways, and I think that is the best way to do it.

Professor GILL: This is a study group, and hopefully, we are trying to get to a particular recommendation on a particular point. Picking up on the last points that were raised, I think that a small group of people here should get together and collect all of the data from the trials. We tried it in Paris. I think that systematic collection of data on a standardised form, and then analysis of those data is absolutely essential at this stage.

Dr PAGE FAULK: If you do that you should have a long-term follow-up of the children too.

Professor GILL: Absolutely.

Professor MOWBRAY: I have, as some of you know, advocated that we should have a long-term follow-up, a registry of all children born after active treatment of recurrent abortion.

Dr LOKE: I am speaking as one who is not in the field of immunotherapy. I am speaking merely as a very humble trophoblast scientist. But it seems to me that the basic logic of immunisation—Peter Johnson's protocol is the only one which seems to me to be logical—is to use trophoblast as an immunogenic source. My question to Peter, really, is whether he has considered other sources of tropho-blast material, like for instance first-trimester membranes, rather than term? Or perhaps even cytotrophoblast?

Professor JOHNSON: We have considered other sources. First-trimester mem-branes we cannot get in sufficient purity to convince ourselves about giving that to women. The same applies to cytotrophoblast. We await developments from you in Cambridge with regard to that. The other potential source would be a chorio-carcinoma cell-line, which clearly is not on. They would be the potential sources. So, I think at the moment we are left with the route that we are using. I would concur with the standardised protocol concept; all I would say is that at the moment to make these preparations with sufficient assessment in the study that we are doing requires a tremendous resource implication.

Professor MOWBRAY: Margareta Unander and Howard Carp have a couple of minutes each to add their extra information.

Dr UNANDER: One of the earlier speakers asked for a useful test to choose the women to be immunised. I find myself standing on the same side of the fence as Alan Beer, saying: We already have that test—the test for blocking antibody. I want to show my results to prove that statement.

I have been immunising women with habitual abortion in Sweden since January 1982. So far I have investigated more than 300 couples who fulfilled the criterion for habitual abortion, that is, they had had 3 or more consecutive miscarriages. The mean age of the women was 34 years and they had had as a mean 4.8 abortions when they appeared.

The investigations performed were:
— Blocking capacity of woman's serum in one-way mixed lymphocyte reaction (MLR).
— Activated partial thromboplastin time (APTT).
  (Lupus anticoagulant was determined but in our hands that method gave too little information.)
— Anti-cardiolipin antibodies.

If the woman had anti-cardiolipin antibody, prolongation of APTT or strong blocking capacity she was also checked for anti-DNA, ANA, and complements C3 and C4.

The women who lacked blocking capacity were candidates for immunisation treatment and underwent extended blood grouping.

The women who had blocking capacity may have had an autoimmune aberration with raised anti-cardiolipin antibody levels and were candidates for treatment with prednisolone and aspirin.

The immunisation treatment:

Third party cells given 3 or 5 times before pregnancy, one unit of leucocyte-rich erythrocyte concentrate from one donor each time.

Before those transfusions an "extended blood grouping" was performed, including determination of the following antigens:

ABO	
Rh subgroups	C c D E e
Kell Cellano	K k
Duffy	Fy^x
"High incidence antigens"	Vel Lu Yt Tj^x

Demands on donor blood:	To avoid:
Compatibility of erythrocyte antigens	Immunisation
Hbs-antigen negative	Hepatitis B
Liver enzymes normal	Hepatitis non-A non-B
Anti-HIV negative	AIDS
Storage in refrigerator >72 hours	virus activation, CMV and others

To minimise the risk of AIDS we used only female blood donors when possible and they are donors who had donated blood regularly for several years and were well known to the staff at the blood centre. None of the recipients of their blood had acquired hepatitis.

The transfusion protocol included 3 transfusions given with intervals of about 2 months. Two months after the third transfusion the blocking capacity was investigated. If blocking capacity had been induced the woman was advised to get pregnant, and if not she was given 2 more transfusions. The women were advised to get pregnant after having received 5 transfusions whether they had developed blocking capacity or not.

So far, more than 200 women have completed transfusion treatment. When I introduced this immunisation protocol it was not shown that the blocking antibody was crucial and therefore I immunised both the women with and those without blocking antibody hoping that those with blocking antibody before treatment would comprise a control group. Later I found that some of those women with blocking antibody had high levels of anti-cardiolipin antibody explaining their tendency to abort.

Among 190 women who lacked blocking capacity before immunisation 105 have become pregnant, whereas 17 of 30 women with blocking antibody before treatment have become pregnant afterwards. The prognostic value of the blocking antibody is clear from the following table:

Blocking capacity before transfusions

	No	Yes
No. immunised	190	30
Infants	60*[57%]	0
Ongoing >20 wks	40 [38%]	0
Extrauterine pregn.	2 [2%]	0
Miscarriages	3 [3%]	17** [100%]
	105	17

Total residual abortion rate: $(3+17)/(105+17) = 16\%$

*1 IUGR Caesarean section at 36 weeks
1 suspected IUGR Caesarian section at 28 weeks
2 deliveries at week 37
2 deliveries at week 38
1 premature delivery at week 28 − IRDS + cerebral haemorrhages
   — died from pneumonia 9 months old
Malformations: 1 testicular hydrocoele

**About half of those women with blocking capacity before treatment had high levels of anti-cardiolipin antibody explaining their abortions. During subsequent pregnancies they were treated with prednisolone + ASA which has resulted in
7 infants
2 ongoing pregnancies >20 weeks
2 miscarriages.

Eleven of those women with habitual abortion lacked blocking antibody but had raised levels of anti-cardiolipin antibody, 2 of them above 10 units. They were immunised, developed blocking antibody, and subsequently had live infants without any treatment with prednisolone and/or ASA. Thus, not even high levels of anti-cardiolipin antibody prove that treatment with prednisolone is the treatment needed.

According to my experience the women with so called "unexplained habitual abortion" may be divided into three groups.

The first group, about 85% of them, consists of women who lack blocking antibody and who have normal or raised anti-cardiolipin antibody levels. They benefit from immunisation treatment.

The second group of between 5 and 10% comprises the women with strong blocking antibody and high levels of anti-cardiolipin antibody. They suffer from the autoimmune aberration that can be treated with prednisolone and aspirin.

The last group of about 10% of the women have strong blocking antibody and normal or moderately raised anti-cardiolipin values. Their habitual abortion is still unexplained. These women display a very peculiar immunologic pattern and we strongly suspect that there is an abnormality, but so far we have not been able to define their aberration.

Concluding signs and treatments of choice in 254 women with habitual abortion:

Blocking	No.	(%)	Anti-cardiolipin	APTT	Treatment
Absent	207	(81%)	0-2 units	Normal	Immunisation
Absent	11	(4%)	≥3 units	Normal	Immunisation
Strong	16	(6%)	≥10 units	Raised	Prednisolone+ASA
Strong	20	(8%)	0-9 units	Normal	???

Professor MOWBRAY: Can I ask you to tell us—the women who failed, whose second pregnancies were all right, had blocking antibodies. Were those second-trimester losses or first-trimester losses?

Dr UNANDER: A mixture. I have fourteen second pregnancies after immunisation—those who had one child after immunisation and got pregnant again—and none of them aborted. So evidently, in those 14 treatment was still effective.

Professor MOWBRAY: So that gives us two lots of people who say, "don't immunise people who have got antibody when you start".

Dr CARP: Our centre has had an immunisation programme for habitual aborters for the last two years. In that time we have immunised 120 patients. The problem which we constantly face is which patients are suitable for immunisation, and which patients are not. Because as we have heard from this meeting, there is really no laboratory test which can tell us absolutely how to select these patients. Our original criteria for immunisation were patients who shared HLA antigens, and also patients who had reduced mixed lymphocyte reactivity. Using those criteria we very soon found that in our first series, 17 out of 22 patients who had developed anti-paternal antibody succeeded in their subsequent pregnancy, compared to only 4 out of 11 who did not produce antibody. So that criterion became clear to us very quickly—that we had to try to produce antibody. This was compared to only 3 out of 13 controls. Then we had certain problems because we could not find any increased HLA-sharing in our series at all, or any difference in the mixed lymphocyte reactivity to the normal population. We refined the criteria to immunise everybody who came to us with three or more abortions with no other documented cause of abortion. We looked at their clinical histories—at what sort of patients we were treating. We analysed 800 first-trimester abortions in 186 patients (Table 1). We were able to determine the character of the abortion in 413. Only 31 of these pregnancies were abortions of live fetuses, 382 were

Table 1

Retrospective analysis of character of abortion in 186 patients with habitual abortions (Author's series)

	1st Trimester	2nd Trimester	Total
No. pregnancies	800	99	899
No. of abortions of which character could be determined	413	81	494
Live abortions	31	30	61
Missed abortions	382	51	433

Table 2

Prospective analysis of character of 1st trimester habitual
missed abortions (Author's series)

No. of pregnancies assessed	42
Live abortions	6/42
Missed abortions	36/42
Missed abortions with previously detected fetal heart	4/36
Blighted ova	32/36

Figures are irrespective of immunisation.

Table 3

Immunisation results

Patients immunised	120
No. pregnancies	80
Patients pregnant	76

Exclusion criteria

Subsequent ectopic pregnancy	3
Subsequent mole	1
X− match + in advance (all aborted subsequently)	4
Live abortions (all aborted subsequently)	6

Recurrent missed abortion
66 pregnancies
62 patients

missed abortions. We then decided to follow these figures up prospectively. We followed up prospectively 42 pregnancies (Table 2). Only 6 of those 42 were live abortions; 36 were missed abortions. Of those 36 missed abortions only 4 had a previously-detected fetal heart; 32 of them were blighted ova—and I use the term 'blighted' ova, not anembryonic pregnancy, because we don't know at what stage the embryo ceased developing; we don't know whether it was originally there or not. We then followed on from one of James Mowbray's ideas that there may be a very significant difference between the abortion of a live embryo and the missed abortion. We immunised all of them and tried to sort out the results afterwards. We immunised 120 patients altogether which has so far given us 80 pregnancies in 76 patients (Table 3). There were 3 subsequent ectopic pregnancies and one subsequent mole; that is, 4 pregnancies that we had to exclude. We had previously one of our patients who had cross-matched positive in advance, that is a high anti-paternal antibody prior to immunisation. So far there have been 4 patients whom we immunised who have aborted subsequently. We have immunised 6 patients who had had live abortions; all 6 of those aborted again. We then looked at the recurrent missed abortions, and that gives us 66 pregnancies in 62 patients. Now they call this match controls; these figures were not randomised; they were not double-blinded. If we look at our primary aborters with missed abortions, 70% had subsequent successful pregnancies compared to

Table 4

Matched controls

	immunised	%	control %		
1°	33/47	70	5/16	31	P.< 0.05
2°	10/19	53			
XM+	37/55	67			
XM−	4/11	36			
1° aborters preg.	30/39	77			P.< 0.05
becoming XM+ pts.	26/35	74	5/16	31	P.< 0.05

only 53% of secondary aborters (Table 4). When we compare that to our control groups we find that we are getting about 31% in the primary aborters. The figures for secondary aborters are not shown, but the figures for secondary aborters, spontaneously, are about 50% in our series. Immunisation does not seem to make much difference to the secondary aborters in our series. If we look at those XN positive—cross-matched positive—which is the way we detect anti-paternal antibody—again we see that there is a big difference between those who develop antibody and those who are cross-matched negative. When we then look at our select group, the ones who do best, they are the primary aborters who become cross-matched positive. In those, 30 pregnancies out of 39 were successful, that is 35 patients, as shown by patients 26 out of 35 in the last quadrant, which is 77%. We then went on to say, "if we can get 77% in primary aborters who become cross-matched positive, should we extend the immunisation to patients with

Table 5

Chromosomal aberrations and immunisation

Pt.	No. Abortions	Abberation	Outcome
1	3	46XX t(2:7) p33 p25	LSCS 40w. 3800g.
2	3	46XX t(13:15) q12 q15	LSCS 40w. 2800g. Esophageal atresia
3	3	47 XXX	FTND 38w. 2700g.
4	6abs 1 delivery 3 abortions	46 XX t(7:8) p13 q13	not yet pregnant

documented causes for abortion?" The four patients shown here (Table 5) are patients with chromosomal anomalies, the ones which I mentioned yesterday. Now, as we know, patients with this type of balanced translocation can have normal pregnancies afterwards. I think we have all seen them, and we all know that this can occur. The question is whether these balanced translocations should cause habitual abortions at all. Patients 1 and 2 and patient number 4—we can see their histories—3 previous abortions, and patient number 4 with 6 abortions and one delivery. We can see the type of translocation. We immunised those patients. The first 2 patients have delivered, the last one—it says that she is not yet pregnant, however she did become pregnant just before I came here. We don't yet know the result of that pregnancy. There is also a super female whom we immunised, who has also had a normal delivery. We then went on and asked,

Table 6 Uterine anomalies and immunisation

Pt.	No. Abs	Anomaly	Outcome subsequent pregnancy	
1	9	Severe adhesions	1) PROM 27/52	LSCS 950g.
			2) LSCS 35/52	2505g.
2	5	Adhesions at fundus	FTND 38/52	3600g.
3	4	Severe adhesions metroplasty further 2 abortions	live blighted ovum at 10/52	
4	4	T shaped (DES exposure)	FTND 38/52	2550g.
5	4	Septate, Excision of septum Further 2 abortions	presently 28/52	
6	5	Bicornuate	presently 23/52	
7	7	Bicornuate	missed abortion 9/52	
8	5	Bicornuate	Missed abortion (blighted) 8/52	
9	1 delivery 6 abortions	Bicornuate	Missed abortion 10/52	

"what about uterine anomalies?" (Table 6) The first 3 patients are patients who have had severe intrauterine adhesions, and I say severe adhesions which very much distorted the uterine cavity. I am not looking at the odd filmy adhesions. One of these patients had a D & C to separate those adhesions; each of them had 2 subsequent abortions after the D & C. You can see the results. Of the first 3 patients, you can see the patients with adhesions—most of them have had successful pregnancies. In the patient with the T-shaped uterus (number 4)—the same thing occurred. However, with the patients with bicornuate uterus (numbers 6 to 9), we have not been able to achieve successes with immunisation. One patient has succeeded and she has gone as far as 23 weeks. So far, we have had 30 babies born. Our rate of anomalies is 2 out of 30; there have been a number of premature deliveries.

Dr SZULMAN: Dr Carp's remarks give me courage to get up and poke my nose into what is not primarily my metier. I think that if women are to be considered for this type of treatment after 3 abortions, these 3 abortions have got to be very carefully charted in morphologic terms. No textbooks talk about it, and very few pathologists talk about it, but there is a tremendous amount of information that can be gained from careful microscopic examination of the aborted conceptus. And it would seem to me that the primary type of women to be subjected to this kind of treatment would be women who have conceptuses that are uniform with respect to their morphology. In other words, you are reaching out for some kind of common trigger for the 3 abortions that you are going to treat. And that can be ascertained morphologically by those who are interested.

Professor MOWBRAY: I think you are reaching for the stars if you think that you can get histological appraisal of the abortions in the past history of women who present with multiple abortuses. It just isn't feasible.

Professor SZULMAN: Is it not feasible because this material doesn't exist, or because this material can or cannot be gotten hold of? But if you are doing things in a prospective way...

Professor MOWBRAY: But when the patient presents, there is nothing you can do to go back and examine material that isn't available from abortions that occurred over the previous 10 or 15 years.

Professor SZULMAN: But ideally it would be a nice thing to have. And if one embarks on a prospective study, this is something to reach out for.

Dr RUSHTON: Two points which I direct at the last speaker in that there is something in one of the newer textbooks which has just appeared on the pathology of abortuses. It is the new edition of Haines' and Taylor's *Gynaecological Pathology*. The data from Sweden on the group with strong blocking antibodies and positive cardiolipid group, we think on examination of the placenta that we can predict these in the first pregnancy if they have purely anecdotal data. We now suggest on the basis of placental appearance that in the next pregnancy those patients should be treated with aspirin and/or steroids.

Professor MOWBRAY: Can I say that, as of your presentation of a couple of days ago, you were talking about second-trimester, we are talking predominantly about first-trimester in which half the losses have occurred before the eighth week. There is no histology; there is no placenta to see; there is nothing. You are very lucky to be able to get anything out of it.

Dr BULMER: But why is there no histology? There is histology, but it is in the original hospitals. Write to the pathologist and get the blocks; they are often there.

Professor MOWBRAY: The experience of the people immunising is that these women abort at home, at 6, 7 or 8 weeks; they are not in hospital.

Dr BULMER: It should be impressed on people that it is important, even if the specimens are put straight into formalin, that that would be better than doing nothing at all.

Professor MOWBRAY: I quite agree. But we are talking about abortions at home.

Dr BULMER: But can you not impress on the women that if they do abort at home how important it is.

Professor MOWBRAY: We get women who present as recurrent aborters. They have already gone through their abortions. By the time we see them it is too late.

Dr BULMER: The tissues worth looking at are the tissues of the women who are still aborting after treatment. They should be looked at.

Professor MOWBRAY: That is a different matter. They are being looked at.

Dr BULMER: In lots of these women there are blocks in pathology if you ask for them.

Professor HARRISON: Spontaneous abortion is the commonest reason for somebody being admitted. The laboratories would seize up if you did that; you are absolutely right, but the laboratories would seize up. When I curette somebody, I am lucky if I get a report back to confirm that the pregnancy was there.

SECTION 7
OTHER METHODS OF TREATMENT

Use of cervical cerclage in patients with recurrent first trimester abortion

D. K. Edmonds

INTRODUCTION

The aetiology of recurrent first trimester abortion has been discussed at some length and includes chromosomal anormalities, uterine anomalies, infections, placentation problems, morphological abnormalities and immunological problems. However, when these patients are investigated, very often nothing abnormal is found. This situation is particularly frustrating for both patient and doctor.

For many years, cervical incompetence has been recognised as a cause of second trimester abortion, and previous procedures such as dilatation and curettage,[1] or therapeutic termination of pregnancy are cited as traumatic causes of this cervical problem.[1] However, many women with recurrent second trimester abortion have no history of trauma, and are said to have a congenital or developmental problem. Attempts to classify these incompetent cervices have been fraught with criticism as the use of a Hegar dilator is purely subjective and the use of hysterosalpingography (HSG) is subject to the angle of the cervix/ uterus to the plane of the X-ray plate and the degree of pressure generated inside the uterus by the introduction of the radio-opaque medium to outline the cervical canal.[2] The recent use of ultrasound has allowed the first non-invasive assessment of the cervical canal[3] although ultrasound has not been used in this study.

Patients with cervical incompetence show classical cervical changes with painless effacement of the cervix, sometimes associated with bleeding, subsequent dilatation and loss of the pregnancy. The reasons for these changes in the cervical tissue at term are known to be the release of prostaglandins and a hydrophilic change in the cervical collagen. As the cervix effaces, the prostaglandin levels rise and labour ensues.[4]

The competence of the internal os as a protection against these changes occurring is not fully understood, but there does not seem to be any reason why cervical incompetence should be a uniquely second trimester phenomenon. In the first trimester, hormonal changes are considerable and high levels of oestrogen may well affect the cervix, initiating changes in incompetent cervices leading to spontaneous abortion. It was, therefore, deemed reasonable to attempt to use

411

METHODS

A total of 37 patients were recruited into the study between 1983 and 1986. All patients had 3 or more first trimester abortions, with no other pregnancies unless ectopic, i.e. no second trimester abortions, or preterm or term pregnancies. Patients who had a history of an ectopic pregnancy could be included but the ectopic pregnancy could not be included as a first trimester abortion. The range of abortions was from 3 to 9, with a mean of 3.8 pregnancies (Table 1). The

Table 1

No. of Pregnanies	No. of Patients
3	22
4	8
5	2
6	3
7	1
8	0
9	1
	37

average age of the patients was 28.5 years. All patients were investigated fully for recurrent abortion before entry into the study and this included, general history and examination, hysterosalpingography, karyotyping of husband and wife, maternal lupus anticoagulant, infection screen for toxoplasmosis, rubella and listeria monocytogenes and thyroid function. Any patient found to have a congenital uterine anomaly or chromosomal abnormalities was excluded.

Patients were asked to contact the Chelsea Hospital for Women when they had 6 weeks of amenorrhoea and a positive pregnancy test. An ultrasound scan was performed at 7 weeks and the presence of fetal heart activity confirmed. Cervical cerclage was then performed using a modified McDonald technique.[5] A double suture of No 2 monofilament nylon was inserted at the level of the internal cervical os, the bladder being reflected if necessary, and the knots tied, independently, anteriorly. The procedure was performed under general anaesthesia. The patient was then managed routinely for ante-natal and intra-partum care.

RESULTS

All 37 patients recruited had cervical cerclage without complication. One patient subsequently presented with a non-viable pregnancy at 10 weeks and the sutures were removed and evacuation of the retained products performed. Thirty-five patients (94.5%) delivered live infants, the other patient aborting at 17 weeks, having never surpassed 11 weeks previously. This abortion was subsequent to a fall which was followed by spontaneous rupture of the membranes; this patient has subsequently had a repeat cerclage and delivery of a term infant, but this pregnancy is not included in this study.

The obstetric outcome of the remaining 35 pregnancies is seen in Table 2. The only patient who had a serious problem was the patient who was G10 PO + 9, who delivered at 26 weeks gestation. The infant weighed 780 gms and has

Table 2

Obstetric outcome following cervical cerclage

Number of patients	37
Spontaneous abortion	2
Premature delivery	5 (14%)
Live born healthy infant	34 (94%)
Live born infant with cerebral palsy	1

survived, but has severe cerebral palsy and will be permanently handicapped. All other infants were normal singletons, and have developed without complication.

In a retrospective analysis of the HSGs performed, 26 women had no demonstrable abnormalities in the uterine body, 11 had funnelling of the utero-cervical junction, with a measured internal os between 3 and 7mm.

DISCUSSION

The use of cervical cerclage in the problem of habitual first trimester abortion is perhaps unconventional, but the results of this study suggest that cervical incompetence may be aetiological in some cases. The major criticism of this study is that is was not randomised, but attempts to fulfil this were unsuccessful. Patients were invited into a no-treatment group but none would agree, and so randomisation was not possible. In estimating the expected abortion rate from already published statistics, it is difficult to obtain definitive figures. Retrospective studies by Warburton and Fraser,[6] Stevenson *et al*,[7] and Naylor and Warburton,[8] suggest a rate of about 30% after 3 abortions. Prospective studies by Boué,[9] Lauritson,[10] Harger *et al*[11] and Fitzsimmons[12] suggest rates of 33%. Based on this data, an abortion rate of about 12 patients would have been expected. Obviously, this is considerably greater than that found in this series, or in the series published by Ayers *et al*.[13]

In considering the aetiology, analysis of cervical tissue shows this to be 10-15% smooth muscle and 85-90% collagen. There is, however, a marked increase in the fibromuscular component at the internal os, the change being gradual in some cases (over 10 mm), or abrupt in others (1-2 mm).[14] The onset of pregnancy leads to changes in cervical tissue, as previously outlined, and it may be that some women have cervices which are congenitally abnormal in the fibromuscular junction and, as a result, pregnancy changes induce a weakness which leads to the loss of the pregnancy. The association between uterine fusion defects and cervical incompetence is well described, with reliable estimates at 30%.[15] The possibility of congenital anomalies of the cervical tissue alone, with no fusion defect, cannot be excluded, and although no association has yet to be found to infer an environmental influence, the association with *in utero* diethyl stilboestrol exposure in the mother is also well documented.[16]

The use, therefore, of cervical cerclage early in pregnancy in the present study group seems justified. The previous use of cerclage in cervical incompetence advocates the insertion of the suture at about 12 weeks' gestation, and it would seem that this would be too late in first-trimester cases. In the series of Ayers *et al*,[13] the cervix was examined clinically during the first and second trimesters and they discovered that 89% of patients had evidence of effacement during the first trimester without any other signs of threatened abortion.

The obstetric outcome in these patients is important as they are a high risk population. The increased incidence of premature labour is similar to the findings of Ayers *et al.*[13] These studies also looked at the placenta, and commented that 24% had placental abnormalities, 11% having major degrees of placental infarction. I doubt whether these abnormalities explain the obstetric outcome *per se*, but they are interesting observations. The aetiology of pre-term labour remains an unsolved mystery in obstetrics, but it is interesting to note that the incidence is greatly increased in women with uterine fusion defects.[17,18]

Finally, the effectiveness of cerclage in this group is difficult to explain, but perhaps, apart from the establishment of an anatomically 'functional' cervix, there may be a protective element preventing chorioamnionitis, or even a direct effect of elevation of the pregnancy mass away from the cervix which prevents stimulation of stretch receptors in the lower uterine body.

REFERENCES

1. McDonald IA. Incompetence of the cervix. *Aust NZ J Obstet Gynaecol* 1978; **18:** 34-37.
2. Mann EC, McLaren WD, Hayt DB. The physiology and clinical significance of the uterine isthmus. *Am J Obstet Gynecol* 1961; **81:** 209-213.
3. Brook I, Feingold M, Schwartz A, Zakut H. Ultrasonography in the diagnosis of cervical incompetence in pregnancy—a new diagnostic approach. *Br J Obstet Gynaecol* 1981; **88:** 640-649.
4. Liggins GC. Ripening the cervix. *Semin Perinatal* 1978; **2:** 261-271.
5. McDonald IA. Cervical Incompetence as a Cause of Spontaneous Abortion In: *Spontaneous and Recurrent Abortion.* Eds. MJ Bennett, DK Edmonds. Oxford: Blackwell Scientific Publications, 1987; pp.177.
6. Warburton D, Fraser FC. Spontaneous abortion risks in man. *Am J Hum Genet* 1964; **16:** 1-13.
7. Stevenson AC, Dudgeon MY, McClure HI. Observations on the results of pregnancies in women resident in Belfast: abortions, hydatidiform moles and ectopic pregnancies. *Ann Hum Genet* 1959; **23:** 395-403.
8. Naylor AF, Warburton D. Sequential aspects of spontaneous abortion. Collaborative study data show that gravidity determines a very substantial rise in risk. *Fertil Steril* 1978; **31:** 282-288.
9. Boué J, Boué A, Lazar P. Retrospective and prospective epidemiological studies of 1500 karyotyped spontaneous human abortions. *Teratology* 1975; **12:** 11-26.
10. Lauritsen JG. Aetiology of spontaneous abortion—a cytogenetic and epidemiological study of 288 abortuses and their parents. *Acta Obstet Gynecol Scand* (Suppl) 1976; **52:** 1-29.
11. Harger JH, Archer DF, Marchese SG, Muracca-Clements M, Garver KL. Etiology of recurrent pregnancy losses and outcome of subsequent pregnancies. *Obstet Gynecol* 1983; **63:** 574-578.
12. Fitzsimmons J, Jackson D, Wapner R, Jackson L. Subsequent reproductive outcome in couples with repeated pregnancy loss. *Am J Med Genet* 1983; **16:** 583-587.
13. Ayers JW, Peterson EP, Ansbacher R. Early therapy for the incompetent cervix in patients with habitual abortion. *Fertil Steril* 1982; **38:** 177-181.
14. Danforth DN. The distribution and functional activity of cervical musculature. *Am J Obstet Gynecol* 1954; **68:** 1261-1278.

15. Craig CJT. Congenital abnormalities of the uterus and foetal wastage. *S Afr Med J* 1973; **47**: 2000-2011.
16. Kaufman RH, Irwin JF. Diethylstilboetrol exposure and reproductive performance in spontaneous and recurrent abortion. In: *Spontaneous and Recurrent Abortion*. Eds. MJ Bennett, DK Edmonds. Oxford: Blackwell Scientific Publications 1987; pp.130.
17. Bennett MJ, Berry JV. Preterm labour and congenital malformations of the uterus. *Ultrasound Med Biol* 1979; **5**:83-85.
18. Buttram VC. Müllerian abnormalities and their management. *Fertil Steril* 1983; **40**: 159-163.

Discussion

Chairman: Professor R. F. Harrison

Professor GILL: After you did the cerclage, approximately what percentage subsequently aborted compared to what you would have expected in the normal population?

Mr EDMONDS: Two aborted out of the 37 who had cerclage. The difficulty is that when you take out the anembryonic pregnancies, and all the estimates have been done on pregnancies which have been clinically confirmed, you can't quote the 30%. Professor Beer has mentioned this morning 11 out of 51. You just can't quote that as an abortion rate. If you do an ultrasound and find a fetal heart active in the normal population, not a recurring aborting population, only 2% will subsequently abort.

Dr MICHEL: I followed up a group of recurrent miscarriers who received immunotherapy, and in this group, still with an intact fetal heart and a fetal form, the risk of miscarriage is still 2-3%. Actually, one or two of them had the miscarriage after they had amniocentesis.

Mr EDMONDS: What about your untreated control group who were not immunised?

Dr MICHEL: At the time when the double-blind trial was done there was no ultrasound done on these patients because they were all referred back to their obstetrician.

Mr EDMONDS: That's the problem; I don't think that anyone has any data to answer your question about what the risk would be with a positive fetal heart at 8 weeks.

Miss REGAN: We used to say that once you have documented a fetal heart you have a 95% chance of that pregnancy going to term. Now in the normal population I have looked at we have had a 20% abortion rate after documenting a fetal heart.

Professor BEER: Our incidence would be much higher than that, doing ultrasounds from 5 weeks on in the group receiving third party leucocyte immunisation. Although I can't quote exactly, I know that all 21 of those got pregnant again subsequently. We were looking and documenting fetal heart activity a week or two earlier than you.

Dr UNANDER: If "tender loving care" really was so important then I must tell you that among my immunised patients I have more than 20 patients who had previous unsuccessful cerclage by their own obstetricians. They still aborted. In some of them intrauterine fetal death occurred later. Also, the group with strong blocking antibodies were treated exactly the same way as those who lacked blocking antibodies. They were checked just as carefully afterwards. I know there are immunological causes. We know that there is evidence that psychological factors may influence the immune response. But certainly "tender loving care" does no miracles for some of these patients.

Mr EDMONDS: I wouldn't disagree with you that it doesn't solve everybody's problem or we would have a 100% pregnancy rate, but I wonder whether sending a patients back away from the home unit is really giving them "tender loving care"?

Dr DAYA: May I ask at what gestational age the cerclages were performed? If you wait beyond 13 weeks, then you would expect the results that you got.

Mr EDMONDS: Seven weeks.

Dr B STRAY-PEDERSON: We don't perform cerclage on first trimester aborters, so your patients are second trimester aborters.

Dr UNANDER: We don't know what some obstetricians may do sometimes, just in desperation.

Dr ALLEN: In the scan, you were indicating pregnancy all the time between the vagina and the uterus. Presumably, there is a very tight cervical seal in a normal pregnant lady, is there not?

Mr EDMONDS: That particular ultrasound was an example of an open cervix, not a normal cervix.

Dr ALLEN: But you said that you really didn't think that cerclage was necessary!

Mr EDMONDS: I was only showing how ultrasound can demonstrate the incompetent cervix. I didn't use ultrasound routinely on my patients. When we did they were all within the normal range. It had been claimed that something like 30% had an internal os that was greater than 5 mm.

Dr ALLEN: But an internal diameter of 5 mm is a big wide trap for bacteria.

Mr EDMONDS: I agree. Maybe that is why they abort.

Dr ALLEN: Exactly! Do you think that is the case? The human is very unusual among all mammals. She continues to mate during pregnancy, offering a severe bacterial challenge.

Mr EDMONDS: Also a physical challenge. That is one of the theories why cerclage might work. Perhaps by elevating the pregnancy you can get it out of the lower part of the uterus.

Professor CLARK: I am not so sure that we should use this word "tender and loving" when trying to talk about the effect of placebo therapy. The surprise to me was not the result that you got after the cerclage, but that you only had 5 anembryonic pregnancies. Of course the patients knew they were going to get something that might be effective. If you assume that there would be a 30% incidence of pregnancy failure in this group, and that most of them would be anembryonic, then if you calculate the expected number of anembryonic pregnancies, you produce the anembryonic pregnancy rate by x^2 value which exceeds 4. So your belief that your treatment didn't work may not be entirely correct. It may be the anticipation of the treatment that was quite effective.

Professor HOWIE: How did you recruit your patients? I would find it very difficult to recruit in a single practice such a number. Was this a referred group of patients? In some studies, the treatment for the patient has been identified before she becomes pregnant. In other words, you are only putting a stitch in those who had preselected themselves to be favourable.

Mr EDMONDS: They were all referred because I had an interest in this problem. They were all selected in that sense. I am sure a number of them would have aborted if they hadn't come up for the ultrasound scan at 7 weeks.

Early recurrent pregnancy failure: treatment with human chorionic gonadotrophin

R. F. Harrison

SUMMARY

Based upon our present knowledge of the endocrine processes concerned with early pregnancy, the role of exogenous hCG in the prevention of habitual abortion has been examined.

A dose regime has been established administering hCG intramuscularly from earliest diagnosis of pregnancy at intervals until 16 weeks gestation.

An open study using hCG in 32 women showed a 6.2% abortion rate. A placebo-controlled study on 20 women gave a significantly better outcome using hCG ($p < 0.01$). A further placebo-controlled study is ongoing, the extra numbers needed to provide a definitive answer being recruited on a multicentre basis.

Pending the outcome of this study, results to date suggest hCG to be the treatment of choice for habitual abortion where no cause can be found or where a potentially treatable hormonal deficiency is suspected.

INTRODUCTION

Data from conceptual cycles and *in vitro* fertilisation have extended greatly the understanding of the endocrinology of conception, implantation and pregnancy. Wide gaps in our knowledge however still prevail.

Inter-related and inter-dependant endocrine systems are involved.[1] The pre-implantation system mediated by the *corpus luteum* allows initial development. This evolves into the post-implantation system, unique to pregnancy and concerned with its maintenance. Here, control is also initially exerted through the *corpus luteum*. The increased participation of the conceptus leads to the transfer of major neuroendocrine control to the feto-placental unit. The time of transfer varies with different hormones between the 6th to 13th weeks.[2] Although the *corpus luteum* and indeed ovarian endocrine function itself continues,[3] its presence is apparently not necessary for the continuation of the pregnancy.[4] The major neuroendocrine control of gestation remains until delivery with the sophisticated interrelationship between mother and feto-placental unit.

421

Amongst other factors, progesterones and oestrogens have both been found essential for the maintenance of early pregnancy.[5,6] Women sampled sequentially through the early stages of pregnancy reveal circulating plasma progesterone levels to be fairly constant until about the 10th week of menstrual gestation rising slowly thereafter.[7] Plasma oestrone and oestradiol measurements rise early whereas oestriol levels are low until approximately week 13 and then begin to rise incrementally.[8]

In abortion, levels of such hormones may be low.[9] Although this is possibly effect rather than cause, such thinking was perhaps behind the introduction of supplemental therapy. Synthetic oestrogens were initially used, then progestagens, and now "natural" progesterones. Oestrogens have, however, been associated with an apparently increased incidence of vaginal carcinoma and other genital tract defects in the offspring of those who took large doses of the synthetic preparations in early pregnancy.[10] Progestagens have the potential to masculinise the female fetus, are luteolytic[11] and have not been shown to be better than placebo.[12] This final criticism may also be levelled against "natural" progesterone, although when administered as vaginal pessaries such therapy enjoys popularity as a support for the *corpus luteum*, particularly following IVF treatment cycles.[13]

Human chorionic gonadotrophin (hCG) appears as early as the 8th day of gestation.[14] Levels are highest between the 6th and 13th menstrual weeks.[15] Studies have shown that it plays a vital physiological role in the early stages of pregnancy. It stimulates both the *corpus luteum* and early feto-placental endocrine function.[16] It is concerned with the active secretion of oestrogen and progesterone from the *corpus luteum*. *In vitro*, hCG has been shown to stimulate such steroidogenesis.[17] *In vivo* exogenous administration of hCG given to support the luteal phase will raise hormone levels and prolongs the life of the *corpus luteum*.[18]

However, it may well be that the *corpus luteum* is limited in its ability to increase steroid production in response to hCG stimulation.[19] There is a lack of correlation between plasma hCG levels and steroid secretions of oestrogen and progesterone.[20] Indeed, hCG may not need to be present beyond the first few weeks of gestation[21], and in terms of its role in feto-placental function has yet to be defined. A placentotrophic level has however been demonstrated *in vitro*.[22]

Although it is wise to admit that in the present state of knowledge a definitive diagnosis is difficult, the concept of an endocrine deficiency as a major cause of abortion is certainly tenable. Bearing in mind the endocrinology of early pregnancy as at present understood, it would appear logical that, when such an abnormality is thought to be present, the exogenous administration of hCG to stimulate and optimise hormonal production by the *corpus luteum* and feto-placental unit in a live pregnancy[23] would be the most appropriate aproach to therapy.

This hypothesis was examined in the following planned manner.

1. SELECTION OF DOSE REGIME

Little guidance is available. Differing schedules and routes of administration abound. The minimum effective dosage of hCG is therefore unknown.[24]

Intravenous therapy appears more effective with the progesterone secretion response, dose related.[25] However, the blood level of endogenous hCG is 50,000 iu/ml and an injection of 5,000 iu, the dosage most commonly used to influence the ovary in IVF cycles, will increase this by a maximum of 2,500 iu/ml. High dosage can be deleterious.[26] hCG has a long half life,[27] plasma levels fall to normal within 6 days of intramuscular hCG administration.[28]

Any regime must be practical and cost effective. It must commence as soon as possible after the diagnosis of pregnancy and continue through and beyond the vital crossover period from *corpus luteum* to feto-placental unit.[2,29] Therefore, with these factors in mind as well as a "petit morceau" of empiricism, a dosage protocol was devised to use in the habitual abortion situation where an endocrine deficiency was suspected or no other cause for the successive miscarriages could be found. An initial loading dose of 10,000 iu hCG was to be given intramuscularly (im) on diagnosis of pregnancy (if before the 7th week). This was followed by 5,000 iu im administered twice weekly up to week 12, and 5,000 iu im once weekly thereafter up to week 16.

2. JUDGING THE EFFICACY OF THERAPY

Two end points can be used: pregnancy outcome and hormonal levels of target organs.

The outcome of pregnancy is obviously very important. There are however difficulties in using it as the sole scientific measure of success. It has been suggested that 1,078 women with a history of habitual abortion would be needed to prove the value against placebo of an agent which raised the salvage rate by a mere 10%.[30] As the incidence of women with such a problem is low, to assemble such a group in one centre would be almost impossible. In addition, there is a high chance that even after 3 successive miscarriages the next pregnancy could continue successfully without therapy.[31] Indeed, support alone may give a 75% successful outcome.[32] Early diagnosis of pregnancy and ultrasound monitoring may have an as yet unmeasured potent placebo effect, and there is of course no guarantee that the cause for abortion in the same woman is the same as that of her previous miscarriages.

The lack of established reference levels and the wide range of normality in those studies published to date, makes conclusions based on early pregnancy circulating hormonal measurements open to criticism. In addition, the hormones so measured may not reflect the concentration of hormonal activity on site in the reproductive tract, and a single sample may not be representative of the hormonal production or its production rate. Low values of many hormones and in particular hCG[33] have been found associated with abortion, but this could be due to an effect in an already doomed pregnancy rather than the cause of demise.

In the absence of more suitable alternatives, while recognising their shortcomings, both criteria were used as measures of success in step 3:- the clinical studies.

3. CLINICAL STUDIES USING hCG IN HABITUAL ABORTION

The trials, all prospective, concern only women who gave a history of the last 3 consecutive pregnancies ending in spontaneous abortion before the 20th week. Wherever possible all other causes were excluded[31,34,35] by the relevant tests. Other abnormalities were detected in 23% of the population leaving as eligible those for whom no cause for habitual abortion could be found or those where the luteal phase plasma progesterone estimations (days 20 to 24) when measured were in our laboratory lower range (< 16 nmol/1).

After recruitment and following informed consent, all women were asked to contact the hospital for a formal diagnosis of pregnancy and commencement of hCG as above at the earliest possible. Prior to the 7th week when viability is diagnosed by ultrasound detection of fetal heart activity, entry was allowed with a normally formed fetal sac containing a fetal echo.

Mindful of the resources and material available, the hCG hypothesis has been examined in 3 phases. An initial open study was followed by a placebo-controlled trial. These two studies were undertaken in the Rotunda and St James's Hospitals Dublin. Reported in full elsewhere,[36] these results are summarised below. The place of hCG in the treatment of habitual abortion will, it is hoped, be finally settled by the results of the present ongoing multicentre placebo-controlled study below.

a. Open Study

Thirty-two women were involved. Twenty had been fully investigated prior to therapy and no other possible aetiological cause found. Their average age was 30.5 years (19-40) and 16 were nulliparous. The average gestation at the start of therapy was 6 weeks.

Table 1

Open Study of hCG in Habitual Abortion
n = 32.

Non Abortion	Aborted
30	2

Five patients had early vaginal bleeding, but only 2 of the 32 patients aborted (6.2%) (Table 1). Sixteen male children (including 2 sets of twins) and 16 females were born. There was one case of unexplained intrauterine growth retardation, one of severe pre-eclampsia and one intrauterine death. This latter occurred at 31 weeks due to twin transfusion syndrome. Both abortions occurred at 10 weeks. One was spontaneous. The other was a missed abortion found at repeat ultrasound scan.

The successful outcome of 93% is more than comparable with the results quoted in the only other studies published to date that used hCG in habitual abortion.[26,37-39] These were uncontrolled trials and therefore also lacking true scientific validation. Such treatment could also be ascribed to a placebo effect but was sufficiently encouraging to make phase b necessary.

b. Placebo-Controlled Trial

Twenty women were randomly allocated double-blind to either hCG (Profasi, Serono U.K.) or identically packaged placebo (regime as above) from the earliest diagnosis of pregnancy. Ten were in their 4-5th week, with average 6 weeks gestation at start of therapy. None who needed second scans to confirm viability had to be eliminated thereafter. Plasma progesterone was estimated at intervals throughout the drug administration period. Any abortus material recovered was examined morphologically and chromosome cultures attempted.

Table 2

Dublin Studies on hCG in Habitual Abortion

	hCG		Placebo	
	No Abortion	Aborted	No Abortion	Aborted
Open Study n = 32	30	2	NA	NA
Placebo Trial* n = 20	10	NA	3	7
Clinical Therapy to Sept. 1987 n = 13	11	2	NA	NA

*p < 0.01 (Fisher Test)

The pregnancies of all 10 women on active therapy continued (Table 2) whereas 7 of the women on placebo aborted, leaving only 3 going through to term (p<0.01 Fisher Test). Seven male children were born on active therapy and 3 females on each of active and placebo. Average age of those on hCG was 30.7 years (24-40), the successful placebo treated women 33.3 years (28-39), and the unsuccessful 33.4 years (25-39). One case of pre-eclampsia occurred in each group and there was one neonatal death in the active group. This was at 31 weeks due to prematurity in a patient who had ruptured her membranes at 27 weeks. All abortions occurred spontaneously before the 14th week. All aborted material examined was apparently morphologically normal and no chromosome abnormalities were discovered.

Pre-therapy plasma progesterone estimations of the whole group were within the normal range (20-50nmol/1). Mean plasma progesterone level on hCG was 61nmol/1, that of the placebo successes 68nmol/1 and the placebo failures 45nmol/1 (not significant). Little can be read into such hormone results except that plasma progesterone is mainly a reflection of the progress of pregnancy, successful or otherwise. A significant difference was however seen in pregnancy outcome between hCG and placebo. This was a prospective study in a group truly representative of the population that presents to the clinic.[40] Nevertheless, the small number involved leaves the results and their interpretation still open to criticism. In this small select group of women, to obtain sufficient numbers, 30, is beyond the resources of all but specialised centres whose clinic population and data will instead suffer from the bias of pre-selection.

The results were, however, sufficiently encouraging and free of side effects to attempt to increase the power of the data in terms of patient numbers. This led to the present ongoing multicentre placebo trial (phase c, below). This does not include Dublin for, in view of the above results, inclusion of placebo would be considered unethical. However, a further 13 patients to date have been treated with the same hCG regime (Table 2). In 11 (85%) pregnancy has continued successfully.

c. Multicentre Trial

Sixteen centres are involved comparing hCG (Pregnyl, Organon) and placebo. Each are scheduled to recruit a maximum of 12 cases randomised in blocks of six to prevent unequal distribution of medication. A paired sequential design has been used with recruitment, pre-therapy investigation and treatment regimes as before. An additional group with other possible causes of habitual abortion are also being studied as are suitable patients who present uninvestigated in the early stages of pregnancy. Any infants born during the trial will be followed up at regular intervals until the age of 21 with particular regard taken of physical and mental development.

Recruitment to date has been steady. It is hoped that a further 18 months should see the definitive answer as to the efficacy of both hCG and placebo in women with habitual abortion of unknown aetiology or where hormone imbalance is suspected.

CONCLUSIONS

Habitual abortion, a distressing condition, has been ascribed to many differing causes. Some of these have specific effective therapy. In many, no aetiology is found, or diagnostic markers can be found wanting. Responses to placebo are high and whatever approach to treatment success rates appear strangely similar. This would tend to suggest that there is no one single cause or one specific therapy that is universally applicable. However pending the outcome of the multicentre study, results using hCG to date can only lead to the conclusion that it should be the treatment of choice in women with habitual abortion where other specific causes have been ruled out and a potentially treatable hormonal imbalance surmised.

ACKNOWLEDGEMENTS

To Serono and Organon for their help and support with phases b and c of the study respectively.

REFERENCES
1. Davies J, Ryan KJ. Comparative endocrinology of gestation. In: *Vitamins and Hormones*. (Eds) RF Harris, PL Munsen, E Diczfalusy and J Glover. New York: Academic Press, 1972; pp. 233-279.
2. Corker CS, Michie E, Hobson B, Parboosingh J. Hormonal patterns in conceptual cycles and early pregnancy. *Br J Obstet Gynaec* 1976; **83:** 489-494.
3. Mishell DR, Thorneycroft IA, Nagata Y, Mirata T, Nakamura RM. Steroid gonadotropin and steroid pattern in early human gestation. *ATOG* 1973; **117:** 631-639.

4. Navot D. Laufer N, Kopolavic J, Rabinowitz R, Burkenfeld A. Lewin A, Granat M, Margaliot E, Shenker JG. Artifically induced endometrial cycles and establishment of pregnancies in the absence of ovaries. *New Eng J Med* 1986; **314**: 806-808.
5. Allen WM, Corner GW. Physiology of the *corpus luteum*. III. Normal growth and implantation of embryos after very early ablation of the ovaries under the influence of extract of the *corpus luteum*. *Am J Physiol* 1929; **88**: 340-346.
6. McKerns KW. Genetic biochemical and hormonal mechanisms in the regulation of uterine metabolism. In: *Cellular Biology of the Uterus*. Ed. RM Wynn. New York: Appleton-Century Crofts, 1967; pp. 71-113.
7. Harrison RF, Youssefnejadian E, Brodovcky H, Johnston M, Dewhurst J. Secretion patterns of plasma-progesterone, 17 α-hydroxy-progesterone and 20 α-hydroxy-preg-n-4-en-3- one in early normal pregnancy. *Br J Obstet Gynaec* 1978; **85**: 921-926.
8. Harrison RF, Kitchin Y. Maternal plasma unconjugated oestrogens in early human pregnancy. *Br J Obstet Gynaec* 1980; **87**: 686-694.
9. Kunz J, Keller PJ. hCG, HPL, oestradiol, progesterone and AFP in serum in patients with threatened abortions. *Br J Obstet Gynaec* 1976; **83**: 640-644.
10. Herbst AL, Ulfelder H, Poskanzer DG. Adenocarcinoma of the vagina—association of maternal stilboestrol therapy with tumour appearances in young women. *N Eng J Med* 1971; **284**: 878-881.
11. Yovich JL. Stanger JG, Yovich JM, Tuvik AI. Assessment and hormonal treatment of the luteal phase of in vitro ferilization cycles. *Aust NZ J Obstet Gynaec* 1984; **24**: 125-130.
12. Shearman RF, Garrett WJ. Double blind study of the effect of 17-hydroxy-progesterone-caproate on abortion rate. *Br Med J* 1963; **1**: 292-295.
13. Rosenwaks Z. Donor eggs. Their application in modern reproductive techniques. *Fertil Steril* 1987; **47**: 895-909.
14. Lenton EA, Neal LM, Sulaiman R. Plasma concentration of human chorionic gonado-tropin from the time of implantation until the second week of pregnancy. *Fertil Steril* 1982; **37**: 773-778.
15. Harrison RF, O'Moore RR, McSweeney J. Maternal plasma beta-hCG in early human pregnancy. *Br J Obstet Gynaec* 1980; **87**: 705-711.
16. Hanson FW, Powell JE, Stevens VC. Effects of hCG and human pituitary LH on steroid secretion and functional life of the *corpus luteum*. *J Clin Endocrinol* 1971; **32**: 211-215.
17. LeMaire WJ, Rice BF, Savard K. Steroid hormone formation in the human ovary. V. Synthesis of progesterone *in vitro* in *corpora lutea* during the reproductive cycle. *J Clin Endocrinol* 1968; **28**: 1249-1256.
18. Mahadevan MM, Leader A, Taylor PJ. Effects of low dose human chorionic gonado-tropin on *corpus luteum* function after embryo transfer. *In Vitro Fert Embryo Transfer* 1985; **2**: 190-194.
19. Tulchinsky D, Hobel CJ. Plasma human chorionic gonadotropin, estrone, estradiol, estriol, progesterone and 17 α-hydroxy-progesterone in human pregnancy. III. Early normal pregnancy. *Am J Obstet Gynec* 1973; **117**: 884-892.
20. Yoshimi J, Strott CA, Marshall JR, Lipsett MB. Corpus luteum function in early pregnancy. *J Endocrinol* 1969; **29**: 225-230.
21. Csapo AI, Pulkkinen MO, Kaihola HL. Effective estradiol replacement therapy in early pregnancy lutiectomised patients. *Am J Obstet Gynec* 1973; **115**: 759-765.
22. Diczfalusy E, Troen P. Endocrine functions of the human placenta. *Vitamins and Hormones* 1979; **19**: 229-311.
23. Moore RM, Rosen L. *Corpus luteum* of the sheep: functional relationship between the embryo and the *corpus luteum*. *J Endocrinol* 1965; **34**: 233-239.
24. Dukelow WR. Human chorionic gonadotropin: induction of ovulation in the squirrel monkey. *Science* 1979; **206**: 234-235.

25. Garner PR, Armstrong DT. The effect of human chorionic gonadotropin and estradiol 17-β on the maintenance of the human *corpus luteum* of early pregnancy. *Am J Obstet Gynec* 1977; **128:** 469-475.
26. Sandler SW, Braillie P. The use of human chorionic gonadotrophin in recurrent abortion. *S Afr Med J* 1979; **55:** 832-835.
27. Midgley AR (Jnr), Jaffe RB. Regulation of human gonadotrophins. II. Disappearance of human chorionic gonadotrophin following delivery. *J Clin Endocrinol* 1968; **28:** 1712-1718.
28. Marshall JR, Hammond CB, Ross GT, Jacobson A, Rayford P, Odell W. Plasma and urinary chorionic gonadotropin during early human pregnancy. *Obstet Gynec* 1968; **32:** 760-764.
29. Deansley R. The endocrinology of pregnancy and fetal life. In: *Marshall's Physiology of Reproduction.* Ed. AP Parkes. London: Longhall Green. 1966; p.891.
30. Goldzieher JW. Double blind trial of a progestin in habitual abortion. *JAMA* 1964; **188:** 651-654.
31. Chamberlain G. Recurrent miscarriage and pre-term labour. In: *Clinics in Obstetrics and Gynaecology.* Ed. TMG Harley. London: WB Saunders 1982; Vol. 9. pp. 115-130.
32. Overstreet E. The newer progestins in threatened and habitual abortion. *Pac Med Surg* 1964; **72:** 289-292.
33. Dutinger J, Newmark J, Reinthaller A, Riss P, Muller-Tyle E, Fischl F, Bieglmayer C, Janisch H. Pregnancy specific parameters in early pregnancies after *in vitro* fertilisation. Prediction of the course of pregnancy. *Fertil Steril* 1986; **46:** 77-80.
34. Stirrat GM. Recurrent abortion-a review. *Br J Obstet Gynaec* 1983; **90:** 881-883.
35. DeCherney A, Polan ML, Evaluation and managment of habitual abortion, *Br J Hosp Med* 1984; **31:** 261-268.
36. Harrison RF. Treatment of habitual abortion with human chorionic gonadotropin results of open and placebo-controlled studies. *Eur J Obstet Gynaec Reprod Biol* 1985; **20:** 159-168.
37. Utian WH. Human chorionic gonadotropin in the treatment of threatened and recurrent abortion. A preliminary reappraisal. *S Afr Med J* 1974; **48:** 769-771.
38. Vorster CZ, Pannall PR, Slabber CF. Treatment of threatened and habitual abortion with human chorionic gonadotrophin. *S Afr Med J* 1977; **51:** 165-166.
39. Sandler SW. Spontaneous abortion in perspective. A 7 year study. *S Afr Med J* 1977; **52:** 1115-1118.
40. Goldzieher JW, Benigno B. Treatment of threatened and recurrent abortion: A critical review. *Am J Obstet Gynec* 1958; **75:** 1201-1214.
41. Glass RH, Golbus MS. Habitual abortion. *Fertil Steril* 1978; **29:** 257-265.

Discussion

Chairman: Mr D. K. Edmonds

Professor CLARK: Do you think that it is possible to get the right answer for the wrong reason?

Professor HARRISON: Absolutely.

Professor CLARK: hCG preparations may be contaminated with what is called "early pregnancy factor", produced sometime in early pregnancy and potentially important in the success of early pregnancy. Are you using a preparation of hCG where all the "early pregnancy factor" activity has been removed so that you know that the effects are actually due to the hormonal changes?

Professor HARRISON: I would doubt it. We used two commercial preparations. They both, as far as I know, come from the same sources, that is from pregnant women themselves. They are said to be pure preparations, based on mouse data.

Dr UNANDER: I was asked to participate in a study on the immunological effects of hCG around 1980. I sent Dr Helen Morton several preparations of hCG. One contained substantial amounts of "early pregnancy factor", at least in the batches that were sent to her. I don't know if they have changed their preparation methods since then.

Professor GRUDZINSKAS: My only qualification to comment on "early pregnancy factor" is that I come from the country where it was invented, and I think this is not documented anywhere. The phenomenon referred to as "early pregnancy factor" (EPF) is usually considered to be part of the group of psycho-pathological processes that has crept down the eastern coast of Australia! On a more constructive note, the reason that the endocrinologists have this view is because of the heterogeneity of the biochemical description of these phenomena loosely referred to as "early pregnancy factor". So the principal assay for those who are not aware of these phenomena is the so-called rosehead inhibition test, a minefield for all sorts of non-specific effects. There is no doubt that there are some phenomena that occur in the earliest hours and days of pregnancy, that are part of the maternal recognition of pregnancy, but really don't have a part to play in a discussion of the therapeutic effect or otherwise of hCG preparations. What proportion of patients were considered for your studies but were rejected?

Professor HARRISON: Twenty percent at most were excluded. We very seldom find a reason for the patient aborting previously.

Professor BEER: In many *in vitro* fertilisation programmes patients are given Pergonal. Paternal serum is being used in many of these cultures. There are strange effects seen on immunoreactivity—possible growth factor contamination, anti-idiotypes and even antibodies present in the preparation. Anti-idiotype, if it is in the preparation, can act as antigen. So you may be delivering a relevant pregnancy antigen in your preparation that could have an adverse effect.

Professor HARRISON: Are you sure that it is hCG?

Professor BEER: I understand that it is hCG.

Professor MOWBRAY: As I understand it, a patient might get as far as 7 weeks before starting treatment, by about 8 weeks?

Professor HARRISON: It would be very rare to get as far as 8 weeks—7 weeks is more usual.

Professor MOWBRAY: Can you give us a rough percentage again of the number of women who aborted before they entered the trial?

Professor HARRISON: None, because we wouldn't have seen them.

Dr ALLEN: We need more information on how techniques like leucocyte immunisation, "tender loving care", cerclage, or anything else may be working. As you point out, the difference in levels of hCG between your treated and your untreated patients was only the difference between 61 and 45.

Professor HARRISON: And that was using progesterone.

Dr ALLEN: But nonetheless, as you pointed out, Elizabeth Lenton of Sheffield showed beautifully two or three years ago that there is a direct correlation between the concentration of hCG and the concentration of progesterone in the blood of normal pregnant women.

Professor HARRISON: Yes, but she was looking at semi-sequential samples. Nothing should be read into the hormone data.

Dr ALLEN: What is the function of hCG after week 15?

Professor HARRISON: I don't know. It is speculative.

Professor STIRRAT: I am rather concerned about your comments about the multi-centre study. If, in fact, you do an multi-centre study, and you get an interim analysis which shows a clear difference, you should stop it, because if that information gets back to your collaborators, then that might influence the way in which they recruit patients.

Professor HARRISON: I agree entirely.

Professor CLARK: I certainly agree that there is more controversy about "early pregnancy factor". But I don't think there is any doubt that there are immuno-suppressant contaminants in the preparations of commercial origin. When the hCG is purified these contaminants disappear. Contaminating substances may be quite significant biologically, and have to be taken into account.

Dr RHODES: There is a great deal of evidence from a number of animal studies to show that the absolute level of hormone is not important. There are particular times during pregnancy when if the mother receives whatever signal she is receiving of the early recognition of pregnancy she will maintain a normal hormonal profile even with the loss of the fetus. The *corpus luteum* in the sheep will be maintained up to 50 or 60 days, even with no live trophoblast or embryo in the uterus. So it may not be the absolute level of hormone that is particularly important. It may be that you are just reaching a critical point in the pregnancy. It may be important that you give it at 5 or 7 weeks, or at 6½ or at 4 weeks, and once you have got the pregnancy over that particular critical point, then the rest of the pregnancy is dependent on other factors.

Professor KENNEDY: Have you, by any chance, measured the hCG levels in the sera of the women who subsequently aborted and compared it with the levels of those who maintained the pregnancy?

Mr EDMONDS: We didn't in this particular study. The progesterone levels were pre-treatment.

Professor HARRISON: The samples were discarded before analysis.

Recurrent abortion: the role of psychotherapy

B. Stray-Pedersen, S. Stray-Pedersen

Interest and research in the psychological aspects of spontaneous abortion was initiated by Javert in 1947, who found that 19% of women with recurrent abortion had psychological disorders.[1] During the following decade psychological factors in women who aborted habitually were thoroughly studied by Javert's group in New York[2,3] and by another multidisciplinary group in Nova Scotia.[4] These investigations focused primarily on the personality of the women. The New York group found that the subjects with recurrent abortion showed remarkable similarities with respect to underlying personality characteristics and in their relationship to their family members. Their mothers were generally found to be the dominant parental figure, making the patients intensely mother-dependent, while their fathers were more anonymous and "ineffective", often lost to the patient during her childhood either through death, divorce or alcoholism.

Furthermore, most of the women expressed feelings of insecurity towards their husbands. This finding naturally led to speculation about the role of the male partner as a causative factor for the miscarriages, a theory which became further emphasised in 1957[1] when Javert described a markedly higher incidence of abortion among married (10%) than among unmarried women (1%).

The Nova Scotia group reported[4] that the abortion-prone women in addition to being immature and dependent, with a stern father, also could be designated as frustrated individuals with mixed feelings about their feminine role, and with a constant fear of failure. By use of different psychological tests the following personality features were observed in women with recurrent miscarriage: impairment of the ability to plan and anticipate, poor emotional control, tendency to place emphasis on conformity, strong feelings of dependency and great proneness to guilt feelings.[3]

Many of these observations on personality characteristics were later confirmed by other investigators.[5,6] However, in the last decade[7,8] there has been an increasing tendency towards a different interpretation of these psychological aberrations. The conclusion drawn by investigators in the 1960's[2,3,4] was that the personality abnormalities ought to be considered as a causative factor for the reproductive failure. Later investigators[5-8] have apparently felt that seeking the roots of miscarriage in the personality of the woman was to speculative a working hypothesis, or that the putative aetiological role of psychological factors might have been exaggerated. They considered it more reasonable that the personality characteristics observed should be regarded more properly as a result and not as a cause of the pregnancy losses.

A spontaneous abortion, especially early in pregnancy, was until recently believed to be an event of less seriousness emotionally than other forms of bereavement. It is now acknowledged, however, that women who experience abortions may develop intense and serious grief reactions which may highly affect their quality of life.[8,9]

Normally, a grief pattern is considered to comprise the following emotional stages: shock, disorganisation, volatile emotions, guilt, hostility, fear, then the feeling of loss, and finally relief and re-establishment.[10] All these stages of grief, in particular the first four stages, have been observed in women suffering from spontaneous abortion.[9,11,12] These feelings can be intense, but fortunately in most cases short-lived.

A miscarriage is often apt to occur at a time when the woman is emotionally labile or psychologically vulnerable. Her loss might be more profound than recognised by others or even by herself at first.[10] She may find it difficult to go back to her job or meet the public after an abortion because she fears that other people will not understand her grief reactions. She often does not have the opportunity to discuss her sorrow with colleagues or friends since her pregnancy has been a secret and thus unknown to them. The size of the uterus had not been visible, and to society the fetus is a non-person and the miscarriage a non-event.

Many women, even during early gestation, might have developed a mental image of the future baby, composed of fantasies, expectations and hopes, combined with an intense emotional investment.[12] The bonding between the mother and the developing fetus may start early in pregnancy, and the miscarriage may mean that she has not only lost her baby, but also part of herself.[13] The woman who has experienced several miscarriages may also believe that her reproductive organs are diseased, or that her general health is poor. This may have an effect on her own self-esteem and on her opinion of herself as a woman, a wife and a mother. If so, the feeling of guilt and failure will be pronounced. "Why did the abortion happen to me?" "What wrong did I do or not do?"

In an earlier investigation we presented the results of diagnostic screening performed among 195 couples with a prior history of habitual abortion.[13] In the same study we also drew attention to the significance of psychological support "tender loving care" (TLC treatment) on the outcome of the succeeding pregnancies in these women. Since then, 223 new couples have been examined and their later reproductive performance continuously followed. Some new (immunological) tests have been included in the screening programme which otherwise has remained unchanged. The study now reported represents a survey of all couples hitherto examined and followed by us.

THE STUDY
Subjects
408 couples with a history of 3 or more consecutive spontaneous abortions were investigated. Altogether these women had accumulated about 1800 miscarriages, varying from 3 to 13 per woman, all pregnancies being hormonally, sonographically or histologically verified. In 64% the spontaneous abortions had occurred predominantly during the first trimester whereas the remaining 36% had had second trimester losses. The majority of women (70%) could be classified as having primary habitual abortion since they had never experienced a successful pregnancy. The other women (30%) had delivered once or twice prior to their series of abortions (livebirths, premature deliveries or stillbirths) and were designated as having secondary habitual abortion.

Diagnostic screening
This usually started 3 to 6 months after the last miscarriage and included recording of a careful medical and obstetrical history, and physical and gynaecological examinations. In all women hormonal tests such as thyroid function tests, glucose tolerance test and three consecutive measurements of serum progesterone during the luteal phase were performed. About 80 women have been tested for lupus anticoagulant, sperm antibodies and anti-nuclear factor. Specimens of endometrial tissue collected by sterile aspiration procedures and of cervical mucus (swab samples) were examined microbiologically. Chromosomal analyses of both partners were performed, and the husband's semen was analysed. Endometrial biopsies were taken in the late luteal phase and correlated to the progesterone values and to the date of ovulation assessed from the temperature chart. Uterine anatomical features (uterine body, cavity and the cervical canal) were assessed by hysterography and/or ultrasound examinations in the luteal phase, and by careful exploration during the curettage. In 74 couples complete HLA-screening (Class I and Class II antigens) was carried out.

RESULTS
In 50% of the 408 couples varying abnormalities which might be associated with their reproductive failure were identified (Table 1). HLA analyses revealed sharing of antigens in the individual couples (1, 2 or 3 loci) to be a less common phenomenon than among parents of patients undergoing kidney transplantation.

The different abnormalities were observed significantly more often among the primary aborters than among secondary recurrent aborters, and also more frequently in couples who had had second trimester abortions. The frequency of positive findings appeared to be correlated with the number of prior abortions: in women who had suffered from only three repetitive abortions, abnormalities were detected in 43%, whereas 83% of the patients with 7 or more abortions showed positive findings.

In 205 couples (50%) no abnormalities could be identified by the diagnostic screening tests employed.

Table 1

Aetiological factors in 408 couples with
recurrent spontaneous abortion

Factors	No.	
Endocrine disorder	21	5%
Uterine body defect	64	16%
Endometrial infection	33	8%
Cervical incompetence	53	13%
Systemic disorder	6	1%
Genetic factor	15	4%
Other factors	13	3%
Multiple factors	203	50%
Unknown aetiology	205	50%
TOTAL	408	100%

FOLLOW-UP STUDIES

Patients with different abnormalities were treated surgically or medically when possible. Thereafter 138 of the 203 women conceived (Table 2), and 112 (81%) of these pregnancies proceeded uneventfully. The success rates observed in the different aetiology groups are shown in Table 3.

Table 2

Number of recurrent aborters achieving pregnancy
in the follow-up period

Group	Total No.	Women achieving pregnancy No.	%
Multiple aetiological factors	203	138	68
Unknown aetiology	205	158	77
Total	408	296	73

Among the 205 couples in whom no abnormalities could be detected, 158 women (77%) have had further pregnancies (Table 2). The majority (116 women) was offered so-called "TLC treatment" i.e. "Tender Loving Care" by one of us. After diagnostic screening and preconceptual counselling they were requested to report to the hospital immediately if they became pregnant. The treatment consisted of psychological support with weekly medical and ultrasound examinations. The women were advised to avoid heavy work and travelling, and sexual abstinence was recommended. No drugs or hormones were given. They were allowed to live normally when they had passed by 3-4 weeks the critical gestational period in which they had experienced their prior miscarriage. During the remainder of gestation they received regular antenatal care.

As shown in Table 3, 85% of the women who received "TLC" treatment had successful pregnancies, whereas the success rate was only 36% in the non-treated group. This difference was found to be highly statistically significant ($\times = 35.4$ or $p \ll 0.001$).

Table 3

Follow-up study recurrent aborters.
Success rate in next pregnancy.

Group	No.	Pregnancy outcome Miscarriage	Pregnancy outcome Viable fetus	Success rate
Multiple aetiologies	138	26	112	81%
Endocrine	17	3	14	82%
Uterine body defect	40	6	34	85%
Endometrial infection	22	5	17	77%
Cervical incompetence	43	10	33	77%
Systemic disorder	5	1	4	80%
Genetic	11	1	10	90%
Unknown aetiology	158	44	114	72%
"TLC" treatment*	116	17	99	85%
No special care	42	27	15	36%
TOTAL	296	70	226	76%

*"TLC"—"tender loving care"

COMMENTS

Our study shows that recurrent aborters constitute a very heterogenous group displaying a widely varying aetiology. None of these, however, should be regarded as absolute causes, i.e. conditions incompatible with attainment of a normal pregnancy. Moreover, the overall percentage of positive findings recorded as well as the individual distribution of the different aetiological factors, has remained remarkably unchanged when compared with the results obtained in our earlier study.[14] Thus, in only half of the cases with recurrent abortion, possible causative factors can be identified, whereas in the other half the aetiology is completely unknown. This fact merely reflects the lack of knowledge about factors involved in recurrent abortion, and thereby the insufficiency of available diagnostic methods.

In personal interviews with our women with recurrent abortion the majority indicated that they were unhappy and anxious and that they felt personally responsible for their reproductive failure, thus confirming the observations in earlier psychological reports.[7,8,12] The situation is in many ways different from that among women with infertility problems. Women having repeated abortions think that the miscarriage is her fault alone. Her husband makes her pregnant, but she herself fails in carrying the fetus to term. Despite this, marital problems appear to be rare. Only 2% of our couples have separated, or changed partner after the abortions, and this figure is markedly lower than that observed in the general population.

In the varying aetiology group the success rate of the pregnancy after institution of appropriate medical or surgical treatment was 81% with no significant differences between the aetiology groups. Admittedly, many of these women also received psychological support such as preconceptional counselling, close and frequent contact with their physician, with reassurance and encouragement during pregnancy.

In the "unknown aetiology" group the success rate of the "TLC-treated" women was found to be as high as 85%; in the non-"TLC-treated" women only 36%. This difference confirms our earlier notion about the favourable effect of "TLC treatment" on the outcome of subsequent pregnancy, a finding which we originally regarded as rather surprising and totally unexpected.

Several criticisms might be raised against the design of this treatment study, in particular, the selection of patients. The study has not been a double-blind, controlled trial. Although we now consider "TLC treatment" as so effective that it is unethical to withold it. It has for practical reasons to be restricted to those women living within a reasonable distance of our hospitals. On the other hand, the treated and non-treated women in this investigation did not differ with respect to age, marital or socioeconomic status. In our opinion, more attention should be paid to those women who cannot be offered "TLC treatment" because they had not become pregnant after the screening. In the "unknown aetiology group" this has been the case in 23% (Table 2). We are now investigating these couples in order to evaluate possible causes for their conceptional delay and to assess the frequency of involuntary infertility.

The beneficial effect of psychological support in recurrent abortion represents by no means a new observation. Javert[1] reported a success rate of 80% after TLC. Several later authors have emphasised the positive influence of psychotherapy.[3,4,6,7] Some of these investigations also showed that the personality abnormalities earlier observed in many of these patients disappeared or became less pronounced after a successful pregnancy.[3,4] A recent study from St Mary's Hospital, London[15] indicates that recurrent miscarriers display significantly higher levels of anxiety than a group of former recurrent miscarriers who had borne children and a group of normal childbearing women. Their results indicated that increased levels of anxiety are effects of the recurrent miscarriage and that the anxiety levels decline during a successful pregnancy. The investigators recommend that psychological approaches should centre on interventions enabling women to identify sources of anxiety and to provide strategies to cope with these. This should allow for a more comfortable, less anxious pregnancy and even assist in carrying the pregnancy to term.

At this stage we can only speculate about the nature of the effect of psychological support on the preservation of a pregnancy. It has been demonstrated, however, that stress and grief may affect the immunological responses.[16] Furthermore, it has been suggested that emotional factors might interfere with the processes involved in implantation or placentation.[17,18]

In psychosomatic medicine it seems to be well accepted that chronic distortion of emotions and depression of feelings may lead to changes in the hypothalamic, pituitary, adrenal or ovarian interplay. Catecholamines may play a role since they are humoral mediators between emotional centres in the brain and the peripheral autonomous system, and also act directly on uterine contractility and blood flow. Serotonin might be a hormone of interest in this connection since it displays vasoconstrictor potencies in the umbilico-placental vasculature exceeding by far, for example, those of prostanoids and angiotensin.[19] Treatment with serotonin antagonists in recurrent abortion has been reported to have good effects,[20] but more work is obviously needed in order to draw any definite conclusions.

All our women with recurrent abortion have expressed an urgent need for knowledge. They feel that they can better cope with the problem if they are assured that everything has been done which can be done. Information is important in helping the patient to accept reality. They are desperate, and willing to subject themselves to any procedure and treatment which may offer the slightest chance of success. It is very important therefore, that these patients are not left to themselves, but offered a thorough and systematic examination before conception and that the basis for any intervention is considered with great care. These patients are very sensitive to the doctor's handling of their problem, to her/ his attitude, insight and knowledge, attention and especially to her/his ability to engage personally and thereby provide the necessary personal care.

In conclusion, the significance of psychological support in recurrent abortion may raise questions as to the validity of the results in many earlier investigations in which different types of treatment have been attempted. The need for controlled, double-blind studies seems obvious. Our results, however, clearly emphasise the insufficiency of randomising the patients for such studies exclusively at the preconceptional stage without paying attention to the handling of the women during their subsequent pregnancy.

REFERENCES

1. Javert CT. *Spontaneous and habitual abortion*. New York: McGraw-Hill Book Company, Inc; 1957.
2. Mann EC. Habitual abortion: A report in two parts on 160 patients. *Am J Obstet Gynecol* 1959; **77:** 706-718.
3. Grimm ER. Psychological investigation of habitual abortions. *Psychosom Med* 1962; **24:** 369-378.
4. Weil RJ, Tupper C. Personality, life situation and communication. A study of habitual abortion. *Psychosom Med* 1960; **12:** 448-455.
5. Kaij L, Malmquist A, Nilsson O. Psychiatric aspects of spontaneous abortion. II The importance of bereavement, attachment and neurosis in early life. *J Psychsom Res* 1969; **13:** 53-59.
6. Hertz DG. Rejection of motherhood. A psychosomatic appraisal of habitual abortion. *Psychosomatics* 1973; **14:** 241-244.
7. Coghi I, Pancheri P, Connolly AM, Dominici L, Nicotra M, Calella A, Vetrone G. Psychological variables in habitual abortion: A combined diagnostic-therapeutic approach. In: *Emotion and reproduction. 5th intern. congress of psychosomatic obstetrics and gynecology.* Eds. L. Carenza, L. Zichella. London: Academic Press, 1979; pp.289-295.
8. Hertz EK. Psychological repercussions of pregnancy loss. In: *The Young Woman: Psychosomatic Aspects of Obstetrics and Gynecology.* Eds. L. Dennertein, M de Senarchleus. Amsterdam: Excerpta Medica, 1983; pp.292-299.
9. Peppers LG, Knapp RJ. Maternal reactions to involuntary fetal/infant death. *Psychiatry* 1980; **43:** 155-159.
10. Clayton P, Desmarais L, Winokur G. A study of bereavement. *Am J Psychiatry* 1968; **125:** 168-178.

11. Stack JM. The psychodynamics of spontaneous abortion. *Am J Orthpsychiatry* 1984; **54:** 162-167.
12. Seibel M, Graves WL. The psychological implications of spontaneous abortions, *J Reprod Med* 1980; **25:** 161-165.
13. Lumley J. The development of maternal-foetal bonding in first pregnancy. In: *Emotion and reproduction. 5th intern. congress of psychosomatic obstetrics and gynecology.* Eds. L. Carenza, L. Zichella. London: Academic Press, 1979; pp. 1067-1069.
14. Stray-Pedersen B, Stray-Pedersen S. Etiologic factors and subsequent reproductive performance in 195 couples with a prior history of habitual abortion. *Am J Obstet Gynecol* 1984; **148:** 140-146.
15. Purkiss R, Gannon K, Pearce S, Beard RW. Anxiety and recurrent miscarriage— cause or effects. *Br Med J* 1987; In press.
16. Bouberg D, Ader R, Cohen N. Acquisition and extinction of conditioned suppression of graft-vs-host response in the rat. *J Immunol* 1984; **132:** 111-115.
17. Kitzmiller J, Watt, N, Driscoll SG. Decidual arteriopathy in hypertension and diabetes in pregnancy. *Am J Obstet Gynecol* 1981; **141:** 773-779.
18. Althabe O, Labarrere C, Telenta M. Maternal vascular lesions in placentae of small-for-gestational-age infants. *Placenta* 1985; **6:** 265-276.
19. Bjøro K, Stray-Pedersen S. Effects of vasoactive autacoids on different segments of human umbilicoplacental vessels. *Gynecol Obstet Invest* 1986; **22:** 1-6.
20. Polishuk WH, Sadovsky E, Pfeifer Y, Sulzman FG. Prevention of psychogenic serotonin abortion. In: *Psychosomatic medicine in obstetrics and gynaecology. 3rd Intern Congress.* Basel: Karger 1972; pp.189-191.

Discussion

Chairman: Mr D. K. Edmonds

Professor GRUDZINSKAS: Could I ask how long they spend with a patient on each visit, because my crude calculations are that about 15,000 visits over a 5-year period probably breaks down to about 60 visits per week. So how long do you spend with a patient if it is a weekly antenatal check? Also, what sort of out-of-hours service do you provide in the event that anxiety levels go up on Saturday and Sunday?

Dr B STRAY-PEDERSON: I have no idea about the timing of the anxiety levels. The average time which we spend on an individual visit is about 15-30 minutes.

Professor GILL: You showed that by treatment you can correct 95% of genetic defects. How was that done? The whole issue of psychotherapy is a very important one to settle by the appropriate clinical trials. To simple-minded experimentalists this would mean "tender loving care", nothing and regular beating! But there must be a more patient-acceptable way. If these data were to hold up under a rigorously developed clinical trial they have tremendous implications for the basic approach to looking at implantation processes.

Dr B STRAY-PEDERSON: Yes, I agree. Also, 90% of those women with translocations had a successful pregnancy. Some had amniocentesis.

Professor HARRISON: How did you treat them?

Dr RHODES: Are you saying that they were all maternal balanced translocations?

Dr B STRAY-PEDERSON: Yes.

Professor CLARK: This is quite exciting work, and for the humble immunologists here, we are all concerned that it is viewed as throwing question marks on the validity of immunotherapy. One way to deal with that is to approach it empirically and do a controlled trial. If you are dealing with humans you have a very powerful and well developed nervous system, and as we know through the effects of hypnosis and voodoo, it can produce some very dramatic physical effects. We also know that the nervous system can effect the immune responses. It has been shown that you can reactivate immune responses by using a conditioning stimulus and then repeating it in the absence of antigens. In trying to solve the problem of the best treatment with these patients, we must investigate the *underlying* mechanism. Wouldn't that begin to tell us more about how our therapies are working? Currently most of us think we know how our therapy is working, but in reality maybe it is something else.

Dr B STRAY-PEDERSON: I agree with you.

Professor KENNEDY: Do you have any information about the compliance rate to your prescription of "tender loving care", in particular to your prescription for sexual abstinence? Do you have any information to what extent that is actually complied with?

Dr B STRAY-PEDERSON: I don't know, but they are very anxious and will subject themselves to any sort of treatment.

Dr RUSHTON: In relation to the central nervous system and the control of implantation, there is a lot of embryological evidence of the effect on vascularity. Also, in relation to sexual intercourse, it has been shown that the incidence of chorioamnionitis in women who have sexual intercourse while they are pregnant is very much higher than in women who don't.

Professor BEARD: In recurrent miscarriage, the placebo effect has been the one thing, because it is so strong, that has dogged all our experimental efforts to try and discover what is going on. I think now that we have to accept this sort of data showing that there is a strong effect which is being mediated in some psychological way. Instead of seeing it as a confrontation between science and the softer aspects of medicine, we should actually see it as an intriguing problem that needs to be resolved.

Professor HARRISON: Have you looked at any psychological stress markers?

Dr B STRAY-PEDERSON: No. I am not a psychiatrist.

Professor HARRISON: I am slightly worried that you mention the word "psychiatrist". Don't you mean "psychologist"?

Dr B STRAY-PEDERSON: We have had bad experience with psychologists.